AF430877

STRATEGIC PHARMACEUTICAL MARKETING

Second Edition

STRATEGIC PHARMACEUTICAL MARKETING

Second Edition

Raja B. Smarta

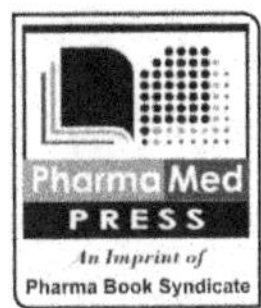

PharmaMed Press

An imprint of Pharma Book Syndicate

A unit of BSP Books Pvt. Ltd.

4-4-309/316, Giriraj Lane,
Sultan Bazar, Hyderabad - 500 095.

Strategic Pharmaceutical Marketing, Second Edition by *Raja B. Smarta*

Published by

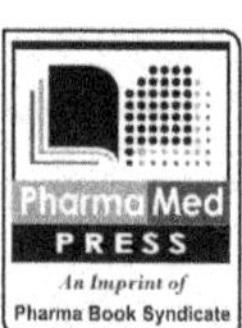

PharmaMed Press

An imprint of Pharma Book Syndicate

A unit of BSP Books Pvt. Ltd.
4-4-309/316, Giriraj Lane, Sultan Bazar, Hyderabad - 500 095.
Phone: 040-23445605, 23445688; Fax: 91+40-23445611
E-mail: info@pharmamedpress.com
www.pharmamedpress.com/pharmamedpress.net

ISBN: 978-93-86819-77-2 (Hardbound)

CONTENTS

CHAPTER 2

Dynamic Pathways

CHAPTER 3

Innovation and Marketing Strategy

CHAPTER 4

Strategic Concepts, Models and Options

CHAPTER 5

Evolution and Change of Gear

CHAPTER 6

Strategic Plus

CHAPTER 7

Force of Segmentation

CHAPTER 8

Positioning Towards Identity

CHAPTER 9

Communication and Promotion Impact

CHAPTER 10

Execution Prerequisites

CHAPTER 11

Core Sales Execution

CHAPTER 12

Marketing Finance

PREFACE

Personally, I am indebted to all students of Pharmaceutical Marketing, Pharmaceutical Executives, all my clients and also the Publisher for the confidence they have reposed in me by giving me this new choice.

In fact, this book is a driving force of their choice, as the original print of **Strategic Pharmaceutical Marketing, First Edition** published by Wheeler is no longer available, which was the only Book on fundamentals of strategic pharmaceutical marketing.

Dilemma

So, I was faced with a dilemma of just reprinting the original book once again with new data or rewriting the entire book and giving it to the publisher, or not writing the book at all as the environment today has undergone considerable change. It is like a dilemma **to be or not to be**. It also forced me to think, **why am I writing this Book** or **revisiting this book of fundamentals.**

Then I realized that the basic transaction between Medical Representative and Physician or Surgeon has still not vanished, although, the essence of transaction is fully changed.

Earlier it was a transaction of new concepts, new products, innovation in marketing, branding, and differentials in positioning but, then it got stuck, with the emergence of generics, making it difficult to differentiate.

However, new customers' transactions took a different mode and basic selling and marketing skills shifted to some extent to the background.

This gave me a thought that why do not I put forward to my readers more about today's environment, about how marketing has changed its **perspectives, perceptions, processes, philosophy** and **practices.** However, as the skill set and the process of selling remains the same, I felt, let me retain the fundamentals of marketing and weave a new story around the new environment, so that, it is useful for those who have given me a **Hobson's choice.** Obviously, many suggestions came and I have incorporated most of them in this book.

My special thanks to all those who provided suggestions, my Students, Pharmaceutical Executives, Management Institutions, Industry Publications and also all of them who are interested in reading this book.

I would also like to make a special mention of my **Interlinkians**, Ms. Shreya Pathare, Ms. Ankita Dhekne and Ms. Crystal Vaz for their interest and assistance in processing this entire manuscript.

A special mention of those demanding clients who have been asking and compelling me to think differently and innovatively. By the grace of God, I could contribute towards bringing something new always, and add value to all our clients.

What's Missing

Pharmaceutical industry has a basic purpose of providing health to medical consumers and patients. Personally, I look, forward to 'Healthy India' which needs support from Health conscious Indians, will of Government and policies to make this happen. In India all plan for their careers and finances but, it is really difficult to find an Indian who plans for his health. I personally think that the missing link is good health and wellness and I would like to contribute in this mission of 'Healthy India' with the help of health and medicines.

Raja B. Smarta

About the Author

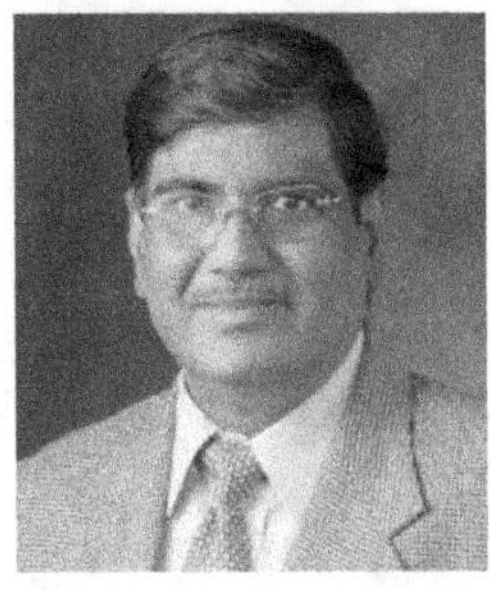 Dr. R. B. Smarta (M.Sc. MMS. PhD. FRSA) is the Founder and Managing Director of Interlink Marketing Consulting Pvt. Ltd. He has been a reputed consultant, corporate trainer and mentor for corporations in Pharmaceutical, Nutraceutical, Wellness, Healthcare and Life Sciences industry for over three decades. Dr. Smarta received his PhD. in Management Sciences in 1982 from University of East Georgia. He is affiliated with IFRSA (Fellow of the Royal Society of Arts) by RSA, UK, CMC (Certified Member of Consultants) by IMCI.

Dr. Smarta is a faculty in leading management institutions namely, JBIMS (Bajaj Institute of Management Studies), NMIMS (Narsee Monjee Institute of Management Studies), IIM (Indian Institute of Management), Indore, and Pharmacy College, Manipal, and a Guide to Ph.D. students. He has been a board member of HADSA which is a part of IADSA (International Alliance Dietary / Food Supplement Associations) along with being an Editor for HADSA's publication Nutrascope.

He has made considerable contribution to International Pharmaceutical Federation (FIP), Delhi Pharmaceutical Trust (DPT), All India Drugs Control officer's confederation, AIDCOC, IPA (Indian Pharmaceutical Association) for their projects inclusive of 'Project Concern'. He has addressed many national and international seminars organized by IDMA, OPPI, Nutra India, FICCI, HADSA - Nutraceutical summits, Nutracon – Hongkong, Strategic Management at IBC–Singapore, FIP at Amsterdam, Ayurvedic Congress etc. Dr. Smarta is an author for two research books, Strategic Pharmaceutical Marketing and Revitalizing the Pharmaceutical Business. He has co-authored for the book (Mega) Market-in German and English and was recently a contributing author for Innovation of Healthy and Functional Foods. His articles have been published in renowned publications like Pharma Pulse, Modern Pharmaceuticals, Pharmabiz, Express Pharma, Hindu, Business Today, Outline Today, etc.

Education

M.Sc. in Organic Chemistry (Drugs) from University of Nagpur (1967)

Ph.D. in Management Sciences from University of East Georgia (1982)

MMS from JBIMS, University of Mumbai (1972)

M.Sc. in Organic Chemistry (Drugs) from University of Nagpur (1967)

MMS from JBIMS, University of Mumbai (1972)

Introduction

As the great philosopher Sun Tzu, author of *Art of War*, observed almost five hundred years before Christ, the smartest strategy of war is not to have a war. This is a strategy which allows you to achieve your objectives without having to fight. It also means that you should make yourself powerful that your competitors lose the moral force to fight you in the market after taking a look at you.

The goal of any marketing strategy is to surpass the competitor. If you are lucky enough not to have any competition, then you must out beat yourself and become stronger. Because you never know when competition will overtake you.

While your competitors are important, they need not be the first thing you think of when devising your strategy. First, comes painstaking attention to the needs of your customer, and close analysis of your company's real degrees of freedom in responding to these needs. Every strategy must encompass a determination to create value for your customers.

Rapid and dynamic changes are taking place in the environment, both in India and globally. Hence it has become necessary to think strategically, understand and adjust to the changes, and plan for the future. For our own survival, we need to be ever watchful of the events taking place. New opportunities and challenges are being thrown up.

We need to regularly scan the environment, match the events and opportunities to our resources and capabilities, and work out strategies accordingly.

We should not let ourselves be swayed by narrow ambitions and short-sighted benefits. It is time we began to think objectively, clearly, where we are heading for, what we want. We need to synthesize the changing times with our goals, to avoid wastage of resources and frustration. We need new strategies, options, and skills to cope with the new competition and new markets. We need to be proactive and develop a vision and focus for the future.

The next decade will witness a power shift between multinationals, and strong national companies in India. The basic struggle will be to cope with the challenges of the new normal world and avoid frustrations. Managers will have to keep themselves busy finding out workable solutions to continuing problems, and will perhaps rely more on their insight and wisdom. The changing global economy and industrial restructuring may bring about the changes and policies in relation to licensing, co-marketing, and so on. The prevalent attitudes of a customer base- doctors, patients, retailers, hospitals, etc.- may itself undergo a change. Are you prepared to meet the challenges?

Those of you who want to become winners will have to aim at developing marketing as a philosophy in your organizations and not look at it as merely another discipline. To make a mark in the changing environment requires an integrated approach of the total organization, right from R&D to providing added value to the products.

In my opinion, India has a space and opportunity for all for the next twenty years. India is the world's best in generics. It is the world's best provider of talents in R&D. It could be that R&D ventures may start in India to optimize the cost of R&D even by multinationals. India is one of the world's best players in terms of 'biotech products'. India is the world's best market with increasing available income. India could become the world's best provider of innovations to the entire world. I can foresee India offering a lot of opportunities for those economically viable pharmaceutical companies- both national and multinational organizations- by 2030.

Reflecting on the substantial changes in the pharmaceutical environment, it has been observed that basics of pharmaceutical marketing have been almost forgotten with them becoming just theories. Having said that, these basics of pharmaceutical marketing are the fulcrum of tomorrow's modern marketing principles. Thus, the question arises, can we resist the 'Basics'?

'Strategic Pharmaceutical Marketing' hence, focuses on the practice of marketing prescription medications. This book highlights the political, economical, social, technological and regulatory perspectives of pharmaceutical marketing, examines consumers and prescribers and explores positive marketing, pricing and distribution strategies. The book provides a detailed explanation of what marketing is as well as provides real-world case studies to demonstrate certain aspects.

The book is written from an industry and academic perspective. It allows pharmaceutical marketers to have a detailed understanding of the functions of pharmaceutical marketing thus, helping them plan their marketing strategies in a more accurate and precise way.

Individuals entering the field of marketing pharmaceutical products-sales personnel, assistant product managers, marketing staff as well as policy makers will achieve an in-depth understanding of the pharmaceutical industry. The marketing models described in the book along with promotion, distribution and pricing scenarios, competitive analysis and market research will benefit the pharmaceutical marketeras a whole.

I would like to call this a 'think book' as opposed to a 'how-to-book' or a 'textbook'. My aim has been to provoke you to think of the surface and latent problems in new ways, and find out different and more imaginative solutions. I have also tried to reflect on the different options for tomorrow to cope with the changing situations.

In chapter zero, I have tried to provide a marketing vision with respect to the changes in the world and the environment, the evolution of the new normal world, marketing perspectives along with challenges revolving around them, steps towards effective marketing along with the essentials of strategic pharmaceutical marketing. Chapter 1 provides a broad overview of the marketing environment and the changes taking place both in India and internationally. This background will enable readers develop an understanding and awareness of the forces which enable to spot opportunities. Chapter 2 provides the essentials of strategic marketing options. Marketing is seen not as an isolated activity but as a corporate goal. Chapter 3 discusses the evolution and dynamics of the physician-patient-therapy interaction pattern. This will help evaluate and identify the customer base and deal with those who are potential adopters or buyers of the product offerings. The important components of strategy and its formulation such as segmentation, positioning, and strategic edge/ advantages are explored in Chapters 4, 5, and 6. Strategies can work if they are properly followed through, and this is the subject of Chapter 7 related to the impact of communication and promotion.

How can we certain that a strategy is being correctly implemented? This issue is discussed in the next two chapters. While chapter 8 discusses the role of policies, tactics, structure and ethics in the successful operation of an organization, Chapter 9 discusses the important aspect of implementation. Chapter 10 helps understand what innovation means to us and how we can work towards exploring innovative marketing responses. The concluding chapter details how financial analysis can help to measure the success of our marketing decisions and responses.

I hope the book will help marketers and CEOs in the pharmaceutical industry bring about synergy in their strategies and operations, by thinking about the options, and looking at innovation as an important ingredient for their progress. I have tried to raise several questions in the book, some of which may have remained unanswered. But if I have been able to provoke some of you to think for yourselves in new directions, I would feel more than satisfied.

CHAPTER 1

Marketing Vision

THE CHANGE AGENT

Long ago, people happily lived under the rule of a king. The people of the kingdom were very happy as they had a very prosperous life with abundance of wealth and no misfortunes.

The king decided to go on a travel to visit places of historical importance and pilgrim centers at distant places. He decided to travel by foot to interact with his people and accompany them. People of distant places were so happy to have a conversation with their king and they were proud that their king was so kind with a good heart!

After several weeks, he returned to the palace. He was quite happy that he visited many pilgrim centers and could see his fellow people leading a propitious life. However, he had a regret.

He had intolerable pain in his feet as it was his first trip by foot to a longer distance. He complained to his ministers that the roads weren't comfortable and were very stony. He could not tolerate the pain as he walked all the way through the rough path.

He said he was very much worried about the people who used to walk along those roads as it would be painful for them too!

He made an order to cover the road of the whole country with leather so that people might feel comfortable, immediately.

The king thought that he had to change this for the betterment and happiness of the people.

His ministers were stunned to hear his order as it would destroy the lives of thousands of cows to get the sufficient quantity of leather and it would cost a huge amount of money also.

A wise man from the ministry came to the king and said that he had another idea.

The king asked - what was his alternative idea. The minister told, 'Why do you want to kill the holy animal cow to cover the road with leather? Rather, you can just have a piece of leather cut in appropriate shape to cover your feet?'

The king was very much surprised by his suggestion and applauded the minister. He ordered for a pair of leather shoes for him and requested the countrymen to wear shoes.

THE ENLIGHTENED SAMURAI

Our era has been dubbed the "Age of Uncertainty," and uncertain it is. Nowadays it is well-nigh impossible to predict very much with accuracy. This only compounds the problems of a company president or manager, who already has more than enough to cope with. Still, this is nothing new. We have faced it before and we will face it again.

A person with strong motivation is actually challenged in our bewildering times, stimulated to use all his skills to overcome odds and come out stronger than before. But others are disturbed and confused by their inability to impose order on their world. This type of manager will never be able to lead his company to prosperity. A manager with longevity must be prepared to weather storms and face unruly situations, undaunted.

It used to be said that a samurai had to be ready to deal with seven foes lying in wait whenever he left his house. He was trained to be prepared to meet death at every corner, and it was this readiness that earned him admiration and respect.

The manager today needs to be even more prepared than the samurai. He must always be conscious of the possibility that his business or he, himself, could topple at any time, as if he were walking a very dangerous tightrope. This is not the time for a relaxed, nonchalant outlook on life or business. The serious manager must keep alert to dangers and his responsibilities even when he is enjoying himself at a party.

A president is charged with the guidance of each and every one of his employees. If he has ten thousand employees, his concern for them has ten thousand faces. Sleep does not come easily and his troubles weigh heavily. Yet the sleepless nights and concern are also what make his life worthwhile. There has never been a company president who has had no worries. Worry and heavy responsibility are part and parcel of the job.

As the environment is consistently changing, pharmaceutical marketers on one hand have to be competent and ready to face any diverse or adverse situation, as society inclusive of business, is looking at pharmaceutical marketing with different perspectives. It's time that pharmaceutical marketers have to look at essentials of strategic pharmaceutical business and ponder over them even before developing strategic intent and direction for their marketing, selling and business.

THE NEW NORMAL WORLD

The world is changing, and is undergoing great shifts, moving towards the new normal. We live in a world where companies like Uber, Airbnb, and Amazon are among a growing number of global companies that did not exist a couple of decades ago, but have rapidly grown, and are thriving across diverse markets displacing some well entrenched players with their disruptive business models. These companies have achieved this by riding the **megatrend of digitization** in an increasingly connected world.

The other megatrend is **sustainability**. Nowadays, companies are realizing the need to develop sustainable business through innovation. Many companies are entrenching sustainability at the very heart of their operations, systems, and processes.

The rise of developing markets is the third megatrend that is shaping the world order. Emerging markets like India, and China along with other developing markets have led global growth in the past two decades and will continue to do so. For that matter, India is making an increasing business impact outside its boundaries across various industries.

Defining Moment

The above mentioned megatrends are disrupting the way the world operates, and is changing the paradigm of how business is conducted.

The interconnected world is witnessing **democratization of entrepreneurship, assertion of developing countries globally,** and **emergence of novel businesses.**

With the aspirations of 1.3 billion people, India stands at a defining moment in its journey to take its rightful place in the world economic order, and also the rapid expansion of Indian businesses in international markets is incredible.

Globally Leveraged Locally Relevant

Consumers are having a high inclination towards their local cultures. Consumers are asking for the best of global offerings and products but at the same time are also very strongly re-experiencing their traditional customs and culture.

Businesses are in dire need to combine global capabilities, and R&D expertise with local consumer insights. Several global brands are discovering the need to adapt their products to suit local demands.

It has been observed that companies can either become mindlessly global or hopelessly local. To manage cross-country operations it is important to find the perfect balance between looking for international leverage with respect to innovation and technology along with having local relevance for meeting consumer needs and aspirations. In order to achieve this balance, it is essential to create the right organization and mindset.

Every Day Great Execution (EDGE)

Enterprises succeed globally when they rapidly convert strategy into action, and plans into P&L across each of the markets.

To meet the needs of the consumers, multinationals use the strength of their global capabilities, and scale and then combine this with the most effective 'route-to-market'. This requires a sharp focus on 'everyday execution' in every single market.

Global leverage often starts with local successes; this applies equally to best practices in executional excellence as well as in product development.

Diversity of Talent

Diversity of talent is the key to global organizations. To compete, and succeed in this dynamic world, companies need talent with international experience, and global mindset. It is important to identify, develop, and retain a diverse talent pool.

Research shows that a more inclusive workforce can boost financial performance, reputation, innovation, and employee motivation. It also companies to better anticipate, and meet the needs of their diverse consumers.

Purpose-Driven and Values-Led Leadership

The reputation, and trust that a company builds with the local communities is its biggest asset. Thus, robust internal systems and processes are very essential for organizations to run not just efficiently but anchored in a set of non-negotiables, and both are equally important.

The values of integrity, responsibility, respect, and pioneering are what motivate, and drive the employees in any global organization.

Therefore, a new kind of leadership that is purpose-driven, and values-led, a leadership that embraces the new mantra of going from 'good' to 'great', would help organizations succeed in this new normal world.

MANAGING THE NEW NORMAL WORLD

Prof. Peter Drucker rightly said long back that at the end organizations will have only two functions with other functions being outsourced. He spoke about **'Innovation' and 'Marketing.** New normal world requires a lot of innovation right from embracing all aspects and trends of the new normal world.

One aspect of this is developing **'Design Thinking.'** Hasso Plattner, Institute of Design at Stanford has developed a framework of design thinking and evolved a paradigm of innovation.

This design thinking process starts with the empathize mode. This mode is the understanding of the people with the context of one's challenge and is the center-piece of the whole process. The problems encountered as a design thinker are rarely your own, they are in fact of a particular group of people, hence, it is important to gain empathy for what is important to them. To empathize, one needs to observe, engage, watch and listen. At the end, one needs to draw conclusions in order to see the bigger picture and grasp the takeaways.

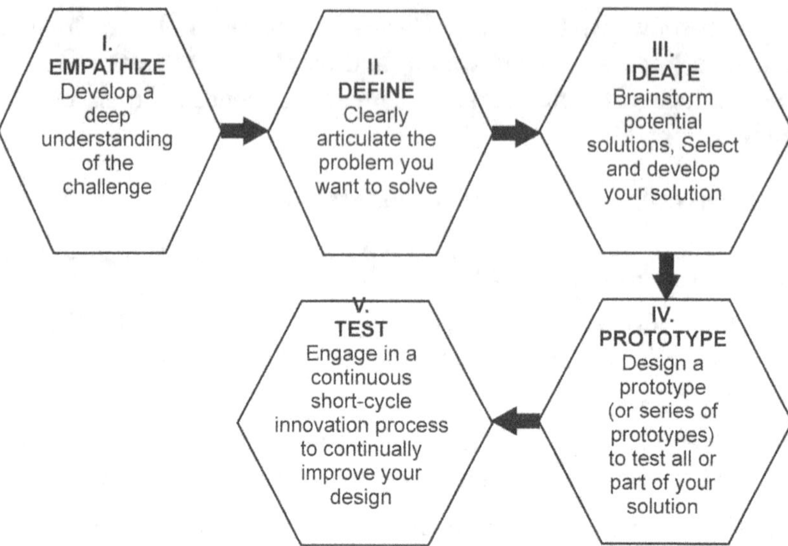

Figure 1.1 Design thinking process

Source: Hasso plattner, institute of design at stanford

Then comes the define mode. This mode is all about bringing clarity and focus to define the challenge taken up. It is essential because it results in one's point-of-view. The point-of-view then defines the correct challenge that needs to be addressed based on newer understandings. To define, one needs to provide focus to the framed problem, evaluate competing ideas, empower teams to take decisions independently and capture hearts and minds of people. At the end one determines the specific meaningful challenge that needs to be taken up.

Third in line is the ideate mode which simply put is idea generation. In this mode one generates solution concepts based on the understanding of the challenge as well as the people. One can ideate with thorough brainstorming, prototyping, body-storming, mind-mapping and sketching. Through ideation one generates all kinds of innovation potential for the determined challenge.

Next is the prototype mode which is the iterative generation of solutions bringing one closer to the final solution. It is important to prototype in order to problem-solve, communicate, test possibilities and manage the solution-building process. To prototype, one needs to start building with the user in mind. Prototyping will help you gain meaningful feedback for the final solution.

The final mode is the test mode. In this mode, one solicits feedback and also provides another opportunity to gain empathy for the people with the context of the design process. The test mode helps one to redefine and refine prototypes and solutions, learn more about the user and also helps to redefine and refine one's point-of-view. In order to follow the test mode it is essential to create experiences and user comparisons.

The process of design thinking is only a framework that can be adapted to one's personal style and type of work. Irrespective of what process is used, it is important to innovate that will ultimately permeate through one's own work.

PERSPECTIVES

Marketing and its Eight Perspectives

Marketing is likely to take a shape of dynamics of business. These dynamics change as marketing evolves and takes shape and includes numerous perspectives.

1. Political Perspective

The political trends are important in any country. They have considerable impact on sales and marketing in stable countries as well. For instance, the United States of America usually expects higher emphasis on social programs and increased government spending when Democrats are in power in the White House. The same applies to liberal governments in the United Kingdom. India but has a focus on 'Make in India', 'Clean India', 'Healthy India' along with other initiatives. These initiative are thus, likely to affect business as well as sales and marketing.

The political trends that affect sales and marketing stances and communication include:

- Trend to align health solutions to political will
- Rising nationalism attitude in using health solutions
- Increase in political terrorism; revolutions
- Rise of socialism to perceive healthcare industry
- Decline of major powers; rise of emerging nations; shifting of power, birth of new powers

- Rise in senior-citizen power
- Instability in places where economy consequences could be important
- Urbanization and creation of new markets

It is important for the marketer to study both domestic and foreign political happenings, reviewing selected published information to get a hang of the political trends and interpret information. It is important to give the voters an economical product that is easily available and affordable at the same time.

2. Economic Perspective

Economic trends that affect business include the following possibilities:

- Depression; worldwide economic collapse
- Increasing foreign ownership of US economy
- Increasing regulation and management of national economies
- Several developing nations become superpowers
- World food production: Famine relief versus holistic management
- Decline in real world growth; or stable growth
- Collapse of world monetary system
- Continuing high inflation
- Worldwide free trade

All companies, irrespective of their size, examine the economic environment in order to plan strategically for sales and marketing, funding and investments. This involves gathering relevant published information, analyzing the information and interpreting it for use in planning. In some organizations, the entire process of dealing with relevant economic information is manual and intuitive. But, many pharmaceutical organizations have put up complete pharmaceutical economics study groups.

Research shows that gathering relevant information (environment scanning) gives rise to several new or modified marketing practices like:

- New marketing targets to improve economy
- Initiating sales training to prepare for group selling
- Cost-effectiveness, cost-benefit studies to support promotional efforts

- New promotional materials emphasizing economic benefits
- Affordability of population
- Disposable income of population
- Consumption and demand need
- Demographic analysis

3. Social Perspective

An important factor of any business environment is the values people behold. Changes in values in the recent years have given rise to massive regulations, deep criticisms, new demands and challenges of the very foundation on which the business rests.

Information pertaining to social trends can be obtained from any published source. The impact of social trends on sales and marketing practices can be analyzed internally or with the help of external consultants. Additionally books as well as analyzing news reports help study the impact.

Sometimes some products face favorable stories, detailing the wonders of the drug, while sometimes some products face unfavorable stories that point out to adverse reactions wherein the company personnel have difficulty in tackling negative publicity.

The key lies in whether the company officials are aware in advance about the story revolving around their product. If the answer is yes, then the company needs to provide as much information as possible. Even of the story around the product is negative, there will at least be access to correct information, leading to fairer coverage.

Research shows that more popular the drug, better the chance for something sensational being aired or printed. More people taking the drug, higher the chances of adverse reactions and unfavorable stories.

Another interesting phenomenon with consumers is that negative publicity about a particular drug may bring favourable attention to it. Consumers who may have never heard about the drug may go ask their doctors because they may think this may be the one that finally works for them. Also, experts state that the consumers of today's times are sophisticated; they may have sympathy for the writer, but know that anybody can have an adverse reaction to anything.

Social view of voters may influence the healthcare policies as well as drug pricing issues. The product needs to be of societal benefit and the companies need to do something for the society at a minimal cost. The society expects benefits like clinical outcomes, good quality and safety.

4. Technological Perspective

It is because of the technological advances in therapy that the pharmaceutical industry is thriving. But it is necessary to bear in mind that changes and advances in technology outside the industry often have significant impact on pharmaceutical marketing practices. For instance, the invention and success of cable television made it possible to utilize a new sales/ educational tool by bringing pharmaceutical programs into the physicians' office or home.

Pharmaceutical industry is clearly technology based and thus, it is necessary to attempt future planning. This planning thus, needs scanning of the environment as well as attempts to identify incipient technological developments.

It is necessary to emphasize that this technological environment is much broader than that within the drug industry itself. For instance, consider rapid growth and even greater potential of laser technology in non-invasive surgery.

The marketing planner must mount a systematic technology scanning program to identify both potential problems and opportunities.

This perspective is very useful as many advances in R&D, drug development, drug delivery and also in quality assurance. The areas of pharmaceutical are changing drastically with specificity and reaching the time to market any product. Business speed is also dependent on technological advances.

The industry regards technological perspective as a space that requires high investment but something that will in turn increase speed and accuracy. The political perspective expects the technological intervention to be transparent in every transaction.

5. Regulatory Perspective

Regulatory perspective applies to every aspect of the marketing mix. It is thus, important to thoroughly understand these regulations as well as comply to them. As a result, the marketer needs to develop and implement creative programs to achieve the marketing objectives. Generally marketers most commonly react to legislation, regulation and edicts. It is however more economical to stay updated with the regulatory environment rather than falling into a legal soup.

Especially in pharma and healthcare there are many regulatory boundaries and they are essential as industry is dealing with 'life' of citizens. The regulatory perspective expects the investments to be low for low price of the product.

6. Ecological Perspective

The ecological perspective says that the imbalance of microbiome in the human body gives rise to diseases. Thus, maintaining the ecological balance is a challenge in itself as it gives rise to diseases which then require new products in the market.

7. Trade Perspective

The challenge here is the All India Organisation of Chemists and Druggists (AIOCD) which needs to grant permissions to every company for launching new products in the market. Also, the challenge is the chemists not wanting to stock more products due to high investment which then requires the company to book orders.

8. Unionization Perspective

Unionization of field force and unionization of manufacturers both is a challenge in the marketing environment as perspectives of the union as well as the trade is different today.

PERCEPTIONS

Perception of Pharmaceutical Marketing

To perceive and understand what is happening in pharmaceutical marketing, we need to ask a simple question: how do doctors decide what product to prescribe? This is a surprisingly complex issue, and to understand this we need to think about the four main players wielding pressure: the patient; the funder (which in the UK means the National health Services (NHS)); the doctor; and the pharmaceutical company.

For patients, things are relatively simple: you want a doctor to prescribe the best treatment for your medical issue. Or rather, you want the treatment that has been shown, overall, in fair tests, to be better than all the others. You will probably expect your doctor to decide the treatment and trust him along with hoping that there are systems in place to ensure that the treatment proceeds systematically and properly, because getting involved in every single decision yourself would consume a lot of time.

Our next players are the funders, and for them, the answer is also realtively simple; they want the same thing as the patient, unless it is expensive. For common drugs, and common decisions, they might have a pre-determined 'pathway' that dictates to General Practitioners (more commonly than to hospital doctors) which drug is to be used, but besides those simple rules for simple situations, they rely on doctors' judgments.

Now we come to our central player in the individual treatment decision: the doctors. They need good-quality and correct information, but they need it, significantly, under their noses. The challenge facing the modern world is not lack of information, after all, but information overload, and even more precisely, what Clay Shirky calls 'filter failure'. Initially, say in the 1950s, medicine was driven almost entirely by anecdote and eminence, in fact, it's only in the past couple of decades that we have gathered good-quality evidence at all, in large amounts, and for all the failures in our current and existing systems, we suddenly now have an over-whelming amount of data. The exciting future, for evidence-based medicine, is an information architecture that can get the right evidence to the right doctor at the right time.

Does this happen? The simple answer is no. Although there are many automated systems for disseminating knowledge, for the most part we continue to rely on systems that have evolved over centuries, like the long, meandering essays in academic journals that are still used to report the results of clinical trials. Often, if you ask a doctor whether they know if one particular treatment is best for a particular medical condition, they'll tell they know it is the best, their answer might scare you.

To be honest, doctors cannot read every scientific article that is relevant to their work. There are tens of thousands of academic journals and millions of academic medical papers in existence, with more produced every single day.

So, doctors frankly will not be going through every clinical trial, about every treatment relevant to their field, meticulously checking each one for the methodological tricks described, diligently keeping their knowledge perfectly current. They will take quick judgments on the basis of their key opinion leaders and on their own clinical experience and these shortcuts can be explored and exploited, with side effects sometimes.

Now let us understand a doctor's prescribing decision from the perspective of a pharmaceutical company. The company wants the doctor to prescribe your product, and it will put in its best efforts to make that happen. The reality is, the company wants sales. So the company publishes and advertises its new treatment in medical journals, stating the benefits but softening the risks and tilting away from unappealing comparisons. Additionally, the company will send out medical representatives to meet doctors individually, and detail the merits of the treatment.

But the company needs to go beyond this. Doctors require ongoing education: they practice for years after leaving medical school, and medicine changes unrecognizably continuously. This education is expensive, and the state is unwilling to pay, so it is the pharmaceutical companies that pay for talks, tutorials, teaching materials, conference sessions, and whole conferences, featuring experts who they know prefer their drug.

Adverts to Patients

The final decision of prescribing a drug lies with the doctors. But in reality the decision of choosing a particular treatment is made between the patient and doctor. This is entirely how a pharmaceutical company would want things to be; but it does not make patients another level to be leaned on, by an industry keen to increase sales.

Celebrity Endorsement

In the 1952 Hollywood movie 'Singin' in the Rain, Debbie Reynolds plays Kathy Selden, a talented singer who hides behind a curtain and covertly provides the sweet singing voice for an on-stage starlet who merely mimes the words. In an interview, Debbie Reynolds suddenly starts explaining that "Overactive bladder affects you because it defects you… effective treatment is available.' The interview didn't mention that she was working for Pharmacia, a company promoting a new treatment for overactive bladder. Accu Check for detecting active blood glucose levels endorsed by cricketer Wasim Akram is an example of celebrity endorsement wherein Wasim Akram being a diabetic himself promotes the portable and easy to use active blood glucose meter.

More than Molecules

The concept that depression is caused by low serotonin levels in the brain is now deeply embedded in popular legends, and people with no neuroscience experience at all will regularly include phrases about it into ordinary discussions of their mood, just to keep their serotonin levels up. Numerous people also 'know' that this is how anti-depressant drugs work: depression is caused by low serotonin, so you basically require drugs which raise the serotonin levels in your brain, like SSRI anti-depressants, which are 'selective serotonin reuptake inhibitors'. But this theory is wrong. The 'serotonin hypothesis' for depression, was always rickety, and the evidence now is incredibly opposing. There is a drug called tianeptine – it is a selective serotonin reuptake enhancer, not an inhibitor, that should reduce serotonin levels – and yet research shows that it is also a pretty effective treatment for depression.

But in popular culture the depression-serotonin theory is proven and absolute, because it has been marketed so efficiently. In drug advertisements and educational material you can see it recycled, simply and plainly, because it makes absolute sense: depression is caused by too little serotonin, therefore our pill, which raises serotonin levels, will fix it. This simple concept is attractive, even though it has little backing in academia, perhaps because it speaks to us of controllable, external, molecular pressures.

Medicalization

Social processes, where the pharmaceutical companies expand the boundaries of diagnosis to increase their market and see the idea that a complex social or personal problem is a molecular disease, in order to sell their own molecules, in pills, to fix it is what sums up the term medicalization. Sometimes it falls apart; because despite the marketing playoffs, these tablets might well do some good.

Patient Groups

Patient groups perform an important and commendable part: they bring patients together, spread information and support, and can help to lobby on behalf of people with the condition they represent.

Many patient groups are funded by the pharmaceutical industry. Basically a patient group requires money and resources to lobby and to support its members and can benefit from specialist knowledge and business know how. A pharmaceutical company offers this and then it has its own requirements: it wants to spread friendly messages for its brand, in a regulatory environment that prevents direct advertising to patients. It also wants to be seen as generous and socially responsible, like any other company.

Doctors and their Diagnosis

Sometimes you feel that are doctors becoming interpreters of pathology tests and re-engineering the results of all tests inclusive of MRI, etc. to treat the patient and search for right diagnosis. Do they diagnose and then ask patients for tests or do they ask the patients for tests based on the symptoms and then diagnose? Which comes first?

What can One Do?

It is important to re-shift or ban drug advertisements that do not intend to serve and inform the general public. If a company really wishes to provide authentic information to the patients then they could probably pay to a central and independent repository that can give grants to the people with good track record of providing evidence-based information to the general public. The general public, patients and the media should be cautious about selling novel medical conditions if they are also into selling the cure. It is essential for drug companies running disease-awareness campaigns to declare that it has plans of developing or marketing a product to treat it. Finally it is also equally important that all the educational materials have the same declarations.

PRE-REQUISITES

Understanding the Industry Structure

The pharmaceutical industry is changing as a result of changes in the environment. These changes are in terms of rivalry, potential new entrants, suppliers, buyers as well as substitutes of products.

The industry existing today can be analyzed by many approaches. One way to do the same is by adapting Michael E. Porter's 'Five-Factor' model. This model provides a suitable and convenient framework for the discussion of several pharmaceutical industry aspects and characteristics.

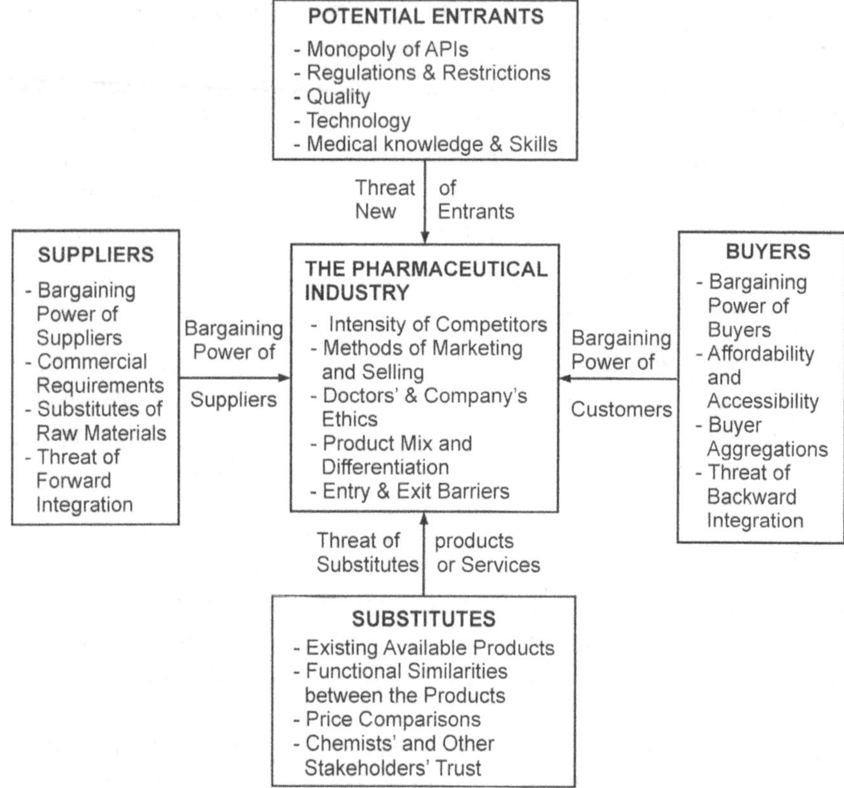

Figure 1.2 Five-factor model for the pharmaceutical industry
Source: Adapted from Michael E. Porter's Five-factor model

As depicted in the model, the degree of rivalry among different organizations in the industry is a function of the intensity of competitors, methods of marketing and selling, ethics related to the doctors and company, product mix and its differentiation, entry barriers and exit barriers. Among these, the intensity of competitors is the most influential.

Competition is enhanced by the threat of entry into the industry which is again restricted by a number of entry barriers. The barriers that restrict this entry are monopoly of APIs, regulations and restrictions imposed by the Government bodies, quality of the products in the product mix, technological involvement along with medical knowledge and skills.

Bargaining power of buyers is the ability to compel the industry to reduce costs or increase certain features, thus commanding profits. Buyers acquire power when they have better affordability and accessibility along with awareness. Additionally, buyer aggregations with threat of backward integration add to the power of the buyer.

Bargaining power of suppliers is the extent to which suppliers of raw materials have the ability to compel the industry to accept high prices or reduced services, thus affecting profits. The factors affecting the power of the supplier include commercial requirements, substitutes of raw materials and threat to forward integration.

Substitute products are another form of competition. These products affect the potential of the industry because of factors like existing available products, functional similarities between the products, price comparisons, chemist and other stakeholders' trust along with the services offered.

Steps in Marketing through Marketing Models

1. The 4 Phase Transaction Model- Conceptual Model

There are many definitions for marketing but the most practical definition is the fact that marketing by nature is transaction with the market. But the question is that how do we identify this transaction with respect to right doctor and right product. This transaction can be identified by market research, medical and clinical knowledge, clinical experience, new diagnosis, new and existing patients along with analyzing database with profiles. The next step is the stimulation of transaction which can be achieved by support to the medical servicemen and stakeholders through product portfolios, concepts, policies, ethics, pricing, media and competition. Facilitating and encashment of the transaction through patients, pharmacies, stockists, distributors, Carrying and Forwarding Agents (C&Fs), entrepreneurs and academicians come next. Sustaining the value of the transaction is the final part of the transaction which ensures the acquisition of a lifetime buyer of the product.

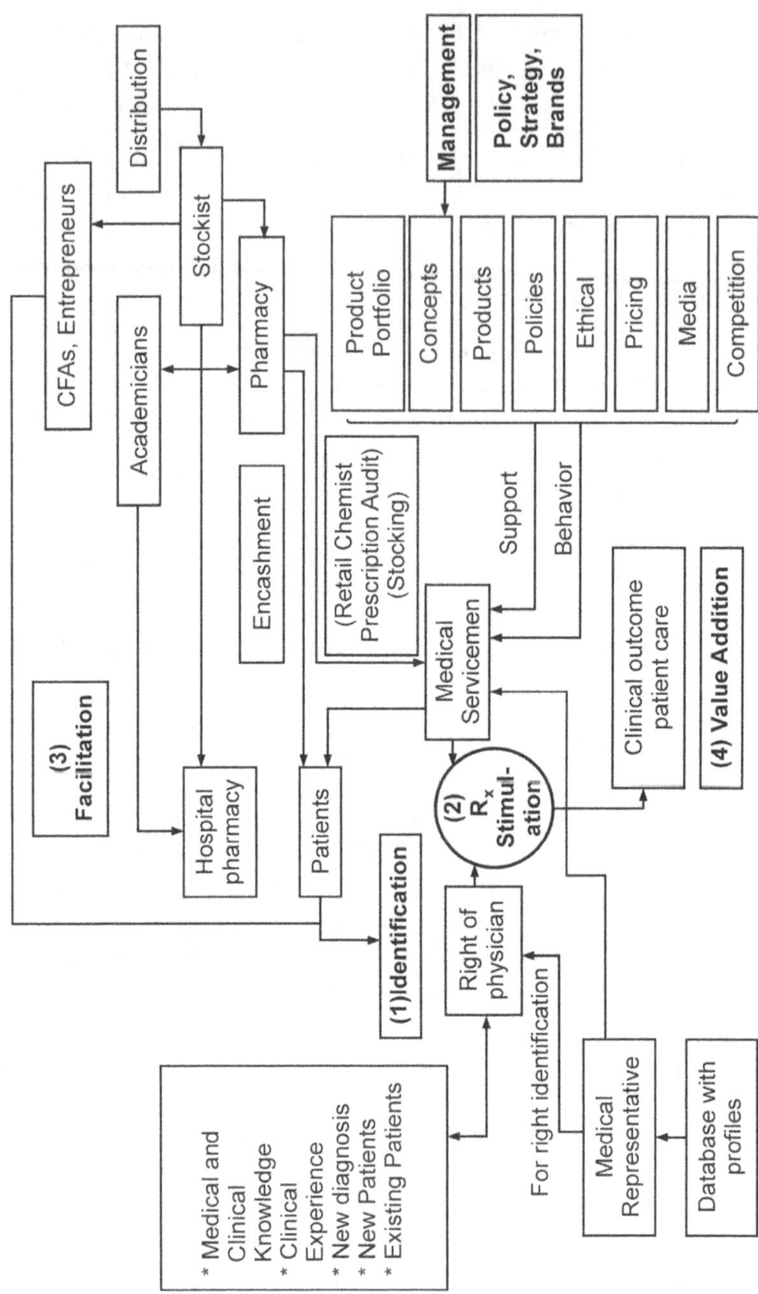

Figure 1.3 The 4 phase transaction model-conceptual Model

Source: Interlink knowledge cell

2. Medical Marketing Model

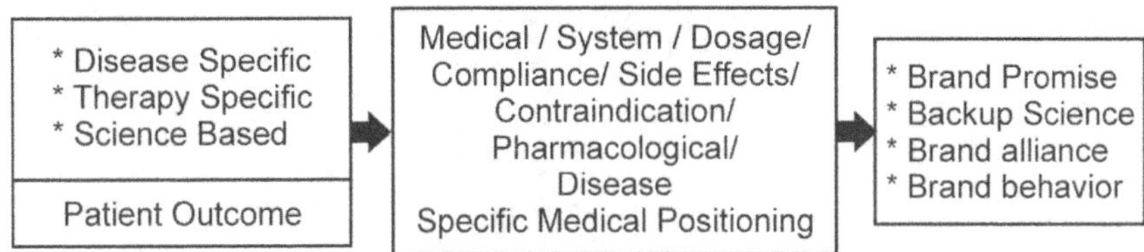

Figure 1.4 Medical marketing model

Source: Interlink knowledge cell

The state today is that most of the drugs are generics and positioning of these generics is difficult. But if you have a medical marketing model then you can look at this positioning through medical positioning first. This medical positioning can be disease specific, therapy specific, science based along with patient outcomes. This is also dependent on what has to be communicated, is it the dosage, the side effects, the compliance or the contraindications. It is important to know what the physician is prescribing and thereby create a lot of differentiation for the product. From this differentiation and medical position brand promise can be created along with some backup science. If necessary in this era of generics, brand alliances can also be considered. Brand behavior is also an aspect that can be looked at by studying post-marketing surveillance and promotional studies through this medical marketing model.

3. Market Projection Model

Marketing projection is dependent on many aspects and these aspects include epidemiological analysis, new diseases, detected and undetected diseases, patient pool and potential. It is important to consider dropouts from a particular study of research of a product while forecasting.

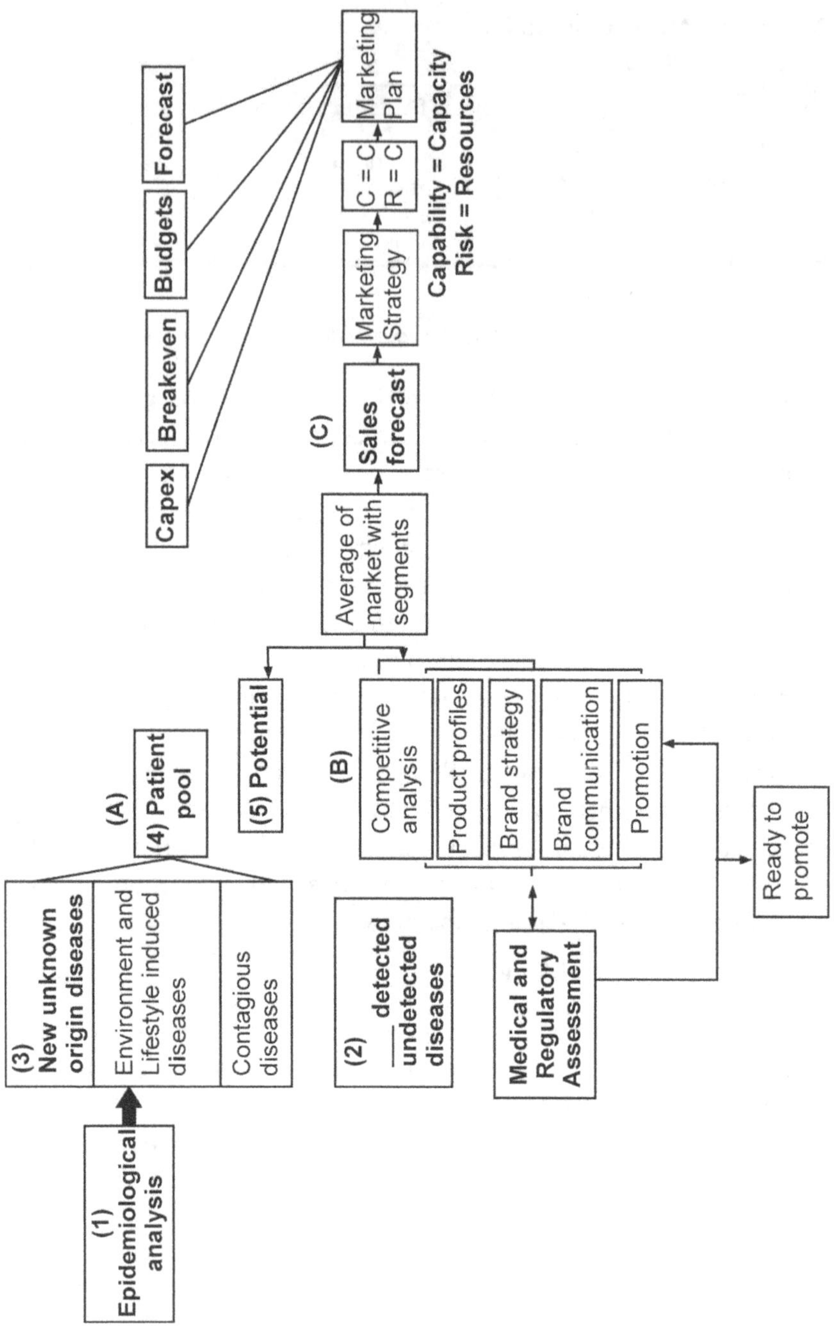

Figure 1.5 Market projection model

Source: Interlink knowledge cell

4. Commercial Model

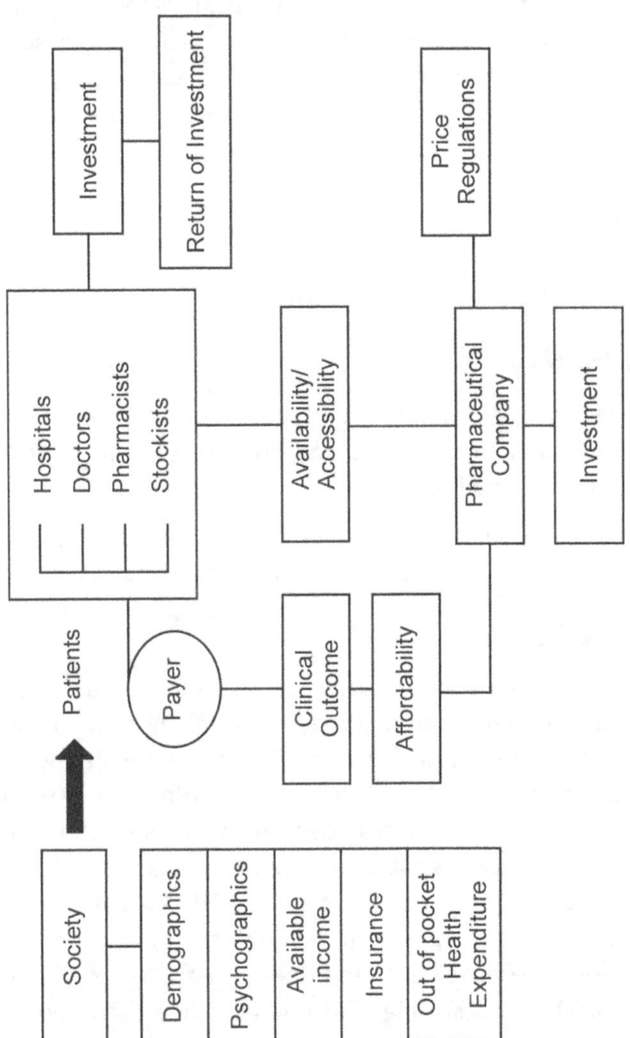

Figure 1.6 Commercial model

Source: Interlink knowledge cell

The commercial model depends on the society. Higher segments of the society do not face the issues of affordability that is there is no price resistance. So it is important to look at the society where the company wishes to operate and to position the product in accordance. It is also important to look at who is the prescriber of the product and his/ her attachments to hospitals, stockists, pharmacists and doctors. So the first commerce of the commercial model takes place at the prescriber level, second commerce at the level of other stakeholders attached to the prescriber, third commerce at the level of availability and accessibility and fourth at the level of investment which then leads to return on investment thus, contributing to profitability.

PROCESSES

The Basics of Strategy and Marketing

Basics of Strategy

In a competitive environment and business variables, the company needs to look at their strengths and engage relevant opportunities to develop a strategy and intent.

Contents are dependent on risk taking ability of the company and the fact that it has brand assets always help double the strategic advantage.

Basics of Marketing

The basics of marketing include understanding the organization's mission and the role marketing plays in fulfilling that mission, setting marketing objectives, gathering, analyzing, and interpreting information about the organization's situation, including its strengths and weaknesses as well as opportunities and threats in the environment, developing a marketing strategy by deciding exactly which wants and whose wants the organization will try to satisfy (target market strategy) and by developing appropriate marketing activities (the marketing mix) to satisfy the desires of selected target markets, implementing the marketing strategy, designing performance measures and periodically evaluating marketing efforts, and making changes if needed.

These activities and their relationships form the foundation on which marketing has been based and thus, has evolved.

New Rules of Marketing

The pharmaceutical industry is experiencing a wave of changes that are prompting the rewriting of the rules of marketing.

Some sales and marketing practices in the pharmaceutical industry are unethical; some research is misused. There is no industry in the world that is snow-white or that is devoid of any problems or issues. There are issues in the food industry, around obesity, in the tobacco industry and in the financial services industry with the global economic crisis. If the problems in the industry are emphasized, and controls are pushed for, then the companies will become more risk-averse, which will then result in less innovation.

Rather than tightening the reins, it is important that companies intensify their marketing efforts while adhering to best ethics-based industry practices that need to be done with awareness of the fundamental changes currently underway within the industry.

New Stakeholders

Launching a new product to any kind of pharmaceutical market comes with its challenges especially with the shifting center of gravity within the industry. The industry is now focused on inputs from a diverse set of stakeholders including regulators, insurance companies, hospital administrators, managed care organizations, nurses, social media, and of course, patients besides individual prescribers.

With the medical representatives having many years of experience dealing with prescribers, have deep insights about the perceptions, preferences and behavior of these prescribers, and thus, know a lot less about the other stakeholders. As a result, getting 'under the skin' of the other relevant stakeholders is a sales and marketing task whose importance is second to none. Adding to this is the fact that newly empowered decision-makers have differing, and conflicting needs and wants. Therefore, it becomes extremely important for any company to position its product that satisfies all the stakeholders. This then becomes a delicate, and new job for pharmaceutical sales and marketing.

But getting these insights right outweigh the challenges faced. For instance, Eli Lilly's erectile dysfunction drug Cialis initially faced long odds in its bid to take on market pioneer Viagra. Dose for dose, Cialis far outlasted Viagra, with a 36-hour window of effectives compared to Viagra's 4-hour one, but physicians considered this a meager advantage. However, the Cialis team, by getting 'under the skin' of its target audience, hit upon a compelling sales point: Having 36 hours to play with allowed couples to have a less pressured, more romantic experience. Contrasting Viagra's positioning as a male performance enhancer, Lilly marketed Cialis as the "couple's weekend pill" helping them to restore intimacy, and reduce stress within their relationships. The creative positioning paid off handsomely: In 2011, sales of Cialis overtook Viagra.

Global Challenges

The rise of developing markets threatens to compound the challenges that face the pharmaceutical companies. The stakeholders may be very different, and the prevalence of diseases might not be the same. Also, the healthcare infrastructure might often not be very sophisticated along with these markets being rather volatile, and difficult to predict. It is not a sure bet, but one has to invest.

In order to achieve a strong foothold in any market in today's times, companies need to commit to building a heavily localized approach that is substantiated by global reputation. Otherwise, the companies risk going the Procter & Gamble way, which sold off its pharmaceutical business in 2009. P&G could not last long in the pharmaceutical industry because of the mere fact that people weren't sure they could trust a soap, and diaper producer with their health.

Speaciality and Niche Markets

The focus of the industry is witnessing a shift from primary care towards speciality, and niche markets. There has been a substantial rise in speciality products. Instead of being marketed to a huge patient population, new pharmaceutical products will most likely follow the footsteps of Novartis' Afinitor, which began as a treatment for kidney cancer but slowly became adopted as a treatment for certain kinds of lung, breast, and brain tumors as well.

The most game-changing trend in the industry is that of personalized healthcare (PHC), an approach that focuses on matching medicines to specific target groups. The shift of approach towards PHC is also necessitated by the increased importance of payers as industry stakeholders. As the speciality drugs are expensive, and targeted towards only a small segment of patients, regulators, and payers are setting the threshold for reimbursement higher, and higher.

Companies are already looking at adapting their marketing strategies in an attempt to claim their niche, but this can backfire if there is no brand recognition. AstraZeneca's Brazilian Iressa, a niche lung cancer drug, lost out to Tarceva, a similar product from oncology giant Roche/Genentech, despite AstraZeneca financing expensive eligibility tests. When the time came for the actual prescription, providing free biopsies to test for the biomarker didn't generate enough goodwill to persuade Brazil's stakeholders to choose AstraZeneca over the better-known brand.

The sales and marketing investments of major pharmaceutical companies has produced outstanding contributions to many critical fields. New stakeholders and new markets hold opportunities for companies to put their best foot forward and succeed at the same time in this rapidly changing world.

Hence, the new rules of marketing look as follows:

1. Patients not the drug or prescription are in focus.
2. Create innovative medical-marketing positioning and communication.
3. Ethics are in the center as we deal with human life.
4. Consider the health care infrastructure and push strategic initiatives to all stakeholders.
5. Use all media inclusive of focused medium of MR (Medical Detailing).
6. Corporate image is equally essential to acquire 'credibility' and develop it.
7. Looking at regulations as facilitators and hindrances to think and proceed.
8. Looking at ROI always in making financial investments.
9. Working towards developing a brand.

PHILOSOPHY AND PRACTICES

1. Philosophy of Marketing

Ethics in Business

Being a business of health and human beings involved in it, ethical dimension of marketing needs to be a major fulcrum of philosophy of pharmaceutical marketing. At the end, it is a business behavior of sales and marketing teams get exposed the moment they deviate from norms of ethics.

Ethics per say, is just decision and thereby action defeating to a situation which a decision maker takes at that moment. It's that moment which is crucial to be on ethics path or deviate from it for immediate gains or competitive edge.

However, it's important to understand that pharmaceutical sales and marketing is not the same as in any other industry selling and marketing, as at the end we are processing health and outcome of health through our products, services, concepts, communications have to keep that safety, efficacy and health solution in focus.

Being a very crucial element of life and creating a thin line difference between health and the patient taking medicines who is not healthy, will get on priority for all policy makers and regulatory, as this is an issue of the population and the country. More important parameters like morbidity and mortality when it comes to human beings have direct impact on how new drugs are invented or devised and how do we as a country, through sales and marketing, address the issue of mortality and morbidity in pharmaceuticals.

As a result, is not only ethics at R&D, product development, quality, quality delivery but also at sales and marketing and final transaction between physicians and pharmaceutical industry needs philosophy of ethical marketing and selling.

Creating New Markets and New Wave in
Patient Centric Satisfaction

Most of the industries have consumers and customers. Even in pharmaceuticals, we have customers as prescribers, insurance companies, other Institutions where supplies are given to arm forces and other services. We also have consumers who are patients or pre-emptive patients. As pharmaceuticals, propagative products, concepts, services and infrastructure for patient healthcare, it's equally important that organization and industry should be attuned towards patient centric healing and satisfaction.

As expressed at many places in this book, we need to be ready to address diversity and adversity and we also need lot of innovation to win over in changing environment.

It's not only important for pharmaceutical sales and marketing to focus on taking the competitors market share or share from growth of the markets, it's going to be consistently important that we improve our competency of sales and marketing teams as well as develop strategies to create new markets for ourselves. It's not Blue Ocean Strategy but it's definitely a new wave strategy for pharmaceutical marketing. The day is not far off where existing pharmaceutical marketing unless it is architectural on basic principles of pharmaceutical marketing, ethics in business behavior and new wave of marketing is crystalized to gather momentum in creating new markets.

> **Blue Ocean Strategy** was developed by W. Chan Kim and Renée Mauborgne. They observed that companies tend to engage in head-to-head competition in search of sustained profitable growth. Yet in today's overcrowded industries competing head-on results in nothing but a bloody red ocean of rivals fighting over a shrinking profit pool. Lasting success increasingly comes, not from battling competitors, but from creating blue oceans of untapped new market spaces ripe for growth.
>
> Blue Ocean Strategy challenges everything you thought you knew about strategic success and provides a systematic approach to making the competition irrelevant.

Selling a Core of Pharmaceutical Marketing

All said and done, whatever we say in literature at least in pharmaceuticals sales and marketing core fabric of sales and selling plays a vital role in creating new transactions and demand for pharmaceutical products. Marketing is definitely cementing itself and penetrating to the center of core which is selling. Unless it is been done meticulously, in an articulate way, sales and marketing in pharmaceuticals would remain two different layers and also bring lot of non-alignment of these two functions. This non-alignment would result in no demand creation and hence strategic impact of marketing will not be visible through selling in the market.

Purpose of pharmaceutical selling is very mobile, as through selling intervention, pharmaceutical companies are providing alternative way in improving quality of life of patients, if they comply with the dosages, indications, contra-indications and prescribers manage other effects to provide that quality to patients.

Objectives of pharmaceutical selling is a process and it's not one time decision but it's a continuous exposure and intervention of pharmaceuticals, medical salesmen with the physicians. In this process of building relationship with the knowledgeable customer like physicians, pharmaceutical medical salesmen must possess skilled and competency to discuss and debate science and also commerce. This is possible only when this pharmaceutical medical salesmen creates trust with physicians. Hence, objective of pharmaceutical selling is creating trust not only with physicians but also with patients, patients families and other stakeholders like pharmacists, stockiest etc.

Besides this trust and increasing quality of patient's life pharmaceutical medical salesmen has overall responsibility, as he is frequently visiting physicians and pharmacists to create value for his own existence in a very competitively dense marketing.

2. Transaction Practice

As core of pharmaceutical marketing is sales and selling, this transaction should not only provide one time prescription generation and also encashment on the same but as the value is generated during the transaction, this mode of transaction should make this sales and process of selling as rain making. No longer will it be a one-time sale but also it will continuously rain.

Lifestyle diseases and other disorders as well as chronic diseases, have a tendency to consume medicines for a long time and that is exactly an important aspect of creating a new process of rain making than only selling as a one-time sale.

Besides selling and rain making definition of product, is also not the same, as it was few years before. Today, any product is also expanded with its packaging, servicing guarantee, warranty, indications, contra-indications and as more regulations are in the offing, the same product would be defined in a different way. This might create fear of uses or limitation in uses or right way to ensure that there is compliance.

As product definition is enlarged, its scope, pharmaceutical sales and marketing should also understand that it's no longer just one ingredient packaged in a capsule or any other galenical form.

3. Safety Practice

In order not to lose focus on sales and marketing, it's imperative that basics of pharmaceutical and marketing like sales drill, segmentation, positioning, targeting has to be in its place otherwise, the same core of pharmaceutical marketing, as it is shifted to selling would go beyond the boundaries of sales and marketing and cross the border of social, political, economic, technological essence of marketing where the controls will be different, measures will be different and rewards will be different. So it is important to stick to basics of marketing, available utilities, barriers of promotions and also to the extent which not only reaches physicians and pharmacists but also to patients not by compelling him to consumer medicines but by making him aware that to keep him healthy he or she needs lot of efforts of compliance and duration of the treatment.

In fact, in the era of generics, products are looking similar from perception point of view except pricing difference. It's important now that pharmaceutical sales and marketers find out how do I differentiate some generics with the help of medical sensibility, meta-analysis and also understanding customer and consumer insights to provide differentiation.

4. Execution Practice

As core of pharmaceutical sales and marketing is shifted to sales, obviously execution becomes the essence of sales. No longer sales management is an issue of relationship with field staff but it is vehemently clear with sales and marketing is devoid of analytics and data management. Number of observations have been studied and also observed that behaviors change on the basis of critical incidences and data points are captured properly through analytics. These analytics become imperative for sales force execution and also efficiency.

5. Business Practice

Not in the beginning and not even at the end, we consider that it's the NGO – a non-profitable or a charitable trust but it is definitely a business, may not be a business like other materials, but it's a business of healing, business to provide health solutions and hence it is requirement of earning decent margin or profit, depending on the tax structure of the country, as this enterprise who is motivated to serve patients, need to survive and remain healthy to provide healthy solutions.

LEARNINGS

With the pharmaceutical marketing environment changing consistently, the pharmaceutical marketers have to be competent and ready to face the diverse and adverse situations.

The world today is moving towards a new normal world by riding the megatrends of digitization, sustainability and rise of the developing markets.

There is a defining moment in the paradigm of how business is conducted with consumers being inclined towards globally leveraged, locally relevant products. To succeed globally, the enterprises need to have:

- Every Day Great Execution (EDGE)
- Diversity of Talent
- Purpose-Driven and Values-Led-Leadership

To manage the new normal world it is important to innovate and one aspect of this is 'Design Thinking', a framework for shifting the paradigm of innovation.

As marketing evolves and takes shape it is important to take in account various marketing perspectives like:

- Political Perspective
- Economic perspective
- Social Perspective
- Technological Perspective
- Regulatory Perspective
- Ecological Perspective
- Trade Perspective
- Unionization Perspective

It is also important to take into consideration the perceptions of marketing to perceive and understand what is happening in the pharmaceutical marketing environment.

The pre-requisite is to understand the pharmaceutical industry structure as it is undergoing significant changes in terms of:

- Rivalry
- Potential New Entrants
- Suppliers
- Buyers
- Substitutes of Products

Marketing in the pharmaceutical industry can be pursued by following the marketing models like:

- The 4 Phase Transaction Model-Conceptual Model
- Medical Marketing Model
- Market Projection Model
- Commercial Model

In a competitive environment and business variables, the company needs to look at their strengths and engage relevant opportunities to develop strategy and intent by following the basics of marketing.

With the pharmaceutical industry experiencing a wave of changes it is imperative for the marketers to follow new rules of marketing keeping in mind new stakeholders, global challenges and specialty and niche markets.

Finally, it is also important to follow the practices of marketing with respect to:

- Philosophy of Marketing
- Transaction Practice
- Safety Practice
- Execution Practice
- Business Practice

CHAPTER 2

Dynamic Pathways

SIRAJ UD-DAULAH, the famous monarch, was once gifted a beautiful painting by another king. Siraj was so happy that he wanted the same painter to do various paintings for him. He commissioned him to paint many paintings including landscapes, portraits, life sketches and graphics. One of them Siraj felt was so beautiful that it deserved to be displayed at the main square of the market so that his subjects too could appreciate the painter's work. The moment it was displayed at the main market, there was praise for the painter from everybody. The painting was indeed a work of art.

Siraj, on the request of his citizens, sent the painter a huge reward. When the ministers went to give him this reward, the painter was sitting gloomily in a corner. The ministers asked him why he looked so sad when he should actually be happy. When they probed him further, he said, 'You know, I have painted a girl holding a bunch of grapes.' 'Exactly,' one of the ministers interrupted, 'Do you know the grapes are so real that even the birds are pecking at them. We can see and feel your greatness. So beautiful and life-like.' The painter replied in a low voice, 'Yes I know this: and so I am disturbed. Do you know, I have also painted a beautiful girl along with the grapes. Does it not mean that the girl is not so natural? You see, I understand that in a sense the painting is beautiful and lively, but something about it is unreal, not alive!" He refused to accept the reward.

The case with the dynamics of marketing in the pharmaceutical industry in India is quite similar. Part of the picture shows how lively the Indian marketing scene is in spite of its many constraints, but the remaining part needs to be handled with courage. We need to accept our inadequacies and find out options and solutions for tomorrow to cope with the challenges and problems of the changing environment.

Alvin Toffler has aptly summarized the process of dynamism and change: 'High speed changes are not chaotic or random as we are conditioned to believe.' He contends that there are not only distinct patterns behind the headlines, but identifiable forces that shape them. It is important for all of us to discern these distinct patters and identify those forces which are likely to shape forthcoming events.

Selling and marketing in the Indian health-care industry has in the last four decades changed its context from 'licensing' to 'marketing'. The future will compel the industry to take a good, hard look at the patterns which are evolving due to the interplay of different forces and amicably push itself towards marketing and innovation.

You should try and find ways to cope with the challenges that these continuing changes are posing. This task can become easier if you try to develop a strategic vision and focus your energy and resources to carve a niche in future. Before we discuss how this can be done, let us get a brief background of the contemporary business scenario as it exists in India today.

REFLECTIVE SCANNING

For seventy years after Independence, the pharmaceutical industry was under the influence of *six* basic forces:

1. *The government* as a force trying to regulate the industry.
2. *The trade* as a force to facilitate the availability.
3. *The medical profession* as a force to stimulate the demand for different types of fixed dosage formulations.
4. *Technology* as a force to create or eliminate competition.
5. *The status of the country* in terms of its industrial development, population, hygiene, health awareness, and per capita income.
6. Influence of *international development and its impact.*

1. The Government

The government started regulating the industry through its industrial policy, drug policy, Drug Prices Control Orders (DPCO), and Bureau of Industrial Costing and Pricing (BICP), which affected the economics of the entire industry.

In the beginning, 'industrial policy' was drafted which continued to be governed by the requirements of compulsory licensing in terms of the Industries (Development & Regulations) Act.

Pricing—particularly the rigid control in price fixation and revision without consideration of actual costs—was the concern of the industry. I distinctly remember that, in 1966-67, Abdec drops (Parke-Davis) which was earlier sold at Rs 7.20 per 10 ml bottle, had to be priced at just Rs 2.70. Alembic also faced similar problems even in the 1980s as most of their products were syrup-based. The sugar price kept on increasing without any increase in prices of fixed doe-syrup combinations.

All bulk manufacturers were required to maintain bulk to formulations ration of 1:2. This made many organizations rethink their product mix.

A Drug Price Equalization Amount (DPEA) was levied as the government felt the prices were unilaterally raised by companies. The government also compelled many organizations to go to court between 1979 and 1987. A large number of companies received notices of recovery of amounts allegedly arising from para 14 of DPCO 1987. A few were even directed to deposit the amounts due from them into the DPEA.

All these changes affected the fabric of the Indian pharmaceutical industry. It has been observed that each DPCO—in 1970, 1979, 1987 and 2013—shook the industry violently, and each time the industry readjusted and met these changes adequately, proving it had a lot of resilience.

Older Indian companies like the Cosme, Mathias Menezes group of companies of Goa (now known as Wallace Group) and the US Vitamin Group of Mumbai started selling medicines in India under the 'licensing' system then prevailing. Initially, they imported finished products from Brown Burg and American Home Products respectively and distributed them in India. Later, they started manufacturing under license of those companies. 'Piptal Drops' was one of the products of Lakeside Laboratories, which was manufactured by Chemo Pharma along with its own products and sold in India. Even TTK distributed and sold products like Ossopan and Ripason, from Rubi Pharma. Till 1993 Criticare imported cancer products under license of Lyphomed USA and sold them in India.

Right from the early days, multinationals have tried to either manufacture or import, and make use of India's large trading network. India is a vast country with a 200-year-old heritage of trading. National and multinational companies took advantage of this and distributed their products throughout India.

As a result, the government established customs duty, excise, and 'octroi' and has now moved towards GST. In the beginning of the 1980s the government also levied 'turnover tax' on traders and manufacturers. It also kept the margin of traders away from the purview of DPCO. This is perhaps the reason why the cost of distribution is the highest only in India.

With the growth of industry, the 'loan license' system was also introduced to cope with the demand of products. The small-scale sector built manufacturing facilities for multinationals and national organizations. This increased the stake of the small-scale industry in pharmaceuticals. Today, 'loan licenses' are restricted as the small-scale units have proliferated beyond imagination to around 16,000.

Lack of support for imposition of a strong patent law, and the absence of an Intellectual Property Act led to the point where companies like Ciba and Hoechst closed their basic research centers in India, and the Indian sector did not invest in R&D. However, as the years passed, awareness and potential impact of the IPR were perceived by the industry. Various companies coped with future challenges by combining their resources to invest in R&D.

2. **Trade**

Trade was the essential focus of many organizations as it provided a greater leverage to them in their growth. During these years many appointed stockists, wholesalers, distributors, and distribution-cum-propaganda agents to promote their products. Sarabhai and Alembic had an open market policy and catered to even small wholesalers of the country directly. Later on, as the business grew, they developed their depots and infrastructure of warehouses. Unichem was the first to develop a distributors' sales force and many others followed suit. Roche and Merck & Co. appointed Voltas as their sole distributors for the entire country while Parke-Davis operated through Spencers in southern India.

Many traders realized the necessity of vertical integration, and expanded their businesses to include manufacturing and selling. Aristo, Alkem, Mohan Pharma (Bangalore), Adroit (Nagpur), and Mcneil (Jaipur) were a few companies that successfully changed their focus of operations from distribution to manufacturing.

As trade gained power and became organized, the All India Organization of Chemists & Druggists (AIOCD) was formed to negotiate with the industry and the government. A new platform of understanding was created among the government, the trade, and the industry to take care of common problems.

During the 1970s the government also felt that co-operative societies should take part in distribution of pharmaceutical products. Rajasthan and Maharashtra took the lead. This experiment, however, failed at the national level.

3. The Medical Profession

The medical profession in India encouraged national and multinational companies to improve their information base initially. As the number of physicians increased, companies became selective, and today, not a single company visits more than one-third of the population of physicians. Physicians responded well to old and new molecules, and also to innovations in marketing and selling. Combiflam is an example of such innovation. Physicians took part in suggesting combinations of different ingredients. Introduction of combinations for tropical diseases is evidence. 'Wotinex' is one such product. When introduction of new molecules was difficult, physicians also accepted "alternative medicines" for a few indications. Liv 52, Gassex and Hepax, are a few examples for liver-related disorders. At the other extreme many irrational combinations were also developed. Classical anti-diarrhoeals were replaced by many irrational combinations.

4. The Technology

Technology has altered substantially for the last few years. Dr. Reddy's Laboratories, Standard Organics Ltd (S.O.L), Kopran, NATCO, Ranbaxy, Cipla, Wockhardt, and many other companies initially changed the quality and price matrix of many bulk drugs. Amoxicillin, Ciprofloxacin, Norfloxacin, Ranitidine, Cimetidine, Dextro-propoxyphem etc., are a few examples of such bulk drugs. These companies practiced 'backward integration/reverse engineering' and used bulk drugs for captive consumption as well as selling to others in India and abroad.

In the early years, Dr. Reddy's Laboratories, through intensive research, have brought about a technological change in the manufacturing processes of many bulk drugs, inclusive of quinolones. This then helped Dr. Reddy's Laboratories reduce the prices of quinolones by half. They also in turn raised the quality to international standards due to which they started global export of their bulk drugs. In fact, they put India, and especially Hyderabad, on the international map for bulk drugs and fine chemicals.

'Backward integration/reverse engineering' continued to be an enabling condition for profitability for a lot of years and would continue to be so, although to a lesser extent than before. The acceptance of (WTO) norms brought in legislations to recognize product patents by 2005. This meant that Indian companies could no longer backward integrate/reverse engineer drugs which have been patented abroad; these skills would only be useful after 2005 only for manufacturing products going off patent. As a result, Indian companies like Cipla, Dr. Reddy's Laboratories, Wockhardt, Sun Pharmaceuticals, among others have initiated investment in product research as opposed to process research. Additionally, these companies are also continuing to hone their backward integration/reverse engineering skills to manufacture drugs going off patent.

USV and Eskayef earlier propagated timed release drugs like DBI, TD and Fessofor. Later NATCO entered the scene and introduced sustained release technology and brought products of day-to-day use in a different form. Theophyllin was one of the drugs they brought in sustained release form. A variety of applications were propagated by Wockhardt through galenical forms of Betadine. A few companies also tried to introduce transdermal technology for a few drugs.

Intravenous manufacturing technology went through enormous changes from glass bottles (McGraw-Ravindra Krishna Keshav Laboratories) to polypropylene bottles (Core Parenteral). Similarly, technology for bottling, liquid manufacturing, capsules manufacturing, and packaging has been tremendously improved, and today 'blister packs' are common place.

Hi-tech baby food processes were evolved. Raptakoss Brett had a monopoly in the manufacturing and marketing of baby food products. Wockhardt also developed a similar technology and launched a few baby food products like Nusobee in India.

Today's world is experiencing considerable technological advancements. There are newer concepts coming up to the likes of bioelectronics, precision medicines, nanodrugs, Health sensors, to name a few. These technological advancements coupled with the shifting behaviors of the patients and healthcare professionals will have a fundamental impact on the future and success of pharmaceutical business.

5. The Health Status of the Country

It is essential to study the health status of the country to understand the potential of therapeutic groups. In fact, India is considered to be a developing country whose socioeconomic, hygienic and industrialization conditions are fast changing. Though the general hygiene is improving, the pollution level has become alarming. Of course, this is more so in urban India. Rural India has been relatively less affected by industrialization, though hygiene has certainly improved there due to the increase in the literacy rate in a few Indian states.

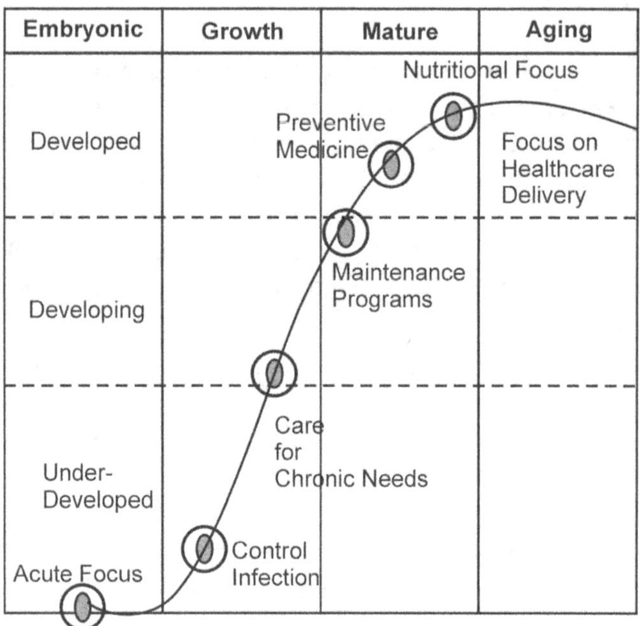

Figure 2.1 Health-care delivery priorities

The above graph (Figure 2.1) will give an idea of the importance of the development level of the country and its needs for different therapeutic groups. Developed countries like the USA where the population is aging, hygiene is at its peak, and the socioeconomic status is quite satisfactory, will require focus on nutrition, psycholeptics, internal medicine and chronic disorders. Developing countries like India, however, require concentration on paediatric problems, acute infections, food-related diseases, and syndromes like worms, anaemia, enteric fever and GI tract disorders, as the hygiene and socioeconomic factors are far from satisfactory.

7. **Influence of International Events**

   Although all international events do not affect India, certain issues do have a direct effect, such as the General Agreement of Tariff & Trade (GATT) and Trade Related Intellectual Property Rights (TRIPS). New chemical entities, new technologies, new diagnostic techniques, alternative medicines, increasing R&D expenditures, open markets, emerging trends of strategic alliances, licensing in, licensing out, new therapies, etc. have already made their presence felt in the Indian scenario. Except GATT and TRIPS, all other issues have already affected Indian markets.

TWO ADDITIONAL FORCES

The late 1980s witnessed the emergence of two more forces—the force of patients', legitimate but recent, and the 'force of medical representatives'. These two forces critically interacted with the other six described earlier and compelled the government and the industry to take a new look at their obligations towards the marketing of pharmaceutical products.

Force of Patients

The state of Kerala and Gujarat were the first to initiate the movement of the Consumer Guidance Society. Owing to the awareness this has brought about, we see today an enormous change in the attitudes of both medical practitioners as well as patients. The Senior Citizens Club in Mumbai has also played an important role in educating patients. Patients have already started becoming as one of the regulating forces of the Indian pharma industry.

1966 saw the birth of the Consumer Guidance Society (CGS). The consumer—patient for the first time could understand that he was no longer at the mercy of the physician or the retailer. He started asserting his rights. He could observe the power of his rights in Kerala and Gujarat as he started demanding the prescribed medicine, and stopped accepting substitute brands. Patients also developed a greater awareness of products banned abroad, and forced the drug authorities to withdraw them from the market. For the first time, patients began to realize their own regulatory power. The communication network in the country has also vastly improved in few years, so much so that patients in each village have been made aware of their rights through various mediums.

Medical insurance: Four subsidiaries of General Insurance Company introduced medical insurance in India in 1986-87 in the form of healthcare financing (Mediclaim) to support the indisposed healthcare industry.

Recent years have seen a liberalization of the Indian healthcare sector to allow for a much-needed private medical insurance market to rise. Due to liberalization and a growing middle class with increased spending power, there has been a rise in the number of medical insurance policies in the country. The Marketing of Health care insurance policies become of crucially important to help people to meet the untoward expenses due to unexpected ailments.

The Government is focused on growing the health insurance net in India and a classic example of this would be the PradhanMantri SurakshaBimaYojana   and   PradhanMantriJeevanJyotiBimaYojana implemented by the Modi Government to expand the reach of the health insurance schemes to the 'below the poverty line' population.

Apart from this, emergence of stand-alone health insurance companies, health insurance products to suit all sections of the society, specialized health insurance products, buying insurance products online, increase in employer oriented schemes including cover for retired employees, payment of premium through credit card, personalized claim settlement, increase in number of distribution channels, value additions in services using technology and shift from health insurance to health care have fuelled the growth of the health/ medical insurance sector in the country.

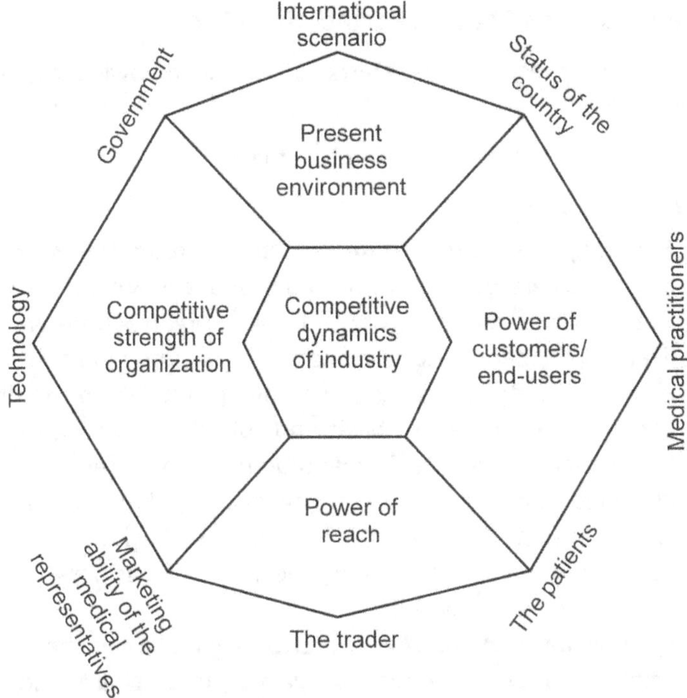

Figure 2.2 Eight cornerstones of dynamics of pharmaceutical marketing

Force of Medical Representatives (MRs)

The Sales Promotion Employees Act (SPEA) which is a part of the Industrial Disputes Act (IDA) in India has created a different negotiating platform for many medical representatives with their organizations. Cipla and U.S. Vitamins Ltd., responded to the practices of the negotiating bodies of medical representatives with the use of alternate media of communication like direct marketing and courier sampling to the physicians. Cipla is still applying and learning from the experience and forging ahead; USV, however, has redesigned its course of action.

This force needs adequate attention from chief executive officers (CEOs), HRD chiefs, and sales and marketing managers. The MRs being a human force, their motivation and development should become an integral part of the marketing mix. Organizations must pay more attention to investing in the development and qualitative improvement of this force and yet give adequate awareness of legal aspects and power to decide at every managerial level.

Shifts and Patterns Shaping Forthcoming Events

We can classify these specific shifts under the following three broad categories.

1. Shifts in Business and Marketing Practices

Business Practices

(i) ***From imports-license to manufacture—franchise—loan license to co-marketing***: Initially finished products were imported under specific licenses and distributed. Later, organizations were given licenses to manufacture in India. A few companies like Walter Bushnell and Elders took many products from different companies on franchise basis and sold them. During the 1980s, Eskayef and Parke-Davis manufactured their few products in Pharmed and Borachem respectively. So, there was a shift to loan licensing. Now Glaxo, UNI-UCB, and Unichem have started co-marketing Citerizine. Thus, the focus of business practice in India has continually shifted.

(ii) ***From volume and market share to profits***: Earlier the focus of a small or a big firm was to gain market share and overall turnover. However, there is a shift from these two issues to profits. Increased competition requires commitment to resources from each operating firm towards increasing or maintaining market share, or increasing turnover. As a result, the focus now is on profits.

(iii) ***From controlled pricing to pricing strategy***: Initially, pricing strategy played a negligible role in pharmaceutical business. All firms were operating under restraints and constraints. This trend was changed by Stangen, who lowered their prices and compelled others to follow them. Today each firm has to work out its pricing strategy for any new product on the basis of many interrelated issues. All firms must make use of "pricing" as an important element in pharma business.

Marketing Practices

(i) ***From 'prescriptions' to 'retailing and prescriptions'***: Earlier, as the brands were limited, prescriptions were serviced by retailers, meticulously. Stocking was done on basis of the prescription strength of every brand. However, as competition became fierce, retailers found it difficult to stock all brands. So retailing assumed importance for individual companies.

In this new environment, the firm must devise methods to strengthen retailing, in addition to generating prescriptions. If retailing is not focused, generated prescriptions are likely to get substituted by similar brands of other companies.

(ii) ***From person-to-person promotion to multimedia approach***: Due to changes in the attitudes of physicians, person-to-person promotion became difficult. It became worst when a consultant started meeting 20-25 MRs within a span of 40-45 minutes on a particular day. Cipla and other firms started promoting their products using direct mail and other marketing approaches to augment person-to-person promotion.

(iii) ***From medically dominated promotion to medico-marketing promotion:*** As the combinations became popular, competition increased and new molecules became scarce, firms started promoting me'-too' products and brands. Concept selling stopped, and brand selling emerged. Medico-marketing promotion had arrived.

(iv) ***From free field staff to bargainable field staff***: Earlier MRs were thought of as ambassadors of their firms, and were responsible for the output of their efforts. Due to increased competition, the emergence and closure of many small pharmaceutical companies in different states of India, and the availability of skilled managerial support, MRs began to feel insecure. The field staff of the small-scale sector followed in the footsteps of the organized sector. The environment too became difficult for the organized sector due to takeovers and mergers.

The Sales Promotions Employees Act (SPEA) was not enacted. By virtue of this, MRs were now considered promotional employees. This act was studied in relation to the Industrial Disputes Act. As a result the status of an MR became confusing. A few groups of MRs called themselves "workers". This is still disputable. The Federation of Medical Representatives Association of India (FMRAI) took shape as a bargaining body.

However, it is up to the individual firms to deal with its MRs, irrespective of their association with these 'bargaining' bodies.

(v) ***From selective capabilities to muscle power capabilities***: Although there were problems at all state levels, most organizations did not stop recruiting MRs to promote their products. Developments on the unionized front posed a challenge to the management of many organizations due to which several organizations recruited hundreds of MRs. Organizations were trying to improve muscle power even by combining their various divisions. Wockhardt merged Tridoss and gathered muscle power to increase its marketing capability.

2. **Shifts in Attitudes of Physicians and Patients**

Physicians

(i) ***From brand loyalty to brand switching***: As the fierce competitive environment offers many choices to physicians, their tendency to try more than one brand is encouraged.

(ii) ***From professional to commercial approach***: Competition among physicians gave rise to many commercial approaches. An example is the insistence on a doctor's part to insert a specific Intra-Occular Lens (IOL) immediately after a cataract operation, without following up on the patient at all to find out if there has been any improvement in his vision.

(iii) ***From individual to group practice***: Many times a team needs to work on a patient, if he requires more investigations and if his case is complex. So group practice, comprising different specializations, was started. This led to polyclinics and easy availability of various specialists.

(iv) ***From symptoms oriented to diagnostics oriented***: The earlier practice and diagnosis were carried out on the basis of the symptoms patients provided or physicians found out. The complexity of diseases known today makes it difficult to diagnose them on the basis of symptoms alone. This is because more than one disease may have similar symptoms. Physicians nowadays have to necessarily diagnose ailments on the basis of certain related diagnostic studies.

Patients

(i) ***From submissive to demanding outlook***: The patient of today is more educated, and more aware of his rights. This has given them the confidence to demand proper treatment from the physician.

(ii) *Increased purchasing power*: Patients are now encouraged by insurance companies, and similar schemes floated by others to improve their purchasing power to treat themselves adequately.

(iii) *Expectation of equal treatment*: No longer do patients tolerate discrimination. They expect similar treatment or care from all physicians and hospitals.

(iv) *From rest at home to hospitalization due to new and advanced life-saving equipments*: At urban and metro towns, this practice has been started. If a patient is critically ill, members of his family and other relatives prefer to admit him to a hospital where he can take rest under observation of qualified physicians and nurses.

3. Shifts in Types of Products

(i) *From technology driven to market driven*: Earlier, investment in R & D and technology used to give new molecules, like Chloromycetin from Parke-Davis and Valium from Roche. Ethambutol and beta blockers were either medically driven or technology driven. As the inflow of new products was reduced, market driven products like Bromhexine plus amoxicillin and Bromhexine plus erythromycin were launched and sold. In fact, except Bromhexine plus tetracycline, no other combination was a pharmacopeal combination. This further led to irrational combinations like addition of salbutamol to cough syrups. A few allopathic and ayurvedic ingredients were also combined to treat indigestion.

(ii) *From concept-based products to Me-Too generic product:* The concept of inhibition of betareceptors was introduced by Imperial Chemical Industries (ICI) with Inderal. Ciba launched Diclofenac, a new entity, as an antiarthritic. Generic antacids were also introduced by many. In each category, a variety of me-too products were launched.

(iii) *From extended life-cycles to short life-cycles*: This trend was due to a technological breakthrough and successive derivatives of single-ingredient new chemicals. Categories like malt tonics, benzo-diazapines, and penicillin enjoyed long product life-cycles. So did Brufen. However, molecules like quinolone derivatives may not enjoy such a life span. We moved from Norfloxacin to Ciprofloxacin to Ofloxacin to Pefloxacin to Lomefloxacin, in only ten years. The shortened life-cycle will destabilize each derivative.

These shifts help us gauge the impact of the changes which have taken place in the pharmaceutical industry. We can plan our actions depending on the severity of the impact.

THE CHANGING CONCEPT OF PHARMACEUTICAL MARKETING

As we have seen, many changes have taken place due to the interplay of eight major forces. Therefore, the concept of pharma marketing has also gone through a process of evolution.

Subtle changes in the marketing concept and practice have fundamentally reshaped pharma marketing in India. Earlier, it was seen as a set of social and economic processes in the form of licensing, franchising, trading, and selling. Although marketing was a widely accepted business function, it was growing out more from a traditional trading and sales management approach, with an emphasis on product planning and development.

The environmental changes compelled all marketing professionals to look at different aspects of the marketing-mix inclusive of pricing, promotion, media mix, distribution, redistribution, advertising, public relations and group selling processes as essential elements in building brands.

Thus, marketing professionals shifted their emphasis to prescription demand, volume (revenues), costs, and profitability. The use of traditional economic analysis to maximize profit by locating the point at which marginal cost equals marginal revenue was replaced with product-mix exercises.

Let us examine how the crucial role of marketing within the organization changed before we proceed to changes in the marketing concept in the external environment.

Role of Marketing Environment

Let us now look at changes in the marketing environment. The basic marketing concepts that relate to the pharmaceutical industry are similar to those of other industries. However, the pharmaceutical industry has its own peculiarities and thus, requires a modified marketing approach.

Till recently, the transaction (call) between the physician and the MR was considered to be the focus of pharmaceutical marketing. It was essential to identify, stimulate, facilitate, and add value to each call to market pharmaceutical products.

Of late, there has been a shift from the focus on 'calls' to one on 'relationships'. Physicians and other customers—retailers, hospitals—need to make long-term commitments to maintain 'brand relationships', as marketing of brands provides updated quality, service and innovation.

Given the increased importance of long-term strategic relationships with both physicians and retailers, organizations are increasingly having to place greater emphasis on relationship management skills. As these skills are present in individuals, rather than being related to organization structures or roles or tasks, key marketing personnel who are able to acquire these skills become increasingly valuable as business assets. These skills can in a way define the core competence of certain marketing organizations that operate as links between their vendors and physicians and retailers in providing value for money. Organizations like Pfizer, Sanofi, Wockhardt, Alembic, Glaxo, and Cadila, and many more take a lot of pride in developing these 'core skills'. They spend a sizeable amount of their revenue in building the relationship management skills of their marketing people. 'Relationship' plays an important role in both trading and selling. However, if this concept is stretched too far, there is a danger of only relationships, and not brands, being established. This is the very antithesis of marketing.

Pharmaceutical marketing, which is essentially 'competence and working capital intensive', needs the development of relationship skills. This is essential not only to achieve brand relationships but also to establish business relationships with debtors. Establishing a relationship should not be the starting point of a call. It should be the outcome of a call. It should result from customer satisfaction.

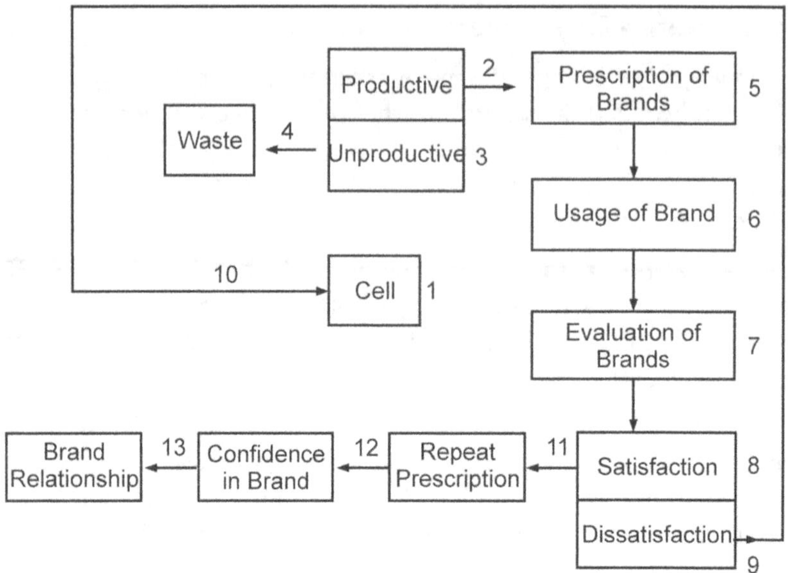

Figure 2.3 'Call' flowchart involving the MR and the physician

In India, unfortunately, the entire marketing process starts with the building of a relationship, and this leads to exploitation by the customer. Alternatively, it ends in submitting to competition.

If you can develop this core competence concept and skills in the marketing of pharmaceuticals in India, you can build marketing capabilities in the business environment.

Role of Marketing within the Organization

Marketing is responsible for building brands and also trustworthy relationships with customers which goes beyond the sale. Its responsibilities differ depending on the stage of the organization, and the strategy it adopts. Cipla, Pfizer, Boots, Ranbaxy, Wockhardt, and Glaxo all appreciated this basic concept and tried to incorporate it in their operations. Cipla introduced multimedia promotion, and Pfizer succeeded in building an old molecule like Tinidazol (Fasigyn) and Piroxicam (Dolonex) through 'positioning'. Boots held its share of Brufen through continuous feedback from their physicians through research. Ranbaxy created a giant product of the decade, Cifran, through a singular focus on one indication. Wockhardt did the same with the unique galenical from IV for Pelox. Glaxo too created history through Zinetac by developing the gastroenterologists' segment exclusively.

Organizations understood that it was their responsibility to focus their efforts on delivering superior value to their customers in the competitive environment. All of them tried to provide value-added benefits through continuous working on quality, R&D, captive bulk manufacturing, marketing capabilities, and competitive prices to doctors through newer and better methods. Internal integration of all facets of business, together with the view of marketing as a basic business philosophy, has changed the role of marketing inside the organization. Marketing has now become an integral part of business.

Torrent was one company which changed the firmly established belief of doctors that national organizations were incapable of providing new chemical entities as this would involve continuous R&D, something only MNCs could afford. Torrent came up with updated well-researched formulations for the first time in India year after year reduced the dependence on MNCs in this respect. Similarly, Dr. Reddy's Laboratories also lent support to the technology upgradation movement; ensuring excellent quality of raw material and basic chemicals for the manufacture of formulations. With leading international organizations buying from them, they emerged as one of the world's most competitive companies and ensured that they provided relative prices, at relative quality, and met the needs of those who wanted to grow through new entities.

Marketing got integrated with organizational strengths and no longer remained only a function. In fact, considering the probable state of affairs in the future, marketing should be a philosophy of the organization and not a discipline or merely a technique. Organizations should start looking inward to develop strengths in delivering better 'value for money' (VFM) in totality.

Although the new articulation of the role of marketing emerged in the latter part of the 1980s, marketing being the principal function of the firm (along with innovation), it became a tool to achieve the main purpose of any business as early as in the 1950s—to create a satisfied customer' (Drucker 1954; Levitt 1960; Mckitterick 1957). Profit was not the primary objective; it was more of a reward for having created a satisfied customer.

In India, we are still struggling to establish the right place of marketing in many organizations. The success stories we have discussed reveal that effective marketing needs vision and focus on the part of the organization and a readiness to integrate them in organizational philosophy.

If marketing is a business philosophy, it needs its due focus on profits. Today profit can be defined as 'future cost' and every marketing executive must ensure that his activities generate profit; profit has five functions to perform.

In order to support:

1. Sudden technology change
2. Economic fluctuations
3. Calamities
4. Employee welfare
5. ROI for entrepreneur or stakeholders and keep organisation on track, profit or surplus needs to be earned.

1. If technology gets upgraded and changed, the organization requires money to quickly shift to new technology. Profit helps this process. Otherwise upcoming competition will take over in no time. Seiko Watches suddenly faced stiff competition from Casio—and it really shook them up. However, Seiko coped with the situation, and Casio withdrew from the watch market. In an altogether different area, McGraw-Ravindra—a giant in intravenous fluids—was also shocked by the changing bottle-packing technology of intravenous fluids.

2. In cases of fluctuation in economic policies, as for instance when the LC opening money went to 250%, the company should have buffer working capital to meet the situation. Profit helps organizations operate in adverse circumstances.

3. Profit helps during calamities like floods, earthquakes, bomb blasts, or riots when organizations need money to survive and prosper.

4. To take care of employees and their welfare year after year, the organization needs surplus. Profit builds this surplus.
5. To earn a return on the investment made by others in the organization. Profit helps boost the morale of the investors.

You will observe how important it is for each marketing activity to focus on *profit* as every activity in marketing is an expenditure or investment.

Those organizations which have knowingly or unknowingly given a vital place to both 'top line' (volume) and 'bottom line' (profits), have integrated the marketing role as a philosophy in the business and have grown well.

STRATEGIC THINKING FOR PHARMACEUTICAL MARKETING

The strategic management arena faces considerable confusion due to the lack of clear understanding of the term strategic thinking.

The term has several and varied meaning but according to Henry Mintzberg (1994), one of the leading authorities in the area of strategic management, by contrast, clearly emphasizes that strategic thinking is not merely "alternative nomenclature for everything falling under the umbrella of strategic management". It is a particular way of thinking with specific and clearly discernible characteristics. In explaining the difference between strategic planning and strategic thinking, Mintzberg argues that strategic planning is the systematic programming of pre-identified strategies from which an action plan is developed. Strategic thinking, on the other hand, is a synthesizing process utilizing intuition and creativity whose outcome is "an integrated perspective of the enterprise." The problem, as he sees it, is that traditional planning approaches tend to undermine, rather than appropriately integrate, strategic thinking and this tends to impair successful organizational adaptation.

Strategic thinking for pharmaceutical marketing includes thinking as well as acting within a certain parameters of assumptions and potential action alternatives and at the same time challenging existing assumptions and action alternatives.

Components of Strategic Thinking

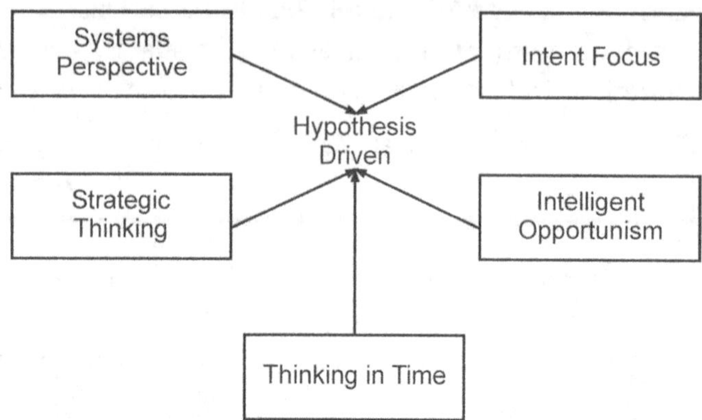

Figure 2.4 Liedtka's model of components of strategic thinknig

(*Source:* Jeanne M. Liedtka: strategic thinking: can it be taught?)

Liedtka (1998) developed a model with identifiable components based on Mintzberg's definition of strategic thinking, which can be applied to pharmaceutical marketing.

The first component of the model is the systems perspective. An individual that thinks strategically must have a mental model of the complete system of creation of value from start to the very end, and should understand the various interdependencies within the chain. It is also important for the thinkers to understand the external business ecosystem and must appreciate the inter-relationships as well. This perspective in turn helps individuals to have a better clarification of their roles and the impact of their behaviors on other parts of the system and on the final outcome.

The second component is intent-focused and intent-driven. This intent provides the focus that allows thinkers within an organization to leverage their energy, to direct their attention, resist distraction, and concentrate to achieve the desired goal. Thus, strategic thinking needs to be driven by the continuous shaping and re-shaping of intent.

The third component is the intelligent opportunism. The essence of this component is the openness to new experience that allows individuals to take advantage of newer and alternate strategies. As a result, it is extremely essential for organizations to consider the contributions of their employees.

The fourth component is thinking in time. It is important for any thinker to drive his strategic thinking by bridging the gap between the current reality and the intent for the future.

The last component is hypothesis-driven. This part embraces hypothesis generation and testing as core activities. It is critical to incorporate creative and analytical thinking through hypothesis generation and testing. The effect of this is an organization that can transcend simplistic notions of cause and effect for life-long learning.

All these components taken together describe a strategic thinker with a comprehensive overview across levels of strategy and end-to-end value system.

THE NATURE OF STRATEGIC PLANNING FOR PHARMACEUTICAL MARKETING

The managerial process of creating and maintaining a balance between the objectives and resources of the organization and the evolving market opportunities is termed as strategic planning. This planning aims at long-term profitability as well as growth. As a result, this kind of planning requires commitments and resources for long periods of time. An error in strategic planning can threaten the growth and the survival of the organization.

One needs to analyze two things for strategic planning for pharmaceutical marketing. Firstly one needs to analyze the main activity of the firm at a given time and secondly one needs to think and plan on reaching the organization's goals. The decisions taken after this analysis will affect the organization's long-run course, the resources allocated, and finally profitability. As opposed, an operating decision, like changing the design of the pack, will not have considerable impact on the long-term financial success of the organization.

Effective Strategic Planning

Effective strategic planning for pharmaceutical marketing involves continual attention, creativity, and management commitment. Strategic planning should not be an annual exercise but an ongoing process because the marketing environment is very dynamic with continuous evolution of the organization's resources and capabilities. Creativity defines sound strategic planning. Marketing managers should establish new strategies based on the assumptions of the changing environment. Ultimately for a successful strategic plan is extremely important to have the top management's support and participation.

Strategic Thinking versus Strategic Planning for Pharmaceutical Marketing

Strategic planning most often takes an already agreed upon strategic route and helps the marketers of an organization to take steps towards realizing that direction. As a result, many are concerned with the extrapolation of present and past as opposed to focusing on how to reinvent the future. Also, being over focused on extrapolation instead of innovation, strategic planning creates an illusion of certainty where certainty is anything but guaranteed. Strategic planning is analogous to single-loop learning normally denotes a programmatic and analytical process carried out within the parameters of achievement.

By contrast, strategic thinking is connected to a creative and divergent process. It is a way that is associated with re-inventing the future and creating a competitive space. Strategic thinking is thus, analogous to double-loop learning that questions the strategic parameters.

Many may think that the dichotomy established between strategic planning and strategic thinking establishes the fact that both these processes are incompatible with one another. But, for a thoughtful strategy-making process, both are as required proportionately and none is adequate without the other in any effective strategy-making regime.

However, the real challenge lies in transforming the strategic planning process in a way that undermines strategy thinking. There ideally needs to be a dialectical thought process of converging and diverging, being innovative as well as judging the implications and being analytical.

THE TASKS OF PHARMA MARKETING

Marketing Strategy

The marketing function in a drug company is responsible for two crucial tasks: to develop a comprehensive business and marketing strategy, and to implement the strategy using various marketing tools and activities.

The development of a business-marketing strategy can be conceptualized at three levels:

First, at the level of the product mix and business portfolios of the company, as resources are always limited and have to be carefully allocated to the opportunities judiciously. Thus, priorities have to be established for the businesses and product portfolios.

The second level involves identifying a specific product mix and developing a marketing strategy at the level of individual products in line with the objectives to be achieved as specified while deciding the product portfolio.

The third level involves the selection of appropriate marketing and selling tools to implement those strategies.

Marketing strategy precedes marketing practice. Prior to the mid-1970s, the marketing approaches were basically centred around what were called the four P's (product, price, place, and promotion). Increased competition has made the strategic dimension of marketing more integrated and important.

It is not reasonable to address the pricing problem before having decided on the target market and the differential advantages of the product. Once the latter is clearly specified, the pricing issue becomes clearer. The case of Norilet (Stangen) is illustrative. Increased competition made it difficult for Norilet to create a niche for itself, but its quality and lowest price did the trick. Decisions regarding selection and determination of the differential advantage are strongly interdependent. A strong differential advantage for one target market might only be a weak differential advantage for another target market.

The differential advantage of a contraceptive product in a developing country like India would be quite different from that in a developed country like the USA. India being an overpopulated nation with a relatively poor literacy rate, and fewer birth control measures, is more than selling a product. It is a concept and message that it needs to put across to its people. So in India, these P's acquire a different dimension.

In the pharmaceutical industry, this process of finding out the differential advantage is sometimes reversed. Discoveries can happen by chance. The strategic marketing tasks then have to be reversed in a given specific environment. The best example is that of Minoxidyl which was invented and introduced as an anti-hypertensive drug; it was discovered that it aids hair growth by accident. The total differential advantage after this accidental discovery was changed overnight. In fact, it became popular later on because it aided hair growth.

The promotion of the utility of eggs as a health food took ten years to succeed, although the government spent a lot of money on the project. India is a country where 'social marketing' is of paramount importance. Awareness regarding diverse areas, ranging from condoms and other contraceptives to the danger of burns during festivals like Diwali, needs to be established, and the necessary social marketing efforts need to be made. It is essential to study these P's; in practice they are all interdependent and therefore need to be integrated.

Marketing Plan

It is extremely crucial to plan as an anticipation of future events. Developing strategies beforehand helps to achieve the objectives and goals of the organization. Similarly, marketing plan constitutes designing activities keeping in mind the objectives of marketing as well as the changing environment of marketing. The basis of all marketing strategies and decisions is marketing planning. All the issues of product lines, channels of distribution, communications and pricing are defined in the marketing plan.

Marketing plan helps to provide a basis on which the actual and expected performance can be compared and thus, is one of the most important activities of business. It also helps the employees and the marketing managers to take efforts towards common objectives. A marketing plan also helps gauge the environment of marketing in conjunction with the internal environment of the organization. Most importantly it enables the marketing manager to enter the market with an awareness of all the problems as well as possibilities.

Elements of a Marketing Plan

Most marketing plans are written as the scope usually is pretty large and complex. Regardless of this, there are some elements that are common to all marketing plans.

These elements mostly include defining the business mission, business objectives, and situation analysis.

Defining the business mission forms the foundation of any marketing plan. Business mission strongly affects the organization's long-term success, growth and survival and should be stated in broader terms careful analysis of anticipated conditions of the environment.

It is very much necessary to state the goals and objectives of the marketing plan before going into intricacies as without these there is no basis to measure the success of the planned marketing activities. The objectives should meet the marketing criteria and the priorities of the organization. These objectives stem from the business mission and penetrate the marketing plan. The objectives thus, form a basis of control to gauge the effectiveness of the marketing plan.

The marketers need to understand the current and potential marketing environment for the product before detailing the marketing activities. This situation analysis is nothing but the SWOT analysis identifying the internal strengths and weaknesses and external opportunities and threats.

Other elements that form a part of this marketing plan include the target markets, budgets, timetable of implementation, marketing research, and advanced strategic planning.

SIX TYPES OF MARKETING

1. Borderless Marketing

Liberalization has opened the doors to multilateral trade. The common focus on customer, value for money, and relationships will result in stronger coordination between the procurement, sales and marketing functions across the world. Such coordination will be essential to serve the purposes of: (i) elimination of boundaries between the various countries, and (ii) removal of the boundaries between the firm and its market environment. In a world of strategic partnerships, it is not uncommon for a partner to be simultaneously a customer, competitor, and vendor, as well as a partner. Thus, it is difficult to keep the traditional marketing management functions distinct in dealing with strategic partners.

Alliances also help remove borders—Ranbaxy, Eli-Lilly, MJ Pharmaceuticals, Torrent-Nova, and Boots have shown the way of borderless marketing. Eli-Lilly came to India with an alliance with MJ Pharmaceuticals in bulk manufacturing and later tied up with

Ranbaxy for promotion of fixed-dose combinations. Torrent started manufacturing and selling human insulin of Nova. Now that Nova is tied up with Boots, human insulin of Nova will be marketed by Boots but will still be manufactured by Torrent.

Alliances could be through franchising a product, selling the rights of a few products, or creating an alliance with companies who have marketing capabilities. All these routes will progress in times to come. Mr. Ajay Piramal's buying over of Nicholas Laboratories and Indian subsidiaries of Roche, Boehringer Mannheim, Rhone Poulenc and Hoechst Research Centre opened up new avenues for better marketing capabilities.

Firms that are unable to achieve extraordinary capabilities in the market, which will help them focus on their customers, will either slowly lose their customer base and altogether disappear, or become highly specialized players. Consolidated Products Ltd. (CPL) in medical products, and Rampion in ophthalmic products are examples of companies operating in 'niche' markets. Moreover, customer focus will require increasingly large investments in information technology.

Personal, specifically targeted, purposeful, and powerful communication will become important. An example of this would be Cipla who, with its predominant focus on direct mailing and marketing through media (other than the MRs), ensured progress even in the absence of cooperation from its MRs. Cipla forged ahead and maintained its position with personal, targeted, special-purpose communications. The experiment of Sandoz for an old product like Visken also showed that if you select your target group properly and address the group with relevant, personal and special-purpose communication, the response rate goes beyond 15%.

When you observe the tie-ups of Coke and Parle, Godrej and Procter & Gamble, and many others, you will agree that in India, 'resources' are an extremely important factor in developing market shares. Therefore, companies may merge, sell and buy to strengthen resources, and then attack markets. The implementation of a market-driven strategy requires skills in designing, developing, managing, and controlling strategic alliances with partners of all kinds, keeping them all focused on the ever changing customer in the borderless marketplace. The same is the case in pharma business. Sun Pharmaceuticals is an excellent example of optimum utilization of resources in a specialty market.

Lack of optimum resources and market penetration led to a new approach towards marketing products—the approach of co-marketing.

2. **Co-Marketing**

While co-marketing is a relatively new concept all over the world, it started in a different way in a nascent form even before the 1970s in India.

Unichem, a pharma company, promoted Saffola oil (of Bombay Oil Mills) to cardiologists as a part of their promotion, while Horlicks (of GSK Consumer Healthcare, formerly known as Hindustan Milk Foods) was promoted by a specially hired team to gather 'endorsement'.

Later on, as the advantages became clear, companies like Johnson & Johnson and Wipro commissioned vendors to promote their baby care products to doctors for 'endorsement'. Glaxo for the first time marketed 'Equal' (a non-sugar sweetener) for GD Searle in India. This is a classic example of co-promotion. The experiment was very successful.

Borderless marketing ensures newer approaches like co-marketing, to focus more on market reach, penetration, and brand share.

The concept of co-marketing is a recent phenomenon in the Indian scene and most companies who have gone in for this arrangement have achieved good results. Some companies, however, enter into co-marketing arrangements after launching their own international brands, an example being that of Sanofi who launched Trental (Pentoxyphyline) and, after a few years, entered into a co-marketing arrangement with Boots (Flowpent).

In another such venture, Sanofi launched Roxatidine in a tie-up with Ranbaxy. Yet another example of co-marketing is that of Sanofi and Astra-IDL together launching Felodipine. Many international companies are considering co-marketing tie-ups not only because they make available more field personnel to promote the molecule but also to counter the threat of generics.

We can expect more co-marketing arrangements in the future.

3. Involvement Marketing

When Claude Hopkins exhibited the 'largest cake in the world', baked with Cotusuet, it was 'existential marketing'. The cake existed, people knew it did, and they knew they should be impressed by the fact that it was the largest cake in the world. When he brought people together to taste the cake, and to compete for prizes by trying to guess its weight, that was involvement marketing.

As all of us know, it is a basic principle of psychology that experience reinforces learning. You can lecture students on the fine art of swimming for hours, but not until they jump into water, try swimming themselves and gulp in some dirty water, can they really take in and understand what you are teaching. Their involvement is essential for getting confidence and converting theory into practice. Involvement marketing provides that experience which leads to better understanding.

Marketers of pharmaceuticals have found that to break through the promotional clutter today demands more than just being there, making aloof announcements and explaining to those who will listen why their products should be consumed. It demands involvement marketing.

There are thousands of pharmaceutical manufacturers in India with hundreds of brands in any prominent therapeutic group, sometimes even for a single molecule. How do you then differentiate your brand in this huge ocean of competitors. How much can you stretch your MRs?

Despite some overlap between the two, there is an important difference between existential marketing and involvement marketing in the pharmaceutical business. The former is what you do to ensure that your brand has a genuine, credible, favorable presence in the mind of the doctor (or) whoever makes the decision. The doctor prescribes the brand and the retailer sells it to the patient. Involvement marketing is what you get your doctors and retailers to do.

Involvement marketing started in a very small way in India by way of brand promotion—Abdec Drops' 'Healthy Baby' contests, Ferradol's milkshakes (provided at hospital gatherings), and Parke-Davis giving away monograms to final year MBBS students at 'specific disease' symposia in medical colleges in the 1960s. In the 1970s, many other organizations came forward and carried involvement marketing further. These marketers realized that it would pay to be involved with what the medical fraternity was doing. Boots (Knoll) would give away 'Oration Awards' for the best presentation in medical conferences. Lupin, Kopran and Cadila started launching almost every product with the involvement of the target group thus forging relationships. Companies established a critical mass for all their new products through such pre-launch involvement activities.

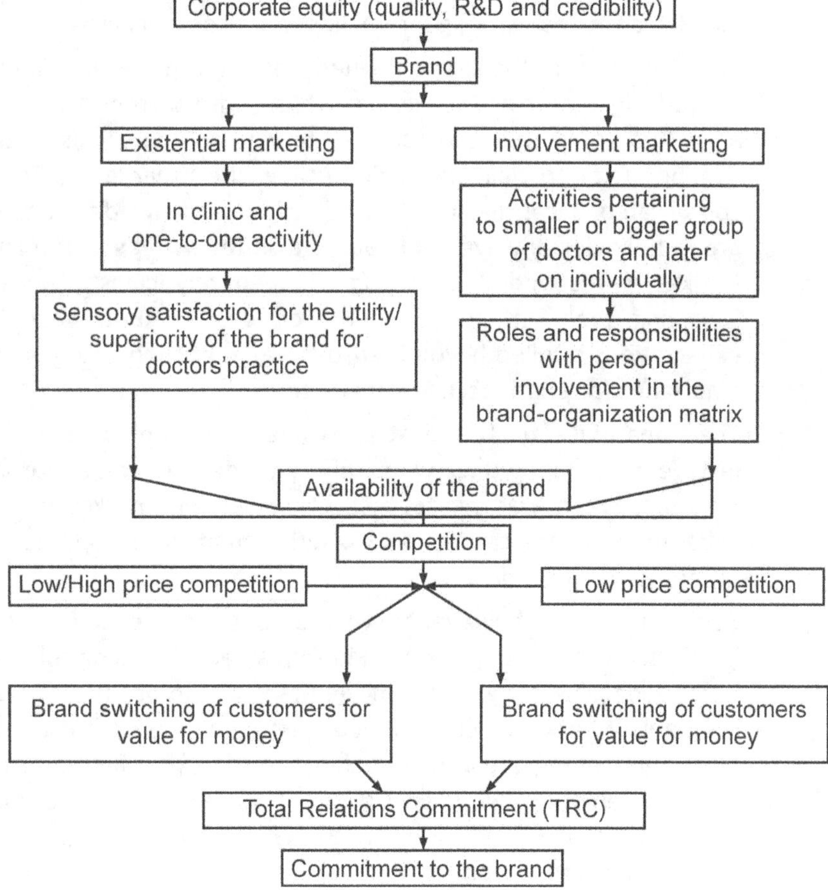

Figure 2.5 Model for total relations commitment (TRC)

In the 1980s, involving the general medical fraternity in product development had become almost a standard industry practice, and marketers came up with a string of innovative ideas through the decade.

- Wockhardt advertised its tonic (Winofit) and antiobesity drug (Flabolin) without the brand name in the local press and asked patients to ask their general practitioners and family physicians what this antiobesity drug was all about.
- Lupin involved chest specialists in the workings of the company. Not only that, it involved them in terms of ownership in Lupin.
- Cipla started working on smaller groups of specialists.

The 1990s was the period when the pharmaceutical industry started to 'demassify' the customer-base, with Torrent, Glaxo, Cipla and lots of other companies targeting individuals. But it degenerated into plain and clinic-to-clinic direct marketing. This was complicated because individual behavior is always different from group behavior. Involvement took a turn to, 'What's in it for me?' Marketers responded by trying to keep physicians pleased by satisfying them in the manner they desired. But when their expectations swelled beyond reasonable proportion, many became a nuisance for pharmaceutical marketers.

The pharmaceutical industry worked on this concept of involvement marketing with different degrees and purposes. Although there was no focus on involvement marketing, these experiments were carried out to differentiate the approaches of different organizations.

Some marketers, however, have the confidence of knowing that involvement marketing is destined to play an increasing role in the years ahead. As the glamour in the market becomes more intense, resistance of doctors will continue to harden, making it even more difficult to get anyone to pay attention to what your brand is saying. Direct interaction with physicians, if based on real customer interests, is the best way to create positive feelings for the organization and the brand.

However, building brands alone is sometimes not enough. Outstanding corporate equity is also a key success determinant. But creating corporate equity means setting up value-building processes, both inside and outside the organization. People appreciate companies that spend millions of dollars on R&D, even if it means that just one of 50 molecules will eventually hit the market. Slowly, the R&D image of an organization is coming to matter more and more in India. This image encompasses the company's vision, its sense of purpose, its dedication and adherence to quality, all of which are key factors in building the overall corporate image. Corporate advertising can do part of the job, but involvement marketing delivers terrific results. The medical fraternity appreciates companies that want to involve them in conquering health problems.

Extra-value strategy: Since involvement marketing costs money, it suffers when the marketer expects to get embroiled in a price war. It is a gigantic task to keep prices at rock-bottom, operating on a paper-thin margin, while still offering extra services, amenities and rewards to keep the customer involved.

Price wars are becoming a reality for several reasons. Competition being fierce is the obvious one. The other is that being cost-conscious is no longer a source of embarrassment, even among the relatively affluent. Everybody is under pressure because of the economic slowdown. But at the same time, doctors are reluctant to compromise on quality and service. After all, they are dealing with the lives of their patients.

A good way to drive your competition crazy might be to formulate an extra-value strategy. A strategy that shifts the focus to a totally different playing field.Glaxo in Cetirizine and Fulford in dermacare products are successful examples when competitors have brands three times cheaper, but they lead their respective markets. There is something to learn from such brands. These two brands have something special going for them. Otherwise, in general, marketers have to figure out how to offer 'gain without pain'. Such marketers are to be found all along the price spectrum, their prices ranging from the lowest to the highest. But they share the same key to success.

Some of the brightest marketers are keeping prices low but not necessarily the lowest, and finding ways to offer value-extras that the lowest-priced competitors can't match. Dr. Reddy's Laboratories started this trend and today everybody is very cautious about pricing any new product. In a market where product patents can't really be protected, it is risky to price a new product at a very high price initially. You are sure to be hit by lower-priced competition within two months, which could swing doctors away from your product. But if the extra value and technology can back you, you can still do wonders at a price that's higher than that of the upstarts.

Playing purely by price (aiming to be the lowest) can prove to be disastrous. With a low price you run risk of setting in a price barrier, and low margins mean that much less money to put into brand building. Happily, most doctors and patients seem to be willing to pay a little more in order to get a lot more. You just need to justify the premium.

4. Beyond Involvement Marketing

Doing what your prospects and customers want could mean having to shake your company to its roots. In conversation with Nestle's former Marketing Director (baby food products), Fabienne Petit summed it up thus: 'I cannot speak with passion about my advertising but I am passionate about my links with the consumer. We are totally committed to our relationship with parents.' So, Nestle has Buitoni, a business unit dedicated to the idea; Buitoni's global strategy is based on a commitment to relationships with the consumer. In fact, it means that the unit will keep reshaping its marketing mix in line with this commitment.

Involvement marketing works only when the company is genuinely passionate about its relationship with its customers. The idea is not alien to pharmaceutical marketers who have made it a point to involve specialists in their areas of specialization. Torrent, for example, committed itself to India's psychiatrists. It promised to provide all that they needed, thus creating the ground for a lasting relationship. That is perhaps what made Torrent what it is today. Lupin has had an edge with chest physicians (tuberculogists in particular), and this treatment area has been a niche it has nurtured quite dedicatedly. Allergan is currently committing itself to ophthalmologists. Worldwide, the company has made eye-care its area of primary focus.

The relationship can start with a small group. But this group can grow to form the critical mass required to set the marketing juggernaut rolling. The core strategy, of course, will depend on organizational strengths and the cost of operations. But one's commitment to relationships can make the difference.

Strategic intent by nature must be sustainable and enduring irrespective of environmental changes. The changes may compel the directional changes of the strategy, but the intent and leadership or ownership ensures that the tactics, or customer-based innovative approaches help the strategy to be effective. However, for such customer-oriented approaches to really work, it is necessary to have the requisite quality and technical inputs. This is where medico-marketing can step in giving specialized knowledge through planned events. But here too the communication has to be creative and innovative.

5. Medico-Marketing

The purpose of medico-marketing is to promote corporate products and services with the help of MRs and by other direct response marketing methods. The purpose of hiring medical advisors, consultants, medico-marketing consultants, MRs, artists, designers, illustrators, or photographers is to help do just that. Yet sometimes there can be a lot of trouble with the creative part of the promotion. I can bet that there's not one marketing director reading this who has not wanted to make the process of designing or copy easier, faster—even less expensive and of course more creative.

Successful marketing and promotion of medical products and services often hinges on the services of several knowledgeable and creative professional companies. Besides hard-core medical knowledge and concepts, it is the designers, copywriters, illustrators, photographers and consultants, who have to translate the marketing objectives into results.

A company can develop interactive literature, manuals, examination papers with affiliation of a few universities or medical colleges use learning models on computers on a one-to-one basis and interact on an individual or on a group basis with selected doctors. Such interaction and education can also provide value-added personal development of the doctors.

(i)   *The medico-marketing model*

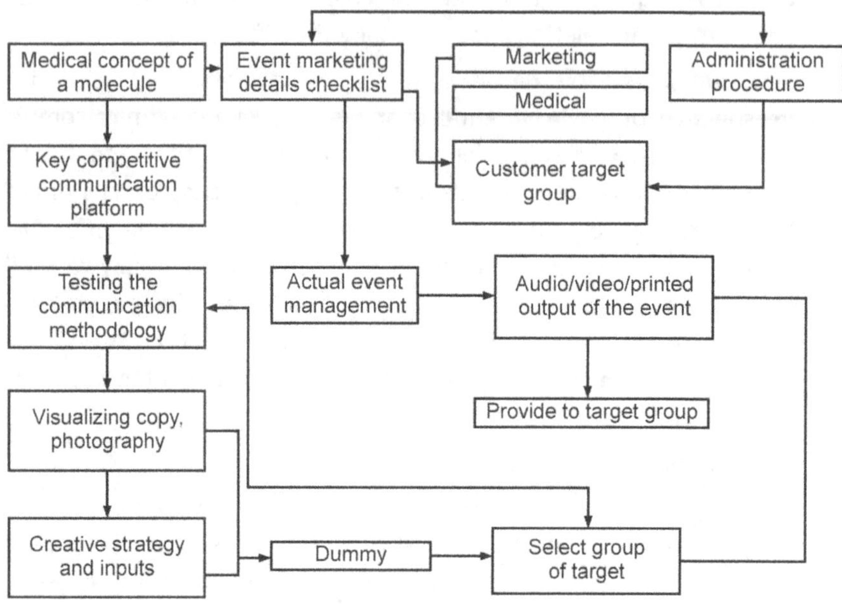

Figure 2.6 A medico-marketing model

Usually the medico-marketing model given in Figure 2.7 is followed by most companies with possibly some variations. Essentially the model aims to provide information on new or existing products by staging events. These events can be one time or on a continuous basis. Sometimes, value-added education and development of personal skills can also be envisaged.

(ii)   *Skills development events*

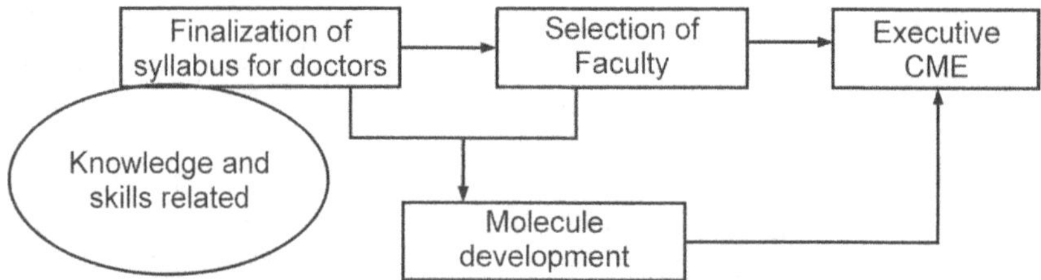

Figure 2.7 The continuous medical education (CME) model

The Continuous Medical Education (CME) model has been successfully used in medico-marketing. The CME model given in Figure 2.7 is self-explanatory.

- ***Managerial events:*** Besides technical and medical skills, physicians also need managerial skills such as time management, assertiveness, patient psychology, parenting, accounting and taxation to succeed in their practice. The process is the same, except that you first need to identify the needs of the group. A few organizations tried to take the lead to impart parenting skills, but for want of continuity and organizational skills this event could not be sustained.

(iii) ***Product launch events:*** Successful medico-marketing requires careful planning and thought. The finest products can go relatively unnoticed if they are not supported by fresh medical insights and innovation. Organizing specialized events can go a long way in drawing the attention of specialists. There can be various types of events depending on the nature of product. But whatever the event, it needs proper organization and management.

- One-time events: Win Medicare celebrated a medico-marketing event for its new product Hepamerz, the hepato-encephalopathy-related product. The medical concept was fully developed with creative communication as the key platform. It was tested by the product management and product development teams with the target group. The creative strategic plan and the inputs for the one-time event were developed with the help of the marketing and sales management teams. An innovative hypothesis, 'liberation of ammonia' to treat hepato-encephalopathy patients was discussed among a gathering of specialists at different regional centers who went away convinced of its efficacy.

- New product events: It has been a regular practice to launch new products with a lot of fanfare. The Upjohris' medical-marketing consultants program for the launch of new products was exceptionally successful. The company took A-class medical practitioners as marketing consultants in a few specific geographic areas and worked through them for a period of two years, including the supervision of pre-launch and post-launch tracking.

- *Concept testing and concentric events:* Prior to staging the event for the launch of Depend, a urinary incontinence brief, Kimberly Clark concept tested and developed the profile of the brand by calling on doctors for four months. It was only at the end of this four-month period that the event was staged to educate users and influencers. Such an exercise ensures success of the event.

- *CME regular events:* A few organizations use the Continuing Medical Education (CME) model to stage CME events in hospitals. Sion Hospital at Mumbai, PG Medical College Hospital, Chandigarh are also some other hospitals in India profess the need of such education for GPs for dissemination of knowledge and understanding of clinical experience. Such CME events are held regularly on periodic intervals. The topics are selected by the organization, the medical council or medical association. Through such continuous events a company can create a critical mass of GPs for its products.

- *CME skills development events:* For developing ophthalmic surgical skills with the use of laser beams, including cataract operations and post-operative insertion of intra-occular lenses (IOLs), the Government of Maharashtra conducted 'eye camps' and invited cataract patients to have themselves operated at subsidized rates. Organizations dealing with ophthalmic products could sponsor such 'eye camps' and help doctors develop their skills to use their products. Such events at regular intervals can also build loyalty to many products like IOLs. The concept is usually to train doctors on the job to use products of the company.

- *International events:* Many surgeons and other specialists always wish to get a first-hand experience in learning new techniques in major international hospitals. For example, diabetologists or endocrinologists would like an opportunity to get exposure at the Joslin clinic. Organizations can sponsor specialists to work in such clinics for specific therapies.

- *Interactive events:* For such events, a few renowned doctors are requested by organizations to come with the medical team of the organization to develop continuous medical education in rural areas of GPs who do not get exposed to urban facilities. Diagnosticians as well as pathological laboratories also conduct such education at rural centers. Organizations can take advantage of such events.

- *Facilitators' events:* Paramedicos and nurses also need development of their knowledge and skills. The Indian Hospital Association (IHA) is trying to organize such educational events in almost all hospitals, though the response from organizations so far has been poor. Manufacturers of products like Betadine and Wokadine can take maximum advantage of such opportunities, to aim at their target customers.

(iv) ***Creativity in medico-marketing:*** To make maximum impact hiring professionals is essential. Good product photography can leave a lasting impression. According to Stan Sholik, medical and macro product photographer, there are three reasons for engaging specialists:

- A specialist can envisage the nature of problems that may be encountered while photographing your particular product. Professional photography can save time and money. The company's reputation will also be enhanced when you are able to pull a creative project together without technical problems. There are quite a few examples of brilliant work done behind the camera in India, such as the video shooting of heart valve operations, by-pass surgery, balloon angioplasty, and so on.

- Many medical photography jobs require sophisticated equipment and techniques. Photography done in the case of the abdominal surgery of Amitabh Bachchan in Breach Candy Hospital and his treatment using Betadine during the critical care at the time of operation was quite impressive.

- A third reason is that a specialist can tell you what can and cannot be done within a given budget. There are surprises.

Beyond specialized technical ability and creativity, you should also look for the personal element in hiring professionals. The creative professional's portfolio and promo material are only a starting point. Technical ability and creativity can be clearly evaluated but they don' tell you if the working relationship will be one you will regret or cherish. Once you have determined that the individual is competent, you need to also ascertain if you will have a satisfactory working relationship.

- A question of rights: The Copyright Act states that copyright belongs to the creator of original works (concepts or ideas are not protected until they become physical work). You can buy as much or as little usage of the images or work as you require. These usage rights must be clearly defined before you begin. When no rights are stated along with the creative fees quoted, then no rights are transferred to you. No buyer wants to go through all the trouble of hiring a photographer or illustrator, creating an image and then find he has no right to use it.

Usage must be clearly stated—whether one-time or indefinite, whether for one medium or several. Physical possession of the original track, transparencies, negatives or artworks does not give you the right to use to work. Keep in mind that the life of the copyright exceeds the life of the creator, so only a written contract of usage rights will protect you from liability now and far into the future. You do not need to buy the copyright unless you want to sell the use of the work to other clients—an unlikely situation. Even after years, the History of Medicine series of Parke-Davis still enjoys copyright protection.

Thus, every creative medico-marketing project needs a focused marketing objective. Do we want to increase sales volume? Brand awareness? Response? Being too scattered or general in your objectives wastes time and money. The best medical marketing campaigns come from how well the piece works, not how great it looks! As one expert says, 'My medical clients are not art patrons! They want to sell their products and services. My design comes after we set marketing objectives, not before.'

6. Brand-Image Marketing

Over time, we have learnt that two people can look at the same thing and see it quite differently. They then describe it to others as they saw it. Opinions are thus formed. Hence, perceptions are based on what a person knows (or thinks he knows). These perceptions often color our judgments. Similarly, what gives shape to the identity of a brand and company is their perceived reality. In a majority of corporate-image-studies, we find that a pharmaceutical corporate is perceived as a high R&D spending company. But the reality is different. Pharmaceutical companies can identify and build their strength by a calibrated strategy to ensure that doctors and customers see them in favorable light.

(i) ***Perception and reality:*** Perception and reality are often the same thing. But in marketing, illusions are created. We are all governed by our perceptions of what we think we know, rather than what is. Most doctors will irrevocably form an opinion if the prescription they write 'bounces' back, even if only once. This could happen because the chemist, feigning unavailability, substitutes the brand. But the deed is done and the doctor will carry a life-long impression about the unavailability of that brand which she/he will communicate to the company MR time and again. What an interplay of perception and reality!

No sane business traveller would travel without proper business arrangement such as confirmed hotel bookings and a fixed appointment to meet clients (or prospects). Yet, companies regularly waste fortunes by launching or upgrading products in complete ignorance of the climate and size of the target market. There are companies such as Unichem and Dr. Reddy's Laboratories which create brands by MRs and promotion and creating an equity. On the other hand, many companies do not even bother about their MR's perceptions, and yet launch new products. They fail miserably with each entry. The success of Sun and Cipla inspired many to follow their practices. Many tried without investing in brand-image marketing and were unsuccessful.

Pharmaceutical companies increasingly face the dual challenge of launching new brands and managing the existing ones in large markets. Questions of market satiation and potential sales keep coming up in strategy meetings. Often these products struggle to demonstrate differences in terms of clinical benefits. Examples include those prescribed for cardiovascular conditions, such as hypertension, infectious diseases and inflammatory conditions.

(ii) ***Creating a brand image:*** Research has shown that there's a direct relationship between a brand's awareness level and its market share. A better brand name is more likely to come up with a better product more often than not. Creating a brand image can bridge the gap between perception and reality. It motivates people and the weaknesses of the brand get automatically addressed.

There are many definitions of a brand, but most seem to concur that a brand is greater than the sum of its parts. A successful brand meets more than just the functional needs of the user. In the case of pharmaceutical products, these go by parameters such as efficacy and side effects. However, traditionally much greater emphasis has been placed on functional or clinical benefits in the management of pharmaceutical brands.

Phensedyl (Rhone-Poulenc) and many other brands faced multidimensional problems in respect of duplication. This helped the organizations take a re-look at their packaging, distribution and other related processes to streamline operations. It only needed the right assessment to promote the strengths of their brand to the maximum in order to defend them against unorganized competitors.

(iii) ***Creating perception:*** Creating a favorable perception is not an exact science. Before a company builds an image, it has to identify its market, inform consumers about its profile and give them compelling reasons to care. Remember, a company's image is the reflection of the people's perceptions.

It is important that the flow of information about the brand is managed and controlled to the highest degree. But more importantly the brand should create a stream of information to raise awareness.

Seven Steps to a Better Brand Image: The type of image a company wants to brandish can be furnished with the following seven steps.

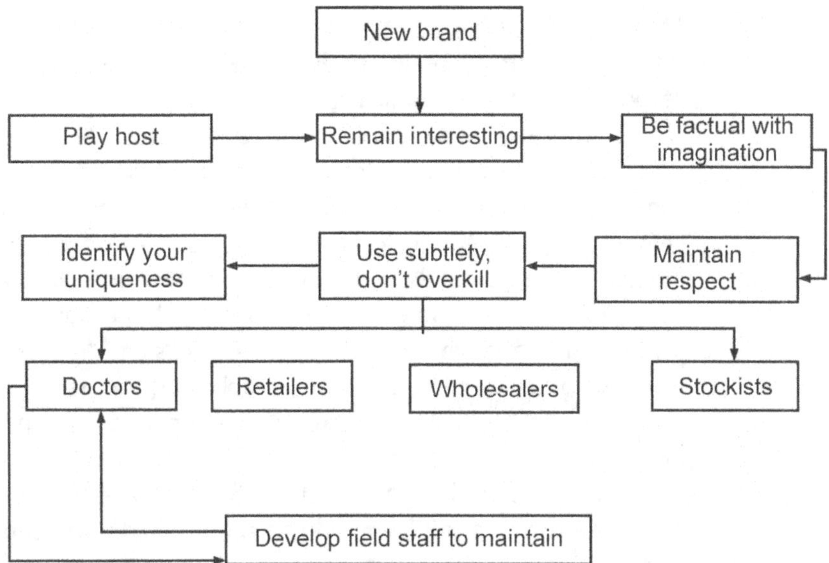

Figure 2.8 Steps to improve brand image

- ***Play host***: Waiting to be called is flattering. But taking the initiative allows one to play host and introduce the brand. Cipla has been doing the same. A small group of doctors is invited and briefed whenever a new brand is being introduced.

- ***Remain interesting***: Respect doctors' schedules, and get to the point straightway. Invite their spouses too and make the presentation short and memorable. The event must be built on the basis of the nature of the brand.

- ***Be factual with imagination***: A little bragging is usually expected, but a person who exaggerates rarely convinces anyone. Factual and realistic information is effective. Case studies, clinical trials, promotional trials, magnificent cure rate of drugs, side-effects and the prescriptions all need to be woven together to create a favorable perception. This has been done by many companies that operate in the fields of oncology and cardiovascular therapies.

- ***Maintain respect***: Someone you are trying to influence favorably should not think of you negatively. A conversation followed by a thank-you note that says 'do call if more information is needed' is usually adequate.

MRs and front-line managers need to be accordingly trained to portray a favorable impression. The rate of response should be predictable.

- ***Use subtlety, don't overkill***: The aim should be that doctors, retailers, wholesalers, stockists become aware of the company and its brand. Service should occur on several levels. Creating a good and lasting image rarely begins with an overkill. A doctor is likely to remember a series of 'history of medicine' pictures by Parke-Davis, a simple but effective reminder of messages at different levels of practice, in contrast to complicated and lengthy presentations. Initially, to create perceptions of and awareness about a company, information should be given in an encapsulated form so that the customer is not burdened with more information than he can comprehend and recall at one time. To make what one has to say more memorable, remember the adage—'Less is more'.
- ***Identify your uniqueness***: The overall strategy may include an advertising or public relations agency handling everything. The manner in which you can reach out to those you hope to influence and from whom you want support, depends on your company's value system and refusal to get baited into reactionary-mode by the competition. It should be consistent with the image.
- ***Develop field staff to maintain quality standards***: If there is a dissonance in the created image and behavior of those who maintain the brand image, you may confuse customers.

In order to succeed in the pharmaceutical business, it is important to develop this seven-step approach and carefully nurture the image of the company. Perceptions are powerful, and, once created, hard to dislodge from the customer's mind. Once the customer is involved, you can then aim to make them loyal to your brand.

ROLE OF R & D AND D & D IN PHARMACEUTICAL MARKETING

R&D activity is very expensive in the drug industry. It has been estimated that 10 to 18% of the sales turnover is spent on R&D in large, research-intensive multinational drug companies. The attrition rate of new substances is extremely high. Most estimates suggest that only one compound out of every 5000—10,000 examined reaches the market. The integration of this expensive, risky and time-consuming R&D activity with the marketing dimension presents unique opportunities and challenges in pharmaceutical marketing to MNCs.

In the case of bulk drugs, the role of R&D has been fully appreciated. The price war on quinolones is an excellent example of what can and what cannot happen if you do not invest in R&D of bulk drugs. However, the scene is changing very fast and all companies will have to abide by the Trade Related Intellectual Property Rights (TRIPS). In a unique experiment, five Indian companies together promoted a group which has invested a sufficient amount in the R&D of bulk drugs to provide adequate security for the future.

The limited knowledge of drug action and disease patterns in human beings led to the development of new products targeted at specific unmet therapeutic needs. This was a difficult task. Most drug research projects were based on screening large numbers of active chemicals, to discover their therapeutic qualities if any. However, as the biological knowledge gap is diminishing, the new 'tailored drug design' approach is becoming more feasible. This approach identifies the key steps in the development of an illness and then aims to develop drugs which can arrest its development at some specific point. The highly successful new drug, Mevacor, launched by Merck in 1987 in the international market and bringing in $ 200 million in 1988, was the result of a very specific effort to produce an anti-cholesterol agent.

On the other hand, Unichem also spent on the design and development (D&D) of a new product and brought out Arkamin H (an anti-hypertension drug) but this did not succeed to the same extent. Similarly, nearly 1500 different natural formulations were examined and tested and a new natural herbal cough formula was evolved by Procter & Gamble in India when they launched Vicks Vaposyrup—an OTC product. But this too did not become a leader. In other words, R&D and D&D efforts require a different marketing thrust, right from identifying unmet therapeutic groups to taking steps to arrest the development of illnesses and fully satisfying the unmet needs.

A trial-and-error R&D approach leads logically to a technological, rather than a market-driven, new -product development process. In this area India is far ahead of other countries. Comblifam (ibuprofen and paracetamol) was one such successful product of Roussel. Many other market-driven products were introduced in India in the 1980s. As more sophisticated methods of chemical synthesis, biotechnology, genetic engineering, computer modeling and other new technologies come into use, the implementation of a true marketing orientation by pharmaceutical companies will be significantly felt.

A new look at emerging market needs will help companies focus their R&D efforts. As R&D requires focus and then application value, many organizations will reorient R&D efforts to match marketing needs. Earlier, marketing and selling were oriented to R&D as they exploited the gaps in medical problems and practices. Even today, major inventions may come through R&D, but tomorrow innovations will come from unmet market needs. Glaxo, Merck, and Takeda exemplify basic differences in orientation. Glaxo is a market-oriented organization, while Merck is technology-oriented, and Takeda excels in making everything better than the originator. Each organization is using its technology to choose a route to meet the needs of physicians. You will also observe that Merck spends far more on R&D than Glaxo does as its basic philosophy is to develop new molecules. Strategy based on R&D strength will ultimately win in competitive markets.

The Next Two Decades

Let us look at what is in store for us in the next two decades.

In view of the global impact on marketing in India, it is likely that fixed-dose formulations will become the core business, and that a variety of *peripheral businesses* will grow around it.

Hospitals have been accorded the status of small-scale units, and are therefore given financial aid. In the next two decades better equipped hospitals will be available to patients. Fortis, Apollo and Wockhardt Hospitals have already come up during the last few years. Many will venture into this area, making product segments like medical products, hospital products, diagnostics, disposables, and hospital equipments grow rapidly.

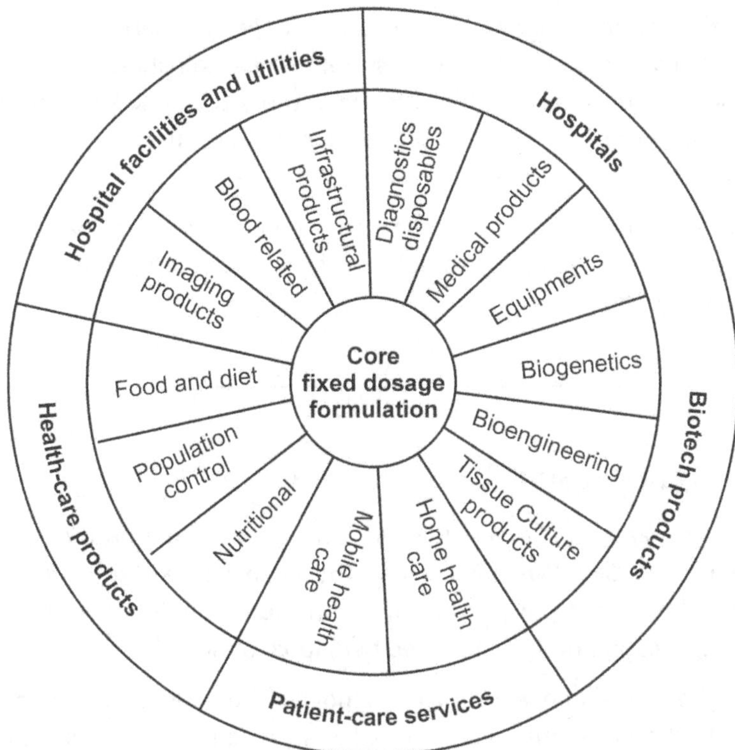

Figure 2.9 Graphic representation of the next two decades of health-care

Also, patients will have increased capacity to pay as privatization of medical insurance schemes has been encouraged by the government. Therefore, it is likely that patients will prefer to be treated in hospitals due to the availability of several private and government health insurance schemes besides Mediclaim.

Patients with chronic ailments or others discharged from hospital may also get care at home. So 'Home Health Care' and 'Mobile Health Care' units may emerge and prosper. Many pilot studies have already been conducted for these services in India.

Biotech products are likely to be widely used in the future, if we build appropriate facilities in hospitals. Biotech, biogenetics and bioengineering products should have an increased demand in India. India being rich in natural resources, tissue culture labs could be so economical here that global companies may look for opportunities to conduct their R&D in this country.

Those pharma companies who are stronger in marketing concepts and abilities may build up support systems like retail pharmacists chains, to ensure better reach of their products to the patients. Food products, nutritional products, and population control products may also have their niches in the market.

The industry which was earlier focused on treating 'sick patients' will expand to cover 'healthy people' with facilities for prophylactic as well as curative care.

CASE

Co-Marketing—Cetirizine[1]

Cetirizine is an anti-allergic molecule, and is a research product of UCB-Belgium. In India, UNI-UCB Ltd had the financial backing of an Indian Pharmaceutical company called Unichem. New to India, UNI-UCB was a small-scale company with a limited field force of 80 MRs.

To effectively launch Cetirizine in India and to gain maximum market share, UCB entered into a co-marketing arrangement with Glaxo, which was the largest Indian Pharmaceutical company, as well as with Unichem.

The bulk drug Cetirizine was manufactured by UNI-UCB in India from the basic stage. The raw material was converted to formulation by UNI-UCB and marketed in the country under the international brand name Zyrtec. The raw material was also sold to Glaxo and Unichem who marketed the tablet formulation under the brand names Cetzine and Zyncet respectively.

UCB-Belgium provided medical, technical and marketing support to its subsidiary, namely UNI-UCB, and also to the co-marketers, Glaxo and Unichem.

This molecule was launched by all the three companies in India in August 1993 through a medical symposium. During the symposium speakers from India as well as Europe spoke of the benefits of Cetrizine.

---

[1] *This case has been contributed by MrGiridharBalwani, Director, UNI-UCB India.*

There was no brand promotion within the symposium. However, all the three companies had put up display panels outside the venues to project all their respective brands, including Cetirizine.

After the conclusion of this symposium all three companies promoted their brands through their own field forces independently. With the inherent advantages of the drug and the combined strength of the three companies, it was expected that they would together achieve a market share of around 20% in the first year. By December 1993, Glaxo had captured a share of 8.4%, Unichem 3.4%, and UCB 0.3%. Overall, UCB had achieved a market share of 12.1%. This is an extremely impressive performance within the short period of five months.

With this level of promotional activity, it was expected that Cetirizine would be a major anti-allergic drug in the Indian market, overtaking worldwide bestsellers like Astemizole, Terfenadine and Loratadine.

LEARNINGS

To cope with the challenges as a result of continuing changes, it is essential to develop a strategic vision and focus one's energy and resources to carve a niche in future.

For seventy years after Independence, the pharmaceutical industry has been strongly affected by six basic forces along with two additional forces viz.

- Government
- Trade
- Medical Profession
- Technology
- Health Status of the Country
- International Events
- Patients
- Medical Representatives

The pharmaceutical industry has also experienced shifts for the last many years which has been broadly classified under three categories in terms of:

- Shifts in Business and Marketing Practices

- Shifts in Attitudes of Physicians and Patients
- Shifts in Types of Products

Due to the interplay of the eight major forces, the concept of pharmaceutical marketing has undergone evolution with changes taking place in marketing in the environment and within the organization as well.

To tackle these changes in pharmaceutical marketing, marketers need to focus on strategic thinking as well as strategic planning for long term growth and success.

The marketing function in a drug company is responsible for two crucial tasks: to develop a comprehensive business and marketing strategy, and to implement the strategy using various marketing tools and activities.

The basic of all marketing strategies is marketing planning which constitutes designing activities keeping in mind the objectives of marketing as well as the changing environment.

Most marketing plans are usually pretty large and lengthy. Regardless of this, there are some elements that are common to all marketing plans viz.

- Business Mission
- Business Objectives
- Situation Analysis

There are basically six types of pharmaceutical marketing:

- Borderless Marketing
- Co-Marketing
- Involvement Marketing
- Beyond Involvement Marketing
- Medico-Marketing
- Brand-image Marketing

It has been observed that the integration of R&D activities with marketing dimensions would present unique opportunities and challenges in pharmaceutical marketing to MNCs.

The next two decades fixed dose formulations will become the core business, better hospitals will be available to patients, patients will have increased capacity to pay due to privatization of medical insurance schemes, emergence of 'Home Health Care' and 'Mobile Health Care', and wide use of biotechnology products.

The pharmaceutical industry which earlier focused on treating 'sick patients' will expand to cover 'healthy people' with facilities for prophylactic as well as curative care.

CHAPTER 3

Innovation and Marketing Strategy

Japanese grocery stores had a problem. They are much smaller than shops in the USA and therefore don't have room to waste. Watermelons, big and round, wasted a lot of space. Most people would simply tell the grocery stores that watermelons grow round and there is nothing that can be done about it.

That is how majority of people would respond. But some Japanese farmers took a different approach. If the supermarkets wanted a square watermelon, they asked themselves, 'How can we provide one?' It wasn't long before they invented the square watermelon.

The solution to the problem of round watermelons was solved as the farmers did not assume it was impossible and simply asked how it could be done. They found out that if you put the watermelon in a square box when they are growing, the watermelon will take on the shape of the box and grow into a square fruit.

This made the grocery stores happy and had the added benefit that it was much easier and cost effective to ship the watermelons. Consumers also loved them because they took less space in their refrigerators which are much smaller than those in the USA meaning that the growers could charge a premium price for them.

When faced with a problem or with changing environment it is important to not assume and innovate in order to find solutions. The more one looks at a particular situation from different perspectives, the more innovative one becomes.

INNOVATION – THE NEW DRIVING FORCE

For any organization, innovation is a distinctive capability which yields competitive advantage and helps performance. Yet, firms often fail to gain competitive advantage from innovation. This is primarily due to the costs and uncertainties associated with the process of establishing innovation, and also because of the difficulties firms encounter in securing the returns from innovation for themselves. The rewards of innovation are often really the value-added effects of products or processes of the firms. Some firms have established value-added processes which stimulate a continuous process of innovation. Other firms can create an architecture that enables them to implement innovative practices effectively.

Continuous Innovation – The Story of Monsanto

Monsanto is an example of a successful firm which has been able to establish a lead in the life-science industry. It made this possible by implementing a continuous process of innovation that we can refer to as Monsanto's law. Monsanto's law takes off from Moore's law in the computer industry. In 1965, Gordon Moore predicted that the computing power of silicon chips would double every 18 to 24 months. The law has been driving the rapid growth and economic value of the computer industry.

Today, the ability to identify and use genetic information in terms of a nonlinear trend in biotechnology is paving the way for incomparable growth in the life sciences. Monsanto has progressed in three areas of genomics – gene sequencing, gene function and genetic improvement. The genomic technologies will continue to double in capability every 12 to 24 months... the Monsanto's law. For Monsanto, innovation in genomic capabilities and creating value-added processes in the organization is critically important to maintain its leadership in the life science industry. One of Monsanto's major pharma companies, Searle, which specializes in the areas of arthritis, oncology, cardiovascular diseases and women's health, is among the industry leaders in terms of its R&D capability. The potential value of Searle's pipeline is approximately seven times its R&D investment compared to an average of two to three times for major pharma companies.

Commercially Viable Innovation

At the same time, business history – especially European business history – is also full of stories of firms which innovated but failed to turn that innovation into sustainable competitive advantage. The British company, EMI, was at one time one of the most effective innovative firms. It was a pioneer in television and a leader in computers. Its music business was at the center of a revolution in popular culture, and its scanner technology transformed radiology. Today, only its music business survives.

Philips pioneered almost every major area of consumer electronics. The company invented the audio cassette and the compact disc and led in the development and manufacture of video cassette recorders. Europe has often enjoyed in innovative lead in aircraft manufacture. The jet engine was invented there and first put into commercial operation by de Havilland. Collaboration between Aerospatiale and the British Aircraft Corporation produced the world's only supersonic passenger aircraft.

Commercial Failure of Innovation

It has been observed that there is no cause for a firm's failure to derive commercial success from innovation. But the reasons why it is difficult to create competitive advantage through innovation fall into three broad categories.

First, innovation is, by its very nature, costly and uncertain unless it is based on proven laws either in an industry or in a parallel industry. It follows that even an innovation that is technically successful may not be profitable.

Second, the process of innovation is hard to manage. Directing innovative companies requires special skills and constant steering towards goals by the leader.

And third, the rewards of innovation are difficult to appropriate. Returns must be defended from competitors, from suppliers and customers, and may accrue to groups within the firm rather than to the organization itself.

The Process of Innovation

Although innovation is costly and uncertain, it nevertheless provides competitive advantage. Managing innovation is costly and risky. When innovation is highly appropriable and timely, the innovating firm emerges as the winner and takes the full kitty. This is frequently the case in the pharmaceutical industry. In such markets, potential participants need to consider carefully whether they wish to enter at all. If there are many players, then it is quite possible that their combined expenditures will exceed the value of the prize for which they compete. If there are few entrants, then large prizes may be available.

STRATEGIES FOR SUCCESS THROUGH INNOVATION

A variety of strategies are available to overcome these difficulties and succeed.

Commitment

An extreme example to show commitment is the tactic of pulling out the steering wheel and throwing it out of the window so that your rivals are left in no doubt whatever of your intention to stay in the game. The problem of commitment, as the extravagance of the example illustrates, lies in making the commitment credible.

Advance announcement of innovative products that have certainly not yet been put in marketable form and may not have even reached a prototype stage has been a regular feature of the recent evolution of the computer industry. It has been such a regular feature, in fact, that such announcements are no longer taken seriously and so have lost their strategic value.

It is difficult for firms to make commitments sufficiently credible, short of legally contracting to supply a product which has not yet been developed. This is decidedly a risky strategy, although it is one which is adopted in the aircraft industry, where there is little doubt that the product can be manufactured and uncertainties mostly relate to its cost.

These competitive issues are much less critical where the process of innovation is specific to the individual firm. This is usually the case when technology is generally available but application in a particular context requires heavy expenditure. Implementation of information technology in the financial services industry provides a good example. General principles are well known and well established. But substantial investment is required in their development and implementation in the context of any particular firm or institution. The use of robotics in the automobile industry has similar characteristics. Tomorrow, we may well be able to quote the example of the use of genomics in the life science industry.

Timing and Cost Effectiveness

Firm-specific innovation normally rests on the local application of generally available knowledge or technology. Success in this, though advantageous, is unlikely to create a sustainable competitive advantage unless the technology is more advanced, or more cost-effective than its rivals.

Spin-off

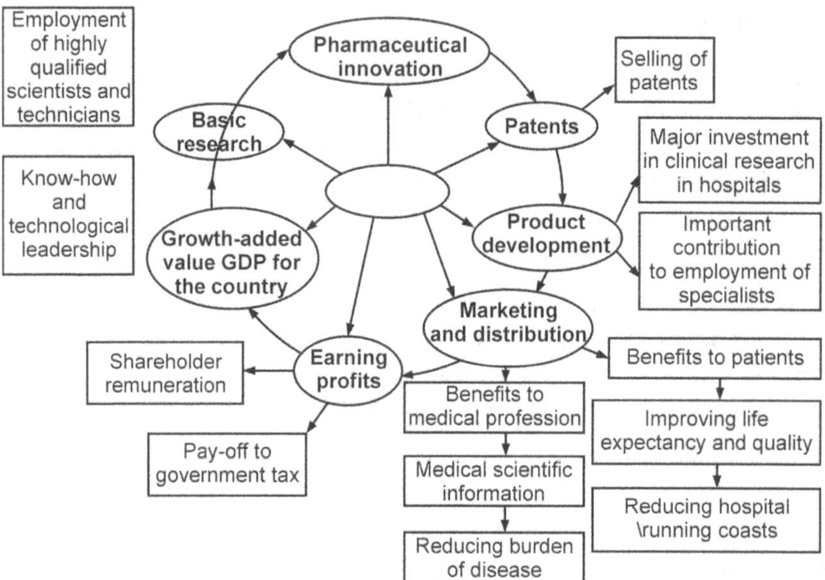

Figure 3.1 Pharmaceutical innovation

The spin-off cycle in the pharmaceutical business starts with a credible commitment to invest in basic research. The major investment in the process of innovation goes from basic research to either the patent development stage or till the stage of product development (See Figure 3.1). At either of these stages, the innovation can be harvested by selling the patent or marketing (commercializing) the product. Many processes, products and patents get lost due to indecisiveness in marketing the innovation considering the prevailing environment. The leader needs to manage this crucial process of commercialization and thereby earn profits through brand management and sales and marketing in order to gain spin-off benefits.

A spin-off strategy, if implemented well, has many benefits. Pfizer not only invested to innovate Viagra, but spent progressively to develop many molecules in hypertension, depression and other areas.

Evolution

The life-science industry is in the process of evolving from the 1980s to the post-2000 period through progressive steps. It really caught up when industry players wanted to develop competitive advantage. Evolution through exploitation of gene therapy and cell therapy is likely to take charge of future innovations. Though the process of 'genomics' will bring about significant changes in the market shares by 2020, it has been estimated that around 20 % of the market will be at the base level and will consist of existing products while the remaining 40 per cent will get captured by new delivery systems, additions, deletions of traditional drugs and remaining 40 % will be captured by 'Genomics'-oriented drugs.

Paradigm Shifts

Drug discovery, or innovation in drugs and medicines, needs paradigm shifts as the industry drivers are changing. Figure 3.2 identifies the major changes taking place in the competitive paradigm due to industry drivers.

Protecting and Exploiting Innovation

The issue of appropriability is fundamental. The central characteristic of a distinctive capability is that it cannot be easily replicated. A fundamental weakness of innovation as a source of competitive advantage is that often it can be easily replicated. The result is that the innovator may be exposed to the costs of innovation and the risks of development and introduction, only to see competitors share – or perhaps dominate – the fruits of success. The results are potentially inefficient as well as unjust, since the prospect of replication reduces the incentive to innovate in the first place. Patents and copyright laws therefore protect innovators, and much innovation is publicly funded – including virtually all fundamental scientific research.

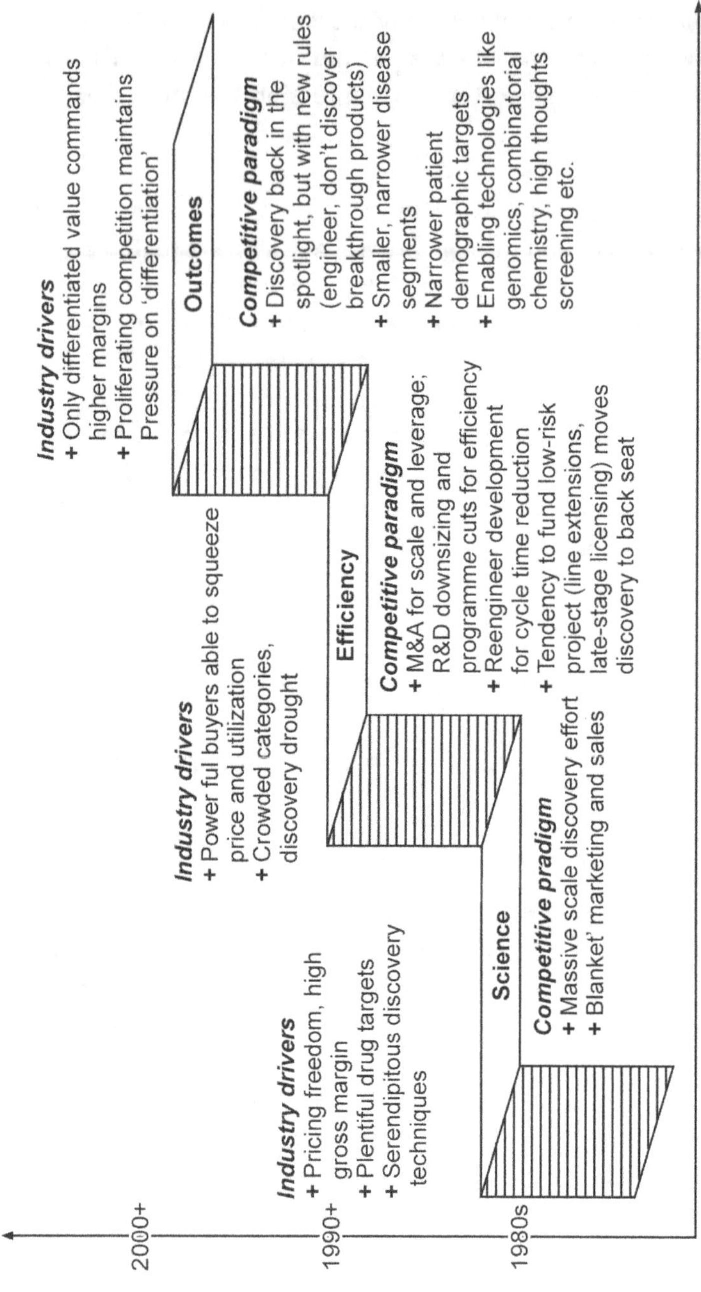

Figure 3.2 Paradigm shifts due to industry drivers

Patent law has been unable to keep pace with the range and complexity of modern innovation, and it is almost a matter of accident whether or not a specific innovation can achieve effective patent protection. Such protection works reasonably well in pharmaceuticals, although even here and there is a well-known science of molecular manipulation, based on the attempt to invent a patent by identifying a compound with essentially the same properties but a distinct chemical composition.

If an innovation cannot be protected by law, it can sometimes be protected by commercial secrecy. This is almost never true of a product innovation. You cannot advertise new products to your customers without at the same time advertising to your competitors. But for modest process innovations, secrecy may aid the innovator. Mostly, however, reverse engineering – working back from the final product to the initial design – gives the imitator an equivalent opportunity.

Innovatization (Innovation + Commercialization)

Neither law nor secrecy is sufficient to allow an innovation to be turned into competitive advantage. Strategy must be used instead.

The most effective way of turning innovation to competitive advantage is to generally deploy it in conjunction with another distinctive capability. Innovation and reputation, field staff competence, architecture, niche marketing, muscle power and so on are often potent combinations.

In other words, it is firms with another distinctive capability that are generally best placed to derive competitive advantage from innovation. But even if this is not possible, innovation can yield competitive advantage with the aid of other strategic tools. The contrast between GSK and EMI demonstrates the difference between success and failure in establishing complementary strategies for the innovation of anti – ulcer drugs. Distribution and manufacturing capabilities are generally important but can be hired or outsourced. If the innovating company does possess these particular attributes, then it is relatively well placed to appropriate the returns to the innovation. This was GSK's position in the UK market, but not in some of the other markets in which it wished to compete. So mergers and acquisition followed.

Strategic Innovation and Markets

There is surfeit of literature on formulation of strategy and any person who has the desire can learn the precepts and conceptualize a framework for formulating a strategy. However, there is little that has been written on the preparation and execution of strategy. Strategy is not merely a cerebral activity. It is practiced-based and an inseparable part of any business. Strategy must be developed on the basis of the operating situation and must be able to provide guidelines for holistic actions that are in accordance with the business objectives.

In business the core of strategy is always dependent on two aspects:

(i)   the competition, and

(ii) one's own objectives.

For both the aspects, one needs to assess one's own capabilities vis-à-vis the competition to develop the strategic edge. In actual operation one needs to reconcile the consequences of these two series of actions which are often in opposition to each other. A good strategy will take a route that can ensure there are no successive actions. Rather, it makes possible the simultaneous application of all actions that can surpass and surprise the competitor. In other words, strategy links together a series of actions that can achieve the business objectives and meet the challenges of competition.

These operating actions from many small and separate campaigns, each of which need regulatory mechanisms to ensure there is no deviation from the ultimate business objective. No portion of any campaign should be separated from the main body unless there is some urgent necessity. It is on this maxim alone that operating actions can deliver strategic results. The best strategy is one that stands always firm and strong and generates energy which propels and motivates its unflinching implementation.

Strategic forces are of changing nature and continually change as the strategy gets implemented. They change depending on the competition and the environment. However, the basic strategy intent must not change. Intent is always based on vision, energy, time, values, speed, techniques, courage, and skill. Leadership or ownership of strategy is an essential component for the success of any strategy. History is proof that success is dependent on the qualities and skills of the leader and the kind of strategy adopted by him or her. Alexander the Great was a visionary, Julius Caeser was an excellent communicator, Gengis Khan was a master of Speed, Napolean was a great revolutionary. US grant was a genius at turnarounds, Frederick the Great of Prussia was remarkably adept at taking calculated risks, Gustarus Adolphus of Sweden knew re-engineering, George Patton was a hard taskmaster. Gandhi never deviated from his path of simplicity and non-violence. All these leaders possessed a variety of qualities and skills far above the normal. They stood steadfast in their beliefs and in their commitment to their strategy to achieve success. They directed their attention at keeping their forces concentrated on the main objective.

Need for Innovation

With far-reaching global changes taking place, to be successful we need to recognize the continual development of new forces and weave them into the major thread of our strategy on a continuous basis. This needs tremendous flexibility, adjustability and innovation. Innovation of existing activities at the core or at the periphery becomes crucial for those who implement. If there is no innovation at the level of every key task and function, the implementers may shy away and leave course midway.

Strategy needs the commitment of those who are responsible for its implementation. It is therefore essential to develop the mindset of the implementers before spelling out the strategy. It is time to come out of our ethnocentric mindset and change to a global one. A global mindset rests on a foundation of openness. It accepts diversity and heterogeneity as a natural and as sources of opportunity and strength rather than as necessary evils. The openness inherent in the global mindset implies an openness to change over time, in one's own culture. To exhibit a global mindset, an organization's management team must be owned with two important features – a deep understanding of the world's diversity and a strong ability to integrate diverse world views. The economic landscape of the world is changing rapidly and becoming more global at a faster pace. This means that for most medium-sized to large companies, market opportunities, crucial resources and competitors lurk not just in their home markets but also increasingly in distant and often poorly understood regions. To take strategic advantage of this globalizing environment, innovation at every level of marketing activity has become imperative.

The institutionalization of strategy is essential for achieving success and strategic endurance. As we have seen, a changing environment often requires the induction and integration of new parallel streams in the mainstream of strategy midway. A good leader should be alert to these changes to take charge of the situation.

Sometimes, the environment may become so turbulent that it compels the leader to refocus the direction of the organization. This phenomenon has been seen earlier in the pharmaceutical industry and continues to happen.

We have witnessed directional changes from formulation to bulk drugs, and back from bulk drugs to formulation. Similarly, in the last few years we have seen oscillations from branded products to generics, and generics to branded products.

Such changes call for a more complete understanding of the industry (Figure 3.3). A spanning of the universe can enable the leader to choose and identify an appropriate strategy and accordingly direct the efforts of the organization without deviating from the central thread.

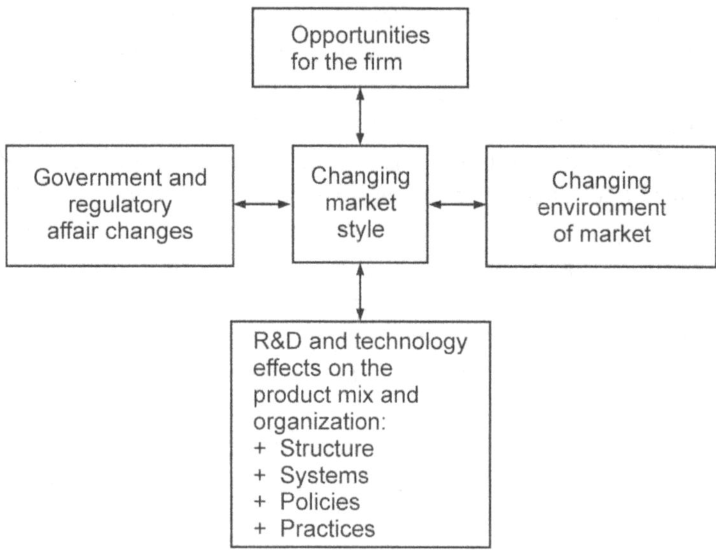

Figure 3.3 Changing marketing structure

Again, in times of change, the ultimate customers modify their attitudes towards products and services. This calls for innovations in marketing strategy that can be beyond conventional marketing approaches and involve the customer.

We will now examine how we can address this crucial aspect of institutionalizing an enduring, long-term marketing strategy.

Institutionalizing an Enduring and Innovative Marketing Strategy

Excellent marketing strategies with a mediocre level of institutionalization have never been successful. This is especially true in a vast country such as India, which needs a high energy for implementation. Every pharmaceutical company today is trying to find formal and informal ways of institutionalizing strategic actions that will take it nearer to the customer. These have inbuilt problems of culture, environment and controls of the organization. But they must serve the company's communication needs to nourish the organization and ensure its effective functioning.

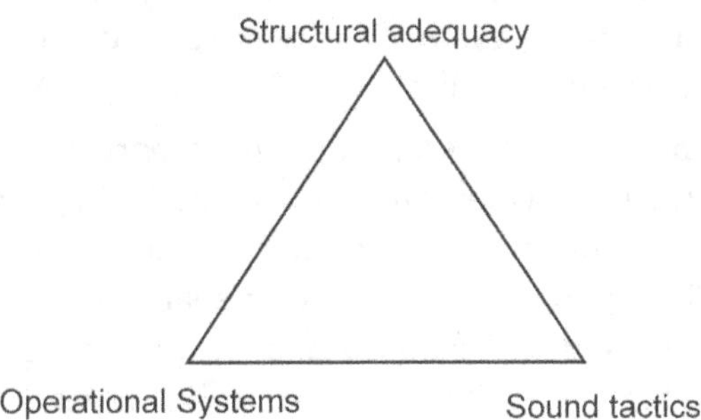

Figure 3.4 Issues affecting institutionalization

The major issues affecting the level of institutionalization of a marketing strategy include structural adequacy, operable operational systems, and most important, use of the right tactics (Figure 3.4).

Structural Adequacy

Old structures are collapsing. Concepts such as one national sales manager with a team of zonal managers and a group of front-line and second-line managers promoting the company only through medical representatives (MRs), and the product management and marketing teams working exclusively on cerebral issues are on their way out.

Deviation has been successful in Cipla, US Vitamin and Sandoz. Each of them utilized different structural approaches to institutionalize marketing strategies. All over the world, the information technology revolution is working towards delayering organizations, making them lean and effective in implementation. How well organizations in India can accept and adapt to this remains to be seen, but organizations that face personnel problems have dropped their usual way of reaching the doctors and retailers, and are designing a 'new structure' to make themselves more effective.

(i) ***Impact of formal structures:*** While institutionalizing strategies, it is important to develop responsibilities at different hierarchical levels and define the roles clearly. If the field force has to report to different managers for its different functional activities, its cohesiveness and efficiency get affected adversely. However, the centralized colonial attitude of the field force has its own defects – it allows only those strategies to be implemented that are in the interest of and accepted by the top person of the field force. The institutionalization then becomes subjective. As a result, 'networking organizations' are coming up to ensure 'institutionalization in spirit'.

There are organizations where the MRs report to the sales manager for their sales activities and to the marketing manager for the support of production promotion. The distribution manager functionally reports to the finance department in the context of outstandings and collections, and to the head of the depot structure for administrative controls. Many entrepreneurial organizations had reporting structures where the institutionalization level deteriorated because marketing activities were not in unison with sales force activities.

This also creates several inter-departmental problems. This does not mean that this kind of structural demarcation and reporting pattern does not work. It can work, provide the leader is capable of coordinating and resolving conflicts through networking.

It is, therefore, important to examine the structural adequacies to enforce strategic actions in the organization, either by developing certain skills in keeping with the culture or by creating an atmosphere of leadership which helps in institutionalizing the basic vision, mission and strategies of the organization.

(ii) ***Impact of flat structure:*** Cipla was trying to make its organization flatter in terms of hierarchy, and was also attempting a new concept of coordination against the earlier one of the reporting to one person in each hierarchy. Teams are more important than individuals. Such structural adjustments and changes are sometimes necessary to deploy the workforce and again cohesiveness in the team to institute strategies. It worked for Cipla, but may not work for others as each company has its own peculiarities.

(iii) ***Impact of flexi-time structure:*** A few organizations have discovered that if they bifurcate working hours, they can intensify the effects of marketing and brand strategies. As a result, one flexi-time team is appointed to work in the morning hours and another in the evening. This system works so well for some organizations that they always launch a new product through such teams. This formal-but-temporary structure is built in such a way that it provides the company an edge. It has also made those organizations effective where there was a problem of coverage of consultants.

(iv) ***Impact of informal structures:*** Wockhardt promoted one of its 'hospital products' through a territory sales force – a set of promoters who, though trained and managed by company managers, were on payrolls of either distributors or an outside agency. This additional set of promoters for focused work in hospitals yielded rich dividends to the organization and helped it gain an edge over its competitors.

(v) ***Impact of product-related structures:*** SOL selected 25 product executives in Hyderabad and gave them products to nurture. It established a link between the product management team and the sales team as they became catalysts in ensuring the institutionalization of strategies. An additional infrastructure of 20-25 product executives was created to comb different specialties. Even Ethnor once tried to segregate its MRs to promote Raricap Syrup and tablets separately to different set of doctors. While the difference of the approach was perceptible, it also created some confusion in the minds of the physicians. So, a company needs to be very careful with product-related structures since it needs to be very careful with product-related structures since it needs systems and policies to back up such structures.

(vi) ***Impact of market-related structures:*** Charak identified the potential of ayurvedic products in the state of Uttar Pradesh and decided to penetrate the state with the help of about 35-40 MRs, besides various media vehicles. The entire structure was developed on market needs. All hospital products and equipment companies also need to design their structures on the basis of markets.

(vii) ***Impact of responsibility-centered structures:*** The sales directors have relatively less freedom in institutionalizing strategies, but control the promotion mix and the costs attached to it to generate a given profit ratio. The responsibility of profit thus lies squarely on these directors. A company needs to strengthen any given structure by examining its adequacy with regard to the strategic actions.

Operable Operational Systems

Whatever structural foundations a company lays to develop its marketing organization, it also needs to develop operational systems to provide feedback and a marketing information system. These systems must help generate adequate information to help the management control and support the activities of the marketing department and the field staff in order to ensure cost-effective institutionalization of the structure.

Operational systems can be formulated and institutionalized in activities of marketing and field staff, product management and distribution personnel. These can be:

- Results of the field staff
- Cost of the field staff
- Promotional efforts
- Strategy implementation by the field staff
- Database generation for marketing efforts
- Activities and results of distributors/carrying and forwarding agents/depots
- Cost of distribution
- Special campaigns feedback
- Special problems/opportunities feedback

The systems can provide information which can be used by the organization proactively.

I have observed that an umpteen number of organizations where systems are classically laid down by the top, but are not adhered to. If non-adherence is tolerated at the cost of results, a stage comes when the senior managers of the organization remain unaware of the systems. Although the forte of multinationals is adherence to an effective system, it has been observed that in India even they have a problem of adherence to systems.

Once the strategy and systems are in place, it is time to look at what tactics you wish to employ to get your plan off the ground.

Sound Tactics

Since the successful execution of a plan often depends more on the tactics employed than on its intrinsic soundness, the developer of a plan should be tactically adept. Many talented young executives have been thwarted in their ambition because they operate under the naïve assumption that 'right is might'. It is not enough to devise wise strategies; they must be implemented with proper tactics.

One of our clients launched an excellent dermatological product to be sold to dermatologists and general practitioners (GPs). Dermatologists were expected to contribute about 80 per cent of the total sales and GPs the rest. The product achieved success, but evaluation showed that 80 per cent of the sales were from GPs and only 20 per cent from dermatologists. At the tactical level, the skills of the field force did not allow proper implementation of the strategy.

In our society, we do not like to discuss the use of tactics; it is not quite acceptable. It gives the impression that one is manipulating people. Indeed, tactics focus on individual skills related to people or situations. Moreover, tactics, when improperly applied, are considered unethical. It is up to an individual to learn tactics through experience. This is, perhaps, one reason that good tactics develop relatively slowly. Tactics are the tools used to carry out the organization's strategies and plans. A skillful manager not only possess a wide range of tactics, but also knows when and how to use them.

Tactics are neither good nor bad, nor are there any perfect tactics. In any situation, there is no one best set of tactics that can be used. Many tactics may work, some better than others. Many may fail, some more surely than others. Many managers mistakenly use the same tactics repeatedly, regardless of situations, because these may have worked for them earlier. Success reinforces the habit and can make you repeatedly use the same tactics mindlessly. There comes a time when tactics do not work, and that is the most critical time. As tools of implementation, tactics should be used like a hammer to drive nails and not smash thumbs. It is up to the manager to learn how to use them properly.

The crucial element is in deciding which tactics to use in a particular situation. This depends on the presence of any one or more cornerstones in a given situation. Take the case of the manager of a field force that is unionized. In making his tactical decision, the manager must decide how to collaborate with the other party in the situation, whether through peers, subordinates, customers or competitors.

A sales manager faces a number of considerations when deciding upon a tactical plan or course of action. There are five critical elements in this tactical model:

(i) **Stakes:** How much money is involved? How much risk is involved? On minor issues, a manger might choose to ignore the adversary. But if the stakes are high, forceful tactics may be needed. Suppose an association of physicians asks you to spend half-a-million rupees on sponsoring an event. There is a possibility of your incurring this expenditure and not gaining much advantage from it; instead, your competitor may display tactical skills and gain from it without spending anything.

An organization spent Rs.2 million on sponsoring a seminar. The sales manager of a competing organization registered for the same conference, along with his medical director. During the day they spent time with their 'core' doctors and in the evening they entertained them. As a result, they built a one-to-one rapport with physicians from all over India in three nights. Then they ensured that all these prominent physicians were adequately followed to yield results, as all of them were selected on their potential. The stake was adequately weighed and the cost-benefit analysis was supplemented by effective tactics.

(ii) **Personalities:** People react to situations in different ways. Some adversaries are belligerent and combative. Some direct actions might prod them into doing exactly what the manager does not want them to do. In such cases, it is better to use various indirect tactics so that there are no personality clashes.

One must also recognize one's own personality characteristics. It would be foolish to try to bluff one's way through if one's acting skills are suspect. Some managers find that their personalities are better suited for dealing with other people on a one-to-one basis rather than in groups. So, they should try to avoid group meetings. Many companies have stopped conducting meetings of large groups of specialists. They now call smaller teams to avoid conflict between two schools of thought held by specialists.

(iii) ***Power bases:*** The power held (or perceived to be held) by both parties plays a pivotal role in tactical selection. The organization that has a strong, unassailable power base can make more forceful tactical moves. On the other hand, an organization that does not possess any power over its environment must use other tactics.

I have come across many organizations that can deal with associations and unions by first establishing an equal power base and then using tactical moves to negotiate. Those who cannot establish power equations loose out as they lack the tactics to negotiate. However, cornerstones like stakes and personalities exert some amount of influence on the power base. The use of different tactics to achieve goals of both the parties satisfactorily is also essential to maintain a relationship. Any tactical move must always achieve a win-win situation.

(iv) ***Urgency:*** In the case of pending collections, it is essential for the company to stop the consignment and recover the payment first. It is sometimes better to recall goods from the transporter, even when the goods have already been delivered to the stockists. Sometimes, when quick action is needed, direct, and forceful tactics may have to be used.

Tactics have different success rates in different situations. Some managers become so enamored with a certain tactic that they try to use it in situations where they do not work. Many managers ignore formal communication techniques and use informal, non-verbal routes. When the going gets tough, it becomes too late and by then they cannot document anything. So, the probability of success reduces.

(v) ***Personal skills:*** Some people can do certain things easily, others cannot. The manager who finds it difficult to detail his product may find other ways of accomplishing the same task. A person who does not talk well resorts to written communication. Managers should use tactics at which they are adept.

(vi) ***Legal considerations:*** Some issues end up as legal liabilities. If an organization ends up with litigation because of, say, having affixed increased price stickers on existing stocks, tactics should be selected carefully. The date should be accurate and the details must be provided to the authorities.

(vii) ***Values:*** The manager's personal values play a key role in tactical selection. The manager should not do things he doesn't feel right about. There are some managers who take up the task of developing subordinates as a challenge. These personal values add to the commitment.

Nani A. Palkhiwala in the introduction to his book. We, the People, states: 'We, as a nation, suffer from fatty degeneration of conscience. The tricolor fluttering all over the country is black, red and scarlet- black money, red tape and scarlet corruption.' Although we are trying to overcome all these aspects, deep-rooted systems cannot be removed overnight. These systems percolate down to all levels of the society, and doctors are not an exception. Palkhiwala further describes two major defects of our society- a lack of sense of fairness and lack of moderation.

The same defects seem to have pervaded many of our pharmaceutical companies. The practices have evolved due to two reasons:

- Stiff competition
- An impatience to deliver results or create sales.

For instance, to alienate its competitors, US Vitamin exclusively sponsored a diabetologists' conference for which they claimed to have spent Rs.4 million on a single conference at Delhi. Since it is really not possible to verify such a claim, the weak and under-confident competitor will develop cold feet.

So, look at your strengths and find innovative ways to match competitive practices that will not drain your resources. Go to your customers and find out what they really need. Innovation is the key. Employ tactics on the basis of the strategic plan.

Natco is one company that did an excellent job in identifying the needs of cardiologists who wanted to be updated through articles of prestigious international journals every month. The company arranged for photocopies of these articles to be circulated among cardiologists. This value addition was highly appreciated by them. Such value addition by understanding the needs of your customers can help you establish a close long-term relationship; forge a strong bond. Because no matter how good your strategy and how strong your tactics, you need to involve your doctors (as also retailers) to convert precepts into practice.

Before we conclude this chapter, let us take a brief look at the forces shaping the Indian pharmaceutical industry and the future scenario. This will give us an idea of the kind of innovation and strategy required to make the industry globally competitive.

FORCES SHAPING INDIAN PHARMACEUTICAL INDUSTRY

India cannot exist in isolation. As the world moves towards initiatives in innovation, India has to follow suit. However, the dynamics of the market in India, and the forces that are likely to shape the Indian pharmaceutical industry will be different for at least the next five to seven years. The forces that will shape industry are depicted in Figure 3.5 and are:

- Core strength of the Indian pharmaceutical industry
- Disease pattern
- Doctors
- Patients
- Alternate medicine
- Health infrastructure
- Information technology
- Health insurance

The core strengths of the Indian pharmaceutical industry include its good blend of Eastern and Western styles of management, well-educated, low-cost, and abundant workforce, low-cost bulk drugs and formulations, large and growing market for the next 25 years, and alternate medicine for masses at low cost.

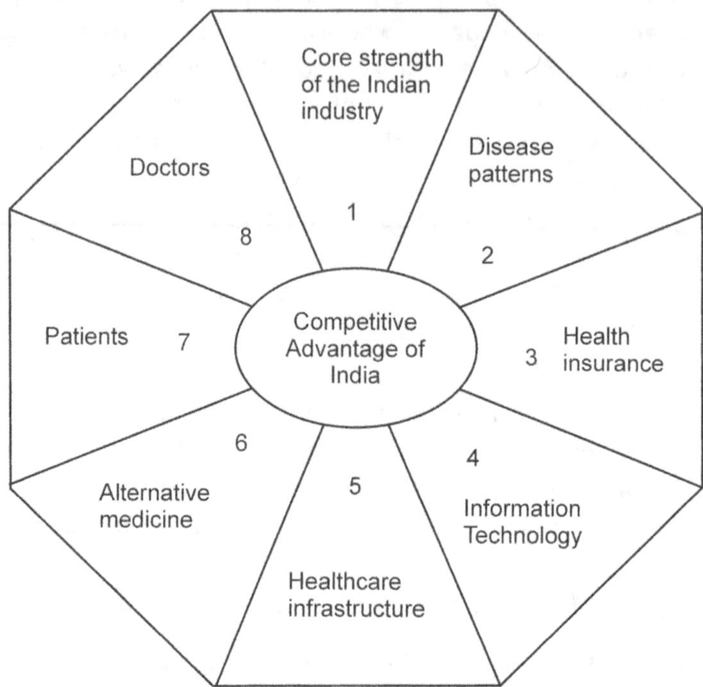

Figure 3.5 Key forces shaping the pharmaceutical industry

Looking at the impact of the eight major forces, one can identify 10 critical success factors which may emerge:

1. Product-portfolio related
    - New products
    - The ability to be the first to enter the market
    - The right kind of portfolio mix as per the prevalent disease pattern
    - The product portfolio base
    - Right positioning
2. Well-trained sales force (MRs)
3. Integration to widen business opportunities
4. R&D efforts to provide competitive advantage
5. Information technology to derive cost advantage and to be customer responsive

6. Good manufacturing practices to provide competitive advantage in terms of quality
7. Strong over-the-counter (OTC) brands
8. Exports – allopathic and ayurvedic products
9. Strategic alliances
10. Business design and strategy

These forces which are shaping industry need to be revitalized through marketing innovation in the next five to seven years. As the forces keep on changing the shape of industry changes, we can slowly go back and forward to innovation and strategy. However, it is very important to develop sustainable and innovative marketing approaches and practices to get results in the pharmaceutical industry.

LEARNINGS

Innovation is a distinctive capacity which yields competitive advantage and helps performance.

It is difficult to create a competitive advantage through innovation because firstly it is very costly and uncertain, secondly the process of innovation is hard to manage and thirdly the rewards of innovation are difficult to appropriate.

A variety of strategies are available to overcome the difficulties surrounding innovation and succeed viz.

- Commitment
- Timing and cost effectiveness
- Spin-Off
- Evolution
- Paradigm Shifts

A fundamental weakness of innovation as a source of competitive advantage is that often it can be easily replicated. Thus, patents and copyright laws protect innovators, including virtually all fundamental scientific research.

The most effective way of turning innovation to competitive advantage is to generally deploy it in conjunction with another distinctive capability.

Strategy is not merely a cerebral activity; it is an inseparable part of any business. Strategy must be developed on the basis of the operating situation and must be able to provide guidelines for holistic actions that are in accordance with the business objectives.

With far reaching global challenges, to be successful, one needs tremendous flexibility, adjustability and innovation. If there is no innovation at the level of every task and function, the implementers may shy away and leave course midway.

In times of change, the ultimate customers modify their attitudes towards products and services with innovations in marketing strategy beyond conventional marketing approaches involving the customer.

The major issues affecting the level of institutionalization of a marketing strategy include:

- Structural adequacy
- Operable operational systems
- Sound tactics

The forces shaping the Indian pharmaceutical industry need to be revitalized through marketing innovations in the coming years by going back and forward to innovation and strategy.

It is very important to develop sustainable and innovative marketing approaches and practices to get results in the pharmaceutical industry.

CHAPTER **4**

Strategic Concepts, Models and Options

There was a person named Nasuruddin who owned a donkey. He used to hire it out to the merchants of his village. The donkey was very strong and could carry a lot of goods on his back, and never irritated the merchants. Within a span of six months, he became popular with the merchants. They started booking him in advance. One of the merchants never paid the hire charges in time. Nasuruddin tried his best to dissuade him from hiring his donkey, but was unsuccessful. Once when the merchant came to ask for the donkey, Nasuruddin told him that the donkey was not at home. Unfortunately, at that very moment, the donkey brayed from inside. The merchant asked Nasuruddin, 'Why are you bluffing? Your donkey is at home! I can hear him. I need him now.' In a split second, Nasuruddin quickly replied, 'Look sir, I don't want to give my donkey to a person like you, who does not believe in men but would rather believe a donkey. I am sorry. . .'

Even when you cannot see any option, there is always a way out. In life, options come from existing situations, provided you are willing to search for a solution. They also come from our reflexes, resources, demands of customers, and expectations of suppliers.

GENESIS

Considering the long lead time in research and development in the pharmaceutical industry, building a market-driven organization demands close integration of the corporate and marketing strategies. It is not possible to build any effective marketing strategy unless it is incorporated in the overall corporate strategy. Together, these strategies should address four crucial issues:

(i)   which customer needs and markets to serve;

    (ii)   how to allocate the company's scarce resources to the selected target customer needs;

   (iii)   what level of risk an organization should take; and

   (iv)   how well are the capacity and capabilities integrated to market any product to fulfill the needs of the target group. We can call this a 'business-marketing strategy', as business is also dependent on customers.

This strategy sets out the way a company elects to relate to its environment and how it expects to excel in its selected products or services. The allocation of a company's resources and efforts must justify the risk it is taking. The business-marketing strategy provides a direction to well-rounded marketing strategies. Marketing strategy is concerned with the product group (portfolio) and product resources across independent strategic business units (SBUs) of the company in a given competitive environment. The selection of target markets and differential advantages of the products that comprise the SBUs is the concern of any product strategy.

ELEMENTS OF BUSINESS-MARKETING STRATEGY

Companies operating in the health-care sector have a multitude of market opportunities: human health products (prescription and OTC drugs), animal health products, hospital products, natural (herbal) products, diagnostic, healthcare services, biotech products, and so on. Each of these opportunities has specific requirements in terms of risk, resources, capacities, and capabilities. It is often possible to find good arguments for investing in each of these market opportunities. Limited resources and competitive pressures usually preclude companies having a presence in all those potentially attractive healthcare markets.

The first strategic decision a company must therefore take is to select those markets in which it wants to participate, i.e. it has to specify its scope and, as a company, recognize its limitations. These decisions define the company's opportunity set. A small opportunity set limits the size and growth potential of the company, but might be realistic given limited resources. A broadly defined *opportunity* set allows for growth and diversification, but requires extensive resources. This also increases the risk of success because of the available resources being spread too thin. You can attract all segments, provided you plan in a phased manner.

Wockhardt in the early 1980s designed a corporate plan to improve its presence in the healthcare market by studying various available options in existing and related markets. They decided to enter different therapeutic groups—hospital products, I.V. infusions, hospital care by building diagnostic centers, bulk products by manufacturing bulk and fine chemicals, OTC high-tech food products and also into veterinary and herbal products. The marketing strategy was integrated in such a way that even for its existing business Wockhardt carefully allocated its resources. The entire process started with the launch of Tridoss (a division of Wockhardt). As its resources increased, Wockhardt then invested in the pre-decided areas. Today, they have a significant presence in all these segments. In fact, in 1993—94, Wockhardt generated additional resources by floating equity shares to grow further and consolidated their position in the healthcare market.

You must pay attention to the *four* basic elements of business-marketing strategy:

1. Risk   R1
2. Resources   R2
3. Capacities   C1
4. Capabilities   C2

While developing any corporate marketing strategy, you must ensure that there is adequate balance between risk and resources on one hand, and capacity and capability on the other (Figure 4.1).

It often happens that, looking at the available opportunity, the management or entrepreneur takes the risk of building objectives out of ambitions, but these objectives cannot be met if resources do not match the ambitious plans. In addition, ambitious objectives require certain 'capacities' in the form of assets. These capacities include the capabilities of those who will implement the programs. So the balance between capacities and capabilities is also very important for any strategy. Besides, corporate strengths must be taken as advantages while working out a marketing strategy. Specifically, a pharmaceutical company must define its scope in terms of opportunity set, or product-market, in accordance with continual environmental changes.

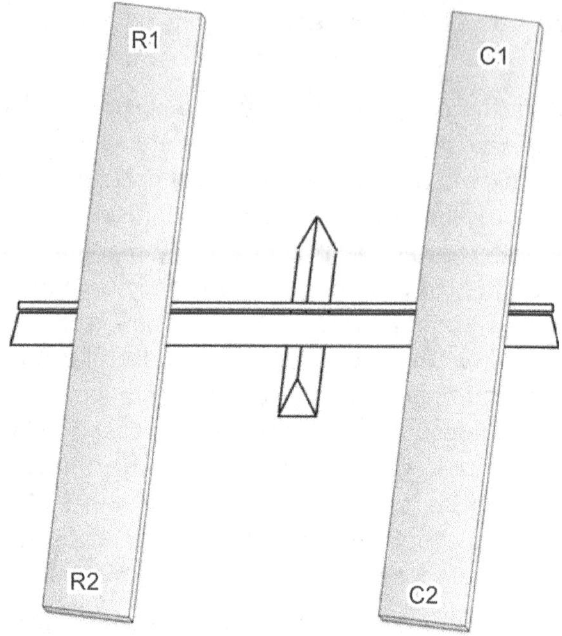

Figure 4.1 Maintain a balance between risk and resources in relation to capacities and capabilities

CORPORATE STRATEGIC OPTIONS

We can identify *fourteen* different options open to Indian firms while developing their corporate strategies:

1. Focusing on strengths
2. Alliances or acquisitions route for new entrants
3. Sustainability
4. Appropriability
5. Diversifications
6. Technological collaborations—Franchises
7. Licensing in—licensing out
8. Identification of markets—Product categories
9. Gaining marketing capabilities
10. Mergers and acquisitions
11. Forward and backward integration with technology
12. Bottom-line strategies
13. Creating an entry barrier
14. Product-market matching

1. Focusing on Strengths

On the international scene initially, Baxter International Inc. derived 90% of its sales from healthcare markets, mostly from the sales of medical supplies and medical equipment. On the other hand, healthcare sales constituted only 9% of the sales volume of ICL. Merck & Co., GSK and Roche Diagnostics, all depended on the healthcare business for over 80% of their income. In contrast, companies like Novartis, Sandoz, and Bayer relied less on the healthcare and pharmaceutical business.

Thus, depending on their individual corporate philosophy and strategy, these companies focused their activities in either healthcare or other businesses.

In the pharmaceutical industry, each one of us must define our own specific objectives at the macro, corporate level in advance, and clearly anticipate the challenges at the division or product level.

2. Gaining Marketing Capabilities

Organizations all over the world have tried to tie up to gain marketing capabilities. Rhone Poulenc tied up with Beecham abroad. This helped Rhone Poulenc to quickly recover the money it spent on R&D. A classic example of such collaboration was observed when an important product like low molecular weight Heparin was given for marketing to a trader in Delhi, M/s Brawn Pharma, although Rhone Poulenc had its own organization in India. You can see how even multinationals are operating with new options. Everybody is exploiting various strategic options.

3. Sustainability

In the future, it will be also important for an organization to sustain itself in existing markets. This is possible if the organization has many specific capabilities, which are stronger than those of other competitors. For example, as a local manufacturer, you may be able to generate business through government negotiations. As a result, business from ESI, Central Government Health Scheme (CGHS), and other tenders can sustain the organization. Other marketers who can hire our contract detailers as a service to existing manufacturers at one-third the cost will once again provide sustainability for those manufacturers. Every organization must identify its sustainable capabilities.

4. Appropriability

Appropriability is the capacity of the firm to retain added value for its own benefits. A firm can distribute added value if it generates any. Reliance Industries created added value for its shareholders by managing the funds so appropriately that each shareholder was happy. Gujarath Ambuja followed. This strength comes out of managing your liquidity and funds and generating added value for customers through price reductions and for shareholders by providing better earnings per share. Similarly many pharmaceutical organizations can provide added value if they manage their funds appropriately.

5. Diversifications

Corporate strategy decision makers define the scope of diversification. Those who are in the core sector of the Indian industry would like to have a presence in health and hygiene as well, since it is an important area.

In India, major industrial groups like the Tatas entered healthcare with Tata Pharma by floating their own operations. Birlas wanted to enter this market with foreign collaboration but had second thoughts at the initial phase itself. Mafatlals, through their Standard Alkali Division, wanted to collaborate with a UK-based company, Syntex. But this venture too was aborted in the initial phase. The Modis began by collaborating with Winthrop and launched Modi-Winthrop which today is called Win Medicare. There are many such examples of diversification.

Those who did not succeed started the diversification process without matching their existing strengths with these new ventures. Those who succeeded could match either the existing strengths or acquired skills and strengths from the environment in terms of people, technology, philosophy, and professionalized business management.

6. Foreign Collaborations for Technology or Franchise

During those days when it was difficult to enter India, Lillys collaborated with MJ Pharmaceuticals and entered the industry by providing manufacturing technology of raw materials and bulk drugs useful for healthcare, while Elders entered the scene with lots of franchises for specific products in India. There are today many such examples around us. Strategic alliance has thus, become a key to survival in the healthcare industry in India as well as abroad. Successful alliances are usually between two equally strong parties. If both the parties are not strong in their specific fields, the alliance does not succeed. What is strategic in strategic alliance is the choice of a partner.

7. Licensing-in and Licensing-Out

Licensing-in and licensing-out arrangements enabled Japanese companies to expand and start wholly owned subsidiaries in a number of major European countries and in the USA. An important strategic factor for large pharmaceutical companies is the extent to which they want to maintain a direct presence in developing countries. Lack of hard currencies and political instability has made some large drug companies reconsider their strategies and strategic partners for licensing-in and licensing-out.

Walter Bushnell, Elder, German Remedies, DupharInterfran Ltd., Wallace, and Win Medicare adopted a novel approach in the Indian industry—they took up a few brands on a licensing-in basis. Such an approach helped national organizations to survive and prosper in the era of patent protection. If an organization has inadequate R&D facilities, and yet wishes to protect itself from patents, it can choose this option to maintain growth.

If it is to adopt such means, an organization must be prepared for FDA documentation and marketing papers. These administrative procedures facilitate the success of such options.

8. Identification of Markets-Product Categories

Multinationals tend to give particular importance to their home markets. However, most large pharmaceutical companies are truly international with production, R&D and marketing activities spread throughout the world market. Recent changes in emerging markets are likely to open up further strategic potential markets for these internationally oriented companies.

Between 40% and 50% of the total sales of large American drug companies come from world markets. Some large pharmaceutical companies still face an important globalization challenge.

Companies like Novartis, Roche, and Sandoz depend heavily on markets in other countries.

Co-marketing, co-detailing, franchising, co-production and loan license agreements have become popular in recent years. All these have tended to reinforce the trend towards globalization. The situation now has changed for India in terms of the generics market share. Generic drugs in India are expected to account for 85% share in the domestic pharmaceutical market by 2020, thus, augmenting the domestic sales.

It will be very important to identify the markets and then decide which products and product categories companies should select to export.

Given the high R&D investments necessary to develop new pharmaceutical products, managers in most companies lean heavily on subsidiaries to adopt global strategies and introduce products in most parts of the world. The tendency towards harmonization of government regulations (especially in EU and the USA) will strengthen control by headquarters even further, or at least put greater emphasis on co-ordination across company borders.

Local subsidiaries are often allowed to adjust the specific target markets and positioning of their products as well as the galenical and dosage forms. More specifically, different functions and activities within functions have to be managed in a flexible manner. Development and clinical trials will need co-ordination and integration as government regulations are harmonized.

As a result of more subsidies and global marketing strategies, a significant source of competitive advantage will be sensitive implementation of strategy bearing in mind local idiosyncrasies of the market, the competition, and the regulations.

9. **Alliances or Acquisitions of New Businesses**

Recent years have seen some major companies from other fields entering the healthcare market. They have done this either through their investments or through alliances via acquisitions. Globally, Kodak initially set up Eastman Pharmaceuticals, but then bought Sterling Drug to bolster their entry. Procter and Gamble entered the OTC area with the acquisition of Richardson Hindustan. Volvo bought shares in Pharmacia, a Swedish pharmaceutical company.

Even in India, the Piramal group first acquired Nicholas Laboratories along with Indian subsidiaries of Roche, Boehringer Mannheim, Rhone Poulenc and Hoechst Research Centreto consolidate its position in the pharmaceutical industry.

10. Mergers and Acquisitions

This is usually a common means of entry into new markets; and plays a central role in all decisions and formulations of corporate strategy. These means basically help organizations to restructure both their capabilities and capacities. Acquiring a 100% export-oriented unit by a progressive growing national domestic company will enhance its capabilities and capacities and help the company to restructure funds, disciplines, activities, markets, etc.

Mergers usually add value if both the firms are complementary. The example of Parle and Coca-Cola demonstrates the value of complementary strengths.

Acquisitions can also sustain exclusivity. The acquiring of Aristrocrat by VIP luggage or Blow Plast provides this advantage of total exclusivity.

These avenues are being exploited and slowly evolving in India.

11. Forward and Backward Integration Strategy with Technology

Ranbaxy, Cipla, and Dr. Reddy's Laboratories, all used the forward integration strategy to take a suitable market share. They maximized their profits by using actively those molecule which they themselves were manufacturing. While they practiced forward integration, Wockhardt, Kopran, and Lupin adopted backward integration, and spent their resources in those molecules which they were selling well. Simultaneously, they also searched for hi-tech processes and products to eliminate the greater degree of competition. All these are proven methods for staying ahead of competition.

12. Bottom-Line Strategies

Owing to changes in the government policy in the last many years, many organizations observed a decline in their profits and their survival became difficult. To meet the situation some Indian companies diversified into agro, herbal, and other related products and instruments. In fact, on the basis of profitability alone they merely adopted a strategy of introducing related products in related markets and made efforts to formulate stronger divisions. Lupin in the 1980s started their Agro Division which by 1989 had a turnover of a mere Rs 9 crore, which then increased to Rs 100 crore, exceeding the turnover and profits of its formulation divisions. This is one of the examples of success in bottom line strategy.

13. Creating an Entry Barrier

Pengloble (Astra-IDL) was launched in Indian when Becampicillin was not available to any Indian organization at the prevailing rates; it was available at nearly double the rate of Astra-IDL. This virtually served as an entry barrier to everybody in the industry who wished to launch Bacampicillin in India then. Many did launch and withdrew, as it was non-remunerative. However, Astra-IDL could not capitalize on this entry barrier to the extent they should have. But the launch was strategically unique. This also opens a new option. You can block others by positioning your product at such a price level which is not at all remunerative for your competitors. This is possible either through control over raw materials as Astra IDL did, or through R&D and technology, at the initial phase of launching.

14. Product-Market Matching

Whatever be the strategic objective, developing successful product strategies will depend on two key issues: target market selection, and differential advantage positioning. Who is the likely target group? What is the product's differential advantage? These questions need to be fully answered specifically. Many marketing strategies fail because the management does not sufficiently and successfully deal with these two key issues.

The marketing dictum that the customer is central and that products have to be developed to satisfy customer needs implies that to satisfy customers, homogeneous target groups have to be identified and offered products to fit their needs. The definition of the target market is important because of the heterogeneity in customer population, the prohibitively high cost of reaching the total population and the impossibility of the product appealing to the entire population simultaneously. The key concept in this context is market segmentation: dividing the market into homogeneous groups of customers to whom individual products can be offered.

Developing a marketing strategy, then, implies selecting one or several segments of the target market(s). On the basis of this concept, many organizations like Cadila, Wockhardt, Cipla, Lupin, Alembic, and Ranbaxy, did launch Alidac, Tridoss, Protec, Pharmanova, Megacare, and Stancare respectively in India in the last three decades, and grew by representing more therapeutic groups and identifying and presenting new products to new target markets with differential advantages to satisfy homogenous customer groups like cardiologists, orthopedics, etc.

STRATEGIC MARKETING OPTIONS

At the moment, in India, the pharmaceutical market structure is fragmented due to the sheer number of firms in each therapeutic group. As changes take place, this structure will collapse and a new 'equal oligopoly' with three or more competitors sharing the major market, and niche players sharing the remaining market will emerge. This means we must look at future markets keeping in mind all structures.

While looking at the options, three major areas emerge:

1. Developing and building brands or markets
2. Maintaining, retaining, holding the brands or markets
3. Defending or withdrawing brands and converting competitive brands or markets

Before selecting a strategy, it is important to assess the competitive position of the firm. The first step in this involves assessing 'market positioning'. This refers to the relevant market's recognition and perception of a firm's position in the market. It may not be valid for other commodities but for pharmaceuticals, this 'perception' gives leverage. Corporate equity is essential for developing marketing strategies. All market perceptions come from the stance of the innovator or follower. This is usually determined by the extent and timing of the introduction of new drugs. Torrent was perceived as an 'innovator' perception and MNCs as 'followers'. All marketing stances stem from these two positions.

Range of Product-Market Strategic Options

The pharmaceutical market itself is very broad and covers a wide variety of markets and options. In general, it can be divided on the basis of several criteria:

- Type of disease (therapeutic groups)
- Type of product (original/generic)
- Severity of disease (acute/chronic)
- Type of prescription behavior [prescription/over the counter (OTC)]
- Need of diagnostics to arrive at diagnosis
- Need of supplementary products for proper nutrition
- Type of encashment behavior at the chemist's shop
- In addition, options like curative and preventive usage, palliative therapies with major course of medicines, long-term usage vis-à-vis short-term usage of any given product, in terms of galenical forms, pharmacological synergy, etc. need to be studied in detail.

All these options can open up new product-market opportunities. Let us discuss them one by one.

(i) ***Type of disease:*** Different therapeutic areas represent different types of opportunities for a pharmaceutical company. Some areas require quick responses from the company as they provide sudden opportunities during and after epidemics, wars and seasonal upheavals.

Some are attractive because the company is usually strong, and maintains a sustainable differential advantage like GSK in anti-ulcer therapies. Some, because there is little competition in terms of number or quality, like the protein supplement of Threptin Biscuits from Raptakos, Brett & Co. Ltd. Some others look at the long-term growth of therapeutic groups, examples being Torrent, and Sun which later tried to capture the market share in the cardiovascular therapeutic group.

A company needs to balance these different options. Diversification in different therapeutic groups itself offers a type of security in addition to providing opportunities for growth. Concentration on existing therapeutic groups implies a certain synergy and economies of scale, and potentially a local dominance over competitors. Syntex and Searle abroad obtained more than 95% of their sales from only three therapeutic areas. In Europe, Boots, Sanofi, and UCB are all reputed to be highly skewed towards a narrow band of therapeutic areas. In India, too, a majority of companies are stronger in three or four therapeutic groups. Earlier, Torrent gained a foothold on the basis of psychotropic range alone and then its expansion into the cardiovascular therapeutic group made a difference. Cadila, Ranbaxy, Sanofi, and Wockhardt are all dependent on three of four major therapeutic groups. Many companies tried to jump on the bandwagon but failed to survive as their field-force orientation and existing customer relationship needed to be established with specific target market doctors. It becomes difficult to train the field force to start afresh with other target market doctors. Few such ventures are successful, unless the expansion is gradual. A (Geneal Physician) GP-oriented company can't launch a cardiovascular group overnight and achieve success. A shift of concentration from GPs to physicians to cardiologists is gradual, and more likely to succeed. Vilco is an excellent example. For many years Vilco tried to establish itself in many areas. It had a turnover of only Rs.0.25 million for more than a decade, with negligible growth. When it focused on herbal preparations like Sensaherb for its existing target market of GPs, it grew.

The disease pattern is dependent on geographical and hygiene factors. In India, we can observe the impact of geographical factors; for example. Mumbai is best patterned for cough, allergic disorders, and other related therapeutic groups owing to its proximity to the coast. Similarly, Bengaluru needs products for allergy and asthma, due to the excessive pollen grains in the environment. Jammu & Kashmir and Andhra Pradesh need anti-ulcerants, as chillies figure prominently in the local diet. Nagpur and Delhi, where there is a high incidence of sun-strokes, need protection of yet another kind in summer. Bihar and UP being relatively unhygienic, poor and backward regions, often have complex disease patterns, requiring frequent use of antibiotics, anti-fungal, anti-septics, hematinics, etc. Madhya Pradesh, Bihar, UP and Mumbai are prone to water-borne diseases. Parts of Maharashtra (Miraj, Sangli, Islampur, Kolhapur and especially

Mumbai) have shown a high incidence of AIDS due to the lifestyle of many.

Industrialized cities and metro cities like Mumbai with their fast-paced life need stress-related therapeutic groups, for treatment of diabetes, cardiovascular diseases, psycholeptics, cancer, and so on.

The people in rural areas, like Gadchiroli (Maharashtra) or Jhumritalayya (Bihar), simply do not have the opportunity to use sophisticated medicines because diagnostic as well as other medical facilities are inadequate. On the other hand, metro cities or even those where people have access to diagnostics, have a market for sophisticated drugs.

Competitively the preference of one brand to another is in proportion with availability. Availability of drugs is dependent on the effectiveness of the distribution channel. Although the actual choice is often influenced by the existing distribution channel structure in a given region, companies can still exercise some choice. For example, in Bihar, firms like Alkem and Aristo are capable of influencing their wholesalers to provide a competitive advantage through availability.

(ii) ***Type of product:*** The sale of generics provides considerable scope for strategic options. Some companies like to believe that their choice depends exclusively on innovation and they totally shun generics. In contrast other companies and many small-scale companies, tailor their cost structure and distribution methods to an exclusively generic orientation. The success of both approaches should make you think. However, other companies are committing themselves more and more to both branded and generic products.

(iii) ***Severity of disease:*** GSK (Betnovate), Boots (Brufen, Froben-SR), US Vitamin (DBITD), Kopran (Vent) chose specialized areas of treatment of chronic diseases such as skin diseases, asthma, arthritis and diabetes. Once generated, prescription can multiply and fetch more dividends. Ranbaxy and Alembic, on the other hand, concentrate more on therapies like those for infectious diseases. You therefore have the option to choose your market on the basis of treating chronic or acute diseases. Worm infestation or amoebic infection may give rise to acute symptoms of helmenthiasis and amoebiasis. If untreated, they can lead to chronic amoebic dysentery or amoebiasis.

(iv) ***Type of prescription behavior:*** The prescription/OTC dichotomy is another important variable. Most large pharmaceutical companies are present in both markets, but for some companies, such as Johnson & Johnson, the OTC business is far more important than for others, say Pfizer and Sanofi. Old, less dynamic therapeutic groups also show a tendency to become over-the-counter (OTC); such as Ferradol, Sharkoferrol, Benadryl, Hepatoglobin, etc. You still observe that these products are less prescribed but purchased repeatedly by patients.

(v) ***Need of diagnostics for diagnosis:*** As diseases are becoming complex, it becomes difficult for doctors to diagnose common symptoms of malaria, typhoid and hepatitis. They require diagnostic analysis. The advantage ofcourse is that the physician can treat patients for the right diseases who can now get faster relief. The opportunities offered by these diagnostics are innumerable. They range from simple diagnostic tests for a variety of diseases from pregnancy detection to cancer detection tests.

(vi) ***Nutritional therapies:*** Total Parenteral Nutrition (TPN) as a part of hospitalization systems for post-operative treatment during convalescence has opened up avenues for a variety of small-volume and large-volume parenterals.

(vii) ***Type of encashment behavior at chemist's shop:*** As trading in India has different dimensions, prescriptions are exchanged for economic reasons in the same therapeutic groups. This is possible when the trader gets more margin on a few brands. It is up to the organization to encash or not to encash the push from traders on the basis of extra margin. It is important to arrive at options which can also capitalize on the push from traders. Products which can be pushed by traders may need evaluation of this option. Those products which are typically prescription oriented may not need this option always.

(viii) ***Curative and preventive usage:*** Depending on the educational background and economic status of a state or part of state, you can chose options for promoting drugs for curative or preventive use. In Maharashtra alone, you can perhaps propagate preventive measures in Mumbai, but in backward areas like Chandrapur you have to necessarily promote curative drugs. The market may not be ready for preventive measures at all.

(ix) ***Palliative therapies with major course of medicines:*** It is usually seen that study of co-prescribed drugs helps us to identify options for a few products. Baralgan is an excellent example of promotion along with anti-diahorreal preparations, as gripping pain is usually accompanied with diarrhea. This option is dependent on the practice behavior of physicians, as well as the accompanied symptoms with major illness. In case of a sprain in the leg, inflammation is usually accompanied with pain. So an anti-inflammatory and analgesic are generally co-prescribed.

(x) ***Long-term Vs. short-term usage:*** Some therapies by nature are long-term like that for arthritis, and some short-term like antibiotics. So the options are open for those who would like to go in for one or both of these therapies.

These different product-market strategic options not only define the boundaries of a company's pharmaceutical business but also dictate the need for necessary resources to optimize the risk of achieving a position of sustainable competitive advantage over competitors.

A pharmaceutical company aiming at introducing a large number of therapeutic categories, with original prescription drugs for acute therapies, distributed directly via drug stores and hospitals, will need very different capabilities from a company which wishes to sell generics in the same markets. While the former will require greater resources in terms of R&D, sales force, production, registration and logistics, the latter will need to invest much less in these areas. Each company can work on its own strengths and find its own niche.

The behavior of dispensing doctors also defines the scope of brands, gelenical forms, dosage forms, and therapeutic groups. The competition among doctors in Basti, Balia and Gonda in UP, for instance, enhances the opportunities for dispensing, while dispensing doctors of Pune, Kolkata, Ahmedabad and Chennai provide a different segment as they need different products to dispense.

FUTURE OPTIONS

Four scenarios exist concerning the future options of pharmaceutical companies. These options help firms to decide their battlefields. 'Niche-speciality players' choose to battle aided by a handful of specialists, 'localized players' depend on their own influence on local markets, a 'manufacturing base' provides options to go out of India, and having 'speciality vendors' throws open options to horizontally integrate the marketing functions. Each option can be strategically developed to build brands.

1. **Niche-Speciality Players**

    The most popular option suggests that the industry will 'shake out' into two tiers of companies: one, a restricted group of large companies with worldwide scope in a broad range of therapeutic areas, and a second group of smaller, niche companies.

    Further supporting evidence for this scenario is the restricted anticipated growth in the USA, UK and Japan, but much greater scope in Asian and developing countries. This implies increasing marketing costs, pressure on margins, threat of generics, increased government intervention, globalization and liberalization trends, and product assortment synergies. The trend of concentration will simultaneously provide opportunities for smaller companies to focus on special markets.

2. **Localized Players**

    This trend towards special markets will see further localization in India. There will be several market zones rather than a single all India market. Since the large companies will not be able to cover all therapeutic categories in all parts of India, profitable market opportunities will continue to exist for smaller, more 'focused companies' like Mohan and Company in Bengaluru, Jenburkt owned by the Bhuta Group in Mumbai, Macmillan owned by three entrepreneuring salesmen in Amritsar, and Mcneilin Jaipur (Rajasthan). As a result of this focus on market zones it was easier for these companies to succeed, keep pace with communications, and concentrate on the major markets with a competitive edge by creating more muscle than a national organization, and having less resource requirements in comparison to national organizations.

Charak (an Ayurvedic company) concentrated in UP with more than 50 MRs and penetrated the market even though it was a national organization. Multinationals may have just half this field force in UP.

3. Manufacturing Base

There may be a third scenario owing to 'rupee power'. Since the relative cost of manufacturing is low in India, it may become a place for manufacturing for the world players provided the labor laws and excise rules are suitably amended to increase productivity. As a corollary, a few organizations have the advantage of small-scale and export possibilities and could do better with 100% export oriented units in formulations. Export of generics in recent times has forced open an option to go all over the world. The same will be the case with bulk and fine chemicals as players like Dr. Reddy's Laboratories, who have gained a reputation of excellence in quality, have made a breakthrough in technology and have an edge over price, push forward their products internationally. In fact, India has really become proficient in exporting bulk and fine chemicals along with generics in recent times.

4. Speciality Vendors

There may be a fourth alternative scenario for the pharmaceutical industry where a number of functions traditionally carried out 'in-house' will be given to outside specialist agencies (J. Zammit-Luica, 1989). R&D will be a major activity in India. MNCs may establish their R&D units in India due to the availability of intelligence at lower cost. Because of the questionable link between research investments and research outputs (Comanor, 1965; Schwartzman, 1970; Angelley, 1973), the task of generating new products might indeed be carried out more efficiently and cost-effectively by a number of university departments and small specialized research institutes or companies. Also such specialized agencies, Contract Research Organizations (CROs) are already carrying out clinical trials and registration requirements more cost-effectively than their pharmaceutical company clients. Being more efficient in terms of size for that function and being designed for such specialized tasks, these agencies provide excellent services. This service of carrying out clinical trials and registration of products is being offered by many specialists in India, and they cover the cost and procure registrations in time. Similarly, the marketing and sales tasks are also being provided by specialized sales and marketing organizations that operate as separate companies. At the moment, professional detailing networks are available outside India. In India, this service is in a nascent state. A few pharmacy colleges of India are already providing this speciality service to pharma companies.

To sum up, the actual configuration of the industry will perhaps be a mix of these four scenarios in India. As we have seen a few companies will graduate to the 'big league'. A few will be perpetual niche players. A few will reduce the cost of manufacturing as well as R&D by conducting these activities in India, and many specialized service organizations will effectively help others to do 'supportive' jobs cost-effectively. Those who do not survive will have to be phased out.

INTEGRATED STRATEGIES, CONCEPTS, AND MODELS FOR BRANDS AND MARKETS

While looking at the limited resources in India, let us first examine the product-mix strategies. In fact, considering the state of hygiene, industrialization, and the tropical nature of our country, we should first define marketing and product-mix strategies.

A frequently encountered typology distinguishes the following *twelve* therapeutic groups in India:

1. Diabetes
2. Cardiovascular
3. Cancer Therapy
4. Anti-infectives
5. Respiratory
6. Pain Control
7. Anti-biotics
8. Internal Medicine
9. Nutritional
10. Herbal Health
11. Adjuvants
12. Others

It has been observed that due to R&D efforts and spent resources, prescribers often think about companies as specialists in specific therapeutic areas. Medical representatives are also usually experts in certain therapeutic categories. For these reasons, product and marketing management functions in pharmaceutical companies are often organized along the lines of therapeutic groups. As such, most secondary data available in the pharmaceutical industry are also categorized in therapeutic groups. Operations Research Group (ORG) also provides information in the same fashion.

Integration of Concepts and Models

Having identified a profitable product-mix and established a presence in growing therapeutic groups, it is important to find out approaches and options available to maintain, retain, defend and withdraw brands. If need be, you should also look at the option of converting competitors' prescriptions to yours.

The range of options for developing marketing strategy emanates from a number of disciplines, including marketing, sociology, economics, financial management, and the new area of strategic management.

The first attempt to form an analytical framework for determining strategic marketing actions—the adoption and diffusion process—was based on the product-life cycle. Wasson and Day have proposed guidelines in this context.

The results of Boston Consulting Group (BCG) studies of cost and price changes in relation to accumulated volume or experience, highlight cost dynamics and their impact on prices, particularly in markets that are growing rapidly. The experience curve gives a new dimension to cost relationships.

The growth-share portfolio model (BCG) has its origin in finance theory, where a variety of risk-return investments are balanced as a portfolio to provide the required return to the investor. When applied to marketing, this concept views products as investments that either require or yield cash according to their position in the portfolio.

McKinsey, Shell Chemicals, and Arthur D. Little developed competition position options and Ansoff pioneered the ROI concept on the basis of the product-market model.

The Profit Impact on Marketing Strategy (PIMS) model and Porters competitive marketing strategy model provided enough insight in developing options for brands.

Let us now integrate these concepts and models.

(i) ***The Life-cycle concept:*** This concept is based on the premise that the life of a product is limited.

It has following characteristics:

1. The sales pattern follows an 'S' curve until sales eventually decline.
2. The inflection points in the sales history denote the stages of introduction, growth, maturity and decline; there is competitive turbulence or shake out once the growth rate declines.
3. The life of the product can be extended.
4. The average profit per unit rises and then falls, over the life cycle.

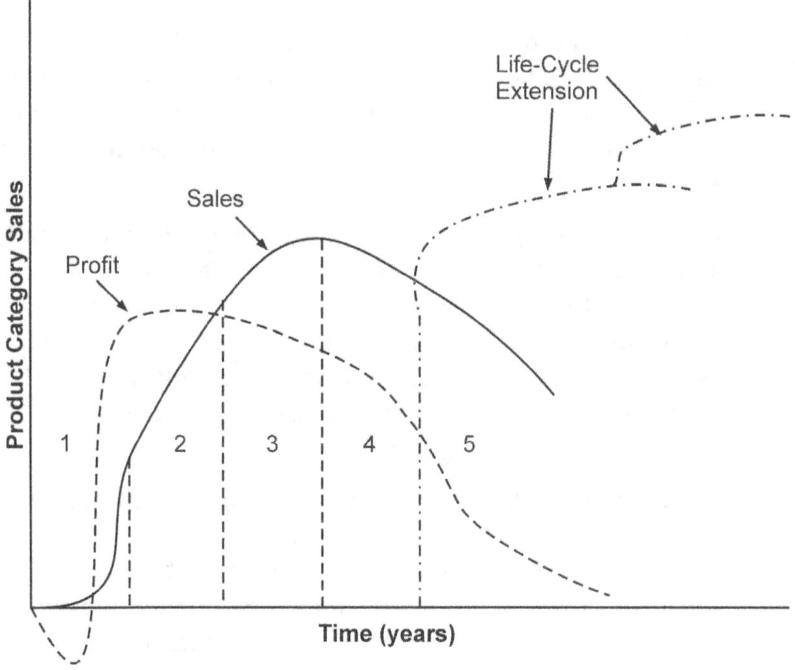

Figure 4.2 States in the life-cycle of a product

Each stage represents different marketing challenges. At the introductory stage the task is to create awareness and achieve acceptance from opinion leaders and early adopters. During growth, the challenge is of establishing brand identification and market position. At the maturity stage, the marketer needs to maintain and improve profit, defend brand position and look for growth segments. During decline, cost reduction, pricing and targeting are important, and planning is done to determine the time of exit.

Although this concept has its limitations in application, it helps us focus on a number of issues that are important for strategic planning:

- It helps change focus at a few stages which we can identify for marketing activities.
- It recognizes a finite limit to the market potential.
- During the introductory phase, profit per unit may decline.
- As the markets mature, you need to change your strategic focus.

Successful products like Septran, Brufen, Becosule, and Terramycin can teach us how products have travelled though all stages in the cycle, and how companies have tried to extend the life cycles of these products irrespective of turbulence in the environment.

(ii) **The adoption-diffusion model**: To survive in the Indian market, it is crucial to ensure a respectable turnover and profits in the first year of launch. Hence, the 'adoption time' becomes a key factor for any new brand. Relevant examples are that of Ketoprofen which did not get adopted, and Pefloxacin which got adopted quickly, in similar conditions prevailing in their respective therapeutic groups.

The adoption-diffusion pattern of innovators, early adopters and laggards should not be considered in parts. In fact, it is important to 'attack' the total early majority of customers, comprising innovators and early adopters, ignoring late adopters initially. This early majority has the potential to provide respectable turnover and profit in the first year. Nowadays, you cannot hope to have high turnover and profit on the basis of dependence on only innovators like specialists; you need the help of the early majority which includes GPs as well. Cifran has been an excellent example of quick adoption from innovators and early adopters, providing early majority to this new quinolone. GPs accepted it as an alternative for Chloromycetin, for enteric fever (typhoid), and the product took very little time to establish itself.

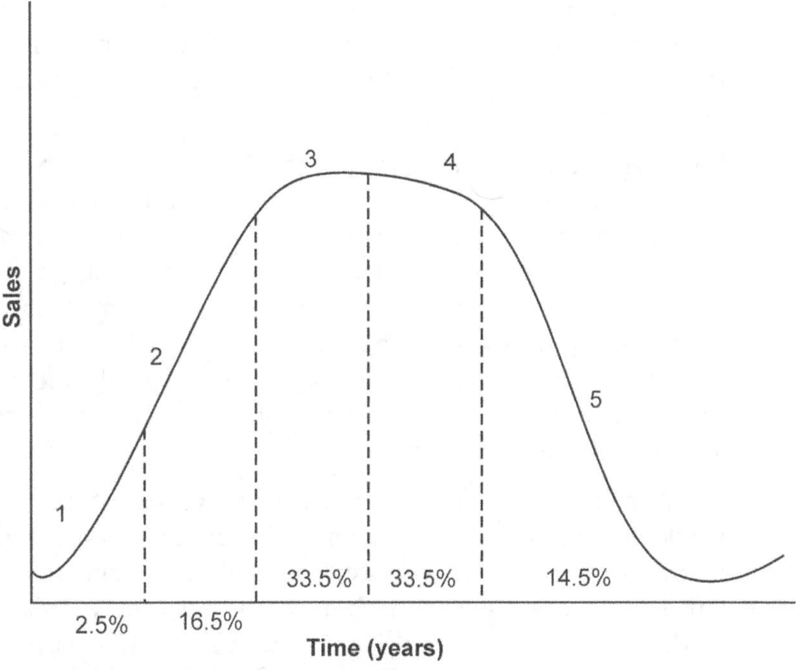

1. Innovators, 2. Early Adopters, 3. Early Majority,
4. Late Majority, 5. Laggards

Figure 4.3 The adoption-diffusion model

(iii) ***The boston consulting group approach:*** In India, certain constraints like the National Pharmaceutical Pricing Authority (NPPA) and the Tariff Commission make it imperative for you to learn how to manage your various brands by taking out cash from each brand. Each brand has to stand on its own merit.

The BCG approach to product portfolio analysis is based on satisfying two company objectives: growth and cash flow. It is essential in Indian conditions to achieve higher growth year after year and manage cash simultaneously. It is possible for growth to hit the liquidity of the organization. In my opinion the BCG approach could be suitable provided you are aware of its limitations. The underlying assumption in the BCG approach is that every company wants to completely finance its growth internally, and therefore always seeks to balance its cash flow. With the higher interest rates in India, many companies are compelled to earn in order to pay interest to banks. Several organizations have to generate external financing, via loans and raising equity, as the cost of capital required to fuel growth, is higher in India.

However, the basic philosophy of the BCG portfolio approach is that some brands will have to generate the much needed extra cash to support the growth of other brands so that the company as a whole can grow without disturbing the cash balance. The future potential of a particular brand is assumed to be controlled by its stage in the life-cycle of its relevant target market with proper investment. It could be an added dimension to BCG thought as Indians simultaneously consider short-term and long-term investments.

Maintaining a healthy cash balance means striking an equilibrium between cash inflows (revenues, contributions, profits) and cash outflows (expenses and investments). Cash inflows are operationalized through the concept of relative market share (RMS). In applying the BCG concept to a particular company, the market growth and relative market share are measured for each brand and, corresponding to the values of these two dimensions, they are placed in a matrix (Figure 2.3). Each brand is then represented by a circle, the diameter of which is proportional to its sales level. There are four names given, one for each of the major quadrants. 'Cash cows' provide cash to excess of their investment needs. 'Dogs' demand little investment (low market growth) but also generate little cash because of their low relative market share. 'Problem children' demand high investments for their struggle in a high-growth market, while their relative low market shares limit their ability to generate profit. 'Stars' generate the contribution (high RMS) that is needed for investments to maintain or improve a strong position in attractive markets.

Based on the BCG concept, specific strategies are recommended according to the brand's position in the matrix.

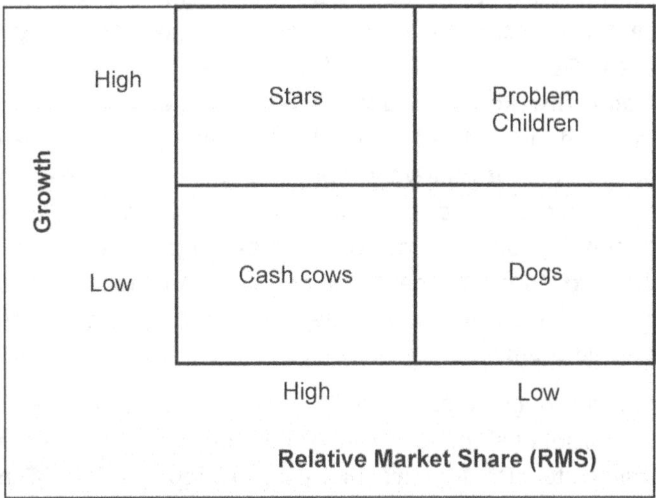

Figure 4.4 The BCG matrix

Coming back to the original objectives of the BCG approach, on the basis of growth and cash balance, a desirable portfolio is identified in which a sufficient number (or proportion) of brands are positioned in high-growth markets so that an adequate number (or proportion) of cash cows exist to fuel the growth of the selected problem children and support all the stars.

(iv) ***Conceptual problems in implementation:*** In the pharmaceutical industry in India, the crucial assumption that cash generation is dependent on the four categories of the BCG matrix is doubtful since the decontrolled category without RMS relationship may have higher cash generation per unit. For example, when Nitravet (Nitrazepam) of Anglo French Drugs (AFD) was launched, it might not have achieved a high RMS in the therapeutic group, but started generating cash right from the first year. After five years, it was providing cash to AFD. You may not be able to classify such products in the BCG matrix. Indeed, a lot of old products in the pharmaceutical industry, even if they have small RMSs, are extremely profitable: very few resources have to be invested and some loyal prescribers guarantee the continuation of substantial sales and profit levels.

Thus, in the context of the India pharmaceutical industry, 'dogs' can be called 'vulnerable cows'. For instance, in our country the old mercurochrome as well as the updated antiseptic Betadine is used. Getting rid of such 'vulnerable cash cows' would be a major mistake in a country like India. They play a major role in the company's future growth, they also provide a secure cash base requiring relatively more cash investment than cash cows do. They tend to be transformed into stars or cash cows, depending on competition. If the competition is strong, they may go through the 'problem child to stars to cash cows' pattern. But if it is negligible, they could become stars or cash cows straightaway.

Another major factor should be considered in India—the *size of the target customers*. If this size diminishes the brands should be disinvested irrespective of their position in the BCG matrix. If you have such a product, you may have to think twice about continuing with it.

Considering this additional parameter along with the BCG approach might help us decide on the investment and cash generation pattern of products or brands.

(v) ***Composite portfolio (COMITE) approach:*** McKinsey, AD Little, and Shell have developed composite portfolio models. Although they differ slightly from each other in approach, their overall philosophy is quite similar. The models propose replacing the market-growth criterion with a more comprehensive market-attractiveness dimension (market-attractiveness in the McKinsey approach and maturity of the market in the AD Little approach). This market-attractiveness dimension is composed of a number of factors, judged by the specific company. The RMS dimension is substituted by a competitive position criterion (in both the McKinsey and the AD Little approach), which includes RMS but also takes into account other factors, judged by the management as important indicators of the competitive position in the industry. If you analyze the success of Combiflam, you will observe that the need to add something to Ibuprofen was so acute (there was a therapeutic gap) that the product had a very high market-attractiveness. Market attractiveness has *five* other major aspects. They are:

- Size of the market
- Growth
- Margin
- Number of major players
- Liability/risk

All these factors were in favour of the launch of Combiflam. Size, growth and margin were attractive. There were few players in the combination market, and the risk was negligible as both the chemical entities had successful penetration. Similarly, the competitive position ensured that the edge over Brufen (the major market leader) was perceived right from the very beginning. It was more than Brufen. The market galloped and within a span of five years, the therapeutic group itself climbed five positions in Operations Research Group (ORG).

Even today, there is a big 'therapeutic gap' for 'new mothers' who do not get attention after childbirth as the child generally becomes the major focus and the new mother takes a back seat in India. You can think of a nutritional product which can help improve the mother's health and also ensure adequate milk for the child. If you start thinking along these lines, you will be able to identify many gaps in today's socioeconomic environment.

(vi) ***The experience curve:*** When you study the cost-dynamics of any brand, you will observe that the average unit cost must go down as time passes. If it does not, then we are not applying our experience to the brand. Economy of scale, minimization of waste sourcing and negotiating for key raw materials to bring down cost, value engineering of the product, all these areas must yield experience benefits. Every product over a period of years must reduce its cost irrespective of increase in inputs. All of you must ensure that the gross contribution of every old product improves with experience, unless there is an upheaval in the market.

(vii) ***ANSOFF's product/market model:*** This model is based on the product-market matrix (Figure 4.5).

Market Product	Present	New
Present	Penetrate	Market Development
New	Product Development	Diversify

Figure 4.5 The product-market matrix

1. As per this model there are two options for any existing product and two others for any new product.
2. Old products have the option to further penetrate the markets by going rural.
3. Another option for existing products to develop new markets was utilized by Brufen, when Piroxicam was launched. Brufen developed new markets by launching a product with higher strength of the ingredient, thus widening its scope.

When you launch a new product in your present market, it becomes essential for you to develop the market for this new product by consistently working on the product or promotion. For instance, Cetirizine was a new product in an existing market. So in the initial phase, companies had to develop the market to use Cetirizine while they ensured market development.

Kopran launched Ciba-Corning instruments in India in all medical colleges and hospitals, and this was a new product in an altogether new market. Kopran had to recruit a new team of promoters as it was not possible for the pharma field force to promote these products in hospitals. A new team of engineers was appointed and different services like L/c opening and ensuring that hospitals received these instruments without delay were adequately provided. After-sales service was an important factor; therefore, spare parts and other technical services were fully managed.

PRODUCT STRATEGIC OPTIONS

Expansion Strategy

An expansion strategy for a product implies increasing its market share or sales volume. To achieve this target five possible routes can be envisaged:

1. Attracting new prescribers to the product category.
2. Increasing the usage rate among current prescribers,
3. Attracting prescribers from competing products,
4. Expanding the market to new segments through new indications, and
5. Devising a retail strategy and increasing the width and depth of distribution.

1. In the early stages of the market life-cycle, an expansion strategy implies convincing prescribers of the validity of the new product category. This was the task for Voveran when it was just introduced in the market; it had to convince prescribers about the therapeutic value of inhibition of prostaglandins. Similar strategies had to be pursued by Combliflam, and Inderal (the first beta-blocker) when they were first introduced in the market.

   Early entrants into the market tend to develop the market by directing their positioning and marketing efforts to new market segments. The launch strategy of Cifran was aimed at educating and continuing the market, initially created by Chloromycetin. Cifran focused its strategy on its better efficiency profile, addressing itself to typhoid cases.

2. The next state is to improve sales and market share by getting each presenter to increase the number of patients on a specific drug, and perhaps by moving the product from the third or second line of treatment to the first line of treatment. This helps increase the usage rate of the product by the same prescribers.

   In mature markets some pharmaceutical companies are pursuing a strategy of turning prescription products into OTC ones, thereby substantially expanding their market without changing the product. FDC for Electral, Parke Davis for Benadryl, and Franco Indian for Dexorange were successful in converting their prescription products into OTC products. Although this particular strategy is not viable in many therapeutic areas, it gives a promising direction to products in low health-risk therapeutic areas, which can move towards major health markets.

3. A state comes when the product gets surrounded by twenty other competitors. In such situations, it is important to work on a 'conversion strategy' by attracting competitive prescribers to your brand. Anybody who is today launching Ciprofloxacin will have to decide on the 'key competitor'—not Cifran but other brands—and then develop a strategy to convert prescribers of that brand to the new Ciprofloxacin product.

4. Both Brufen and Aspirin expanded their markets by developing new segments by promoting Brufen as an anti-pyretic and Aspirin as a preventive to anginal attack owing to its property of platelet aggregation.

5. Retailing strategy was devised by Oriprim DS (Cadila) for the first time in India. It ensured availability, and the product took off quickly.

Maintenance Strategy

The maintenance strategy for a product is not necessarily passive. If a product is a market leader in an attractive market, maintenance implies the use of resources simply to hold the current position. Brufen for anti-arthritic treatment as well as Becosules in the vitamins group have been doing just this. A maintenance strategy usually implies a 'value-added' approach, whether the task is to consolidate market leadership, or to ensure a *status quo* position if one is not the market leader—Beplex Forte of Anglo French AFD, for example, needed this strategy. Such a strategy becomes crucial especially when a drug nears its patent expiry date or is at the end of its product life cycle.

Milking Strategy

'Milking' (or 'harvesting') refers to the strategy of holding back resources and trying instead to generate as much cash revenue as possible within certain constraints. Milking usually implies cost-cutting in operations and capital expenditure, raising the price (if possible) and reducing field force and promotional support (if any). The result hoped for is a gentle loss of market share, which reflects the policy of capitalizing on the position achieved by past investment, restricting the resource input, and 'creaming off' the generated revenue. For instance, industry stakeholders observed that Abbott milked on its Erythromycin in the market, partly because of competition and market conditions, and partly because of the abundance of strong new products which compete for R&D and marketing resources.

Divesting Strategy

If the product has no future, it is quite easy to reduce the investments to zero and let it die a natural death. For example, because of strong generic competition Roche cut off marketing support to its former 'cash cows' Valium and Librium. An active decision to divest, however, is psychologically, socially and politically more painful. This is particularly true if the product has, potentially, a bright future because it is positioned in an attractive market. Yet it is sometimes necessary to divest because spreading resources too thinly can mean failure, and it is often better to concentrate on only a few products. Hence, the pressures of limited R&D resources, field force time, and advertising or promotional funds can make it necessary to divest potentially interesting products and projects; especially where patents are about to expire. In the UK, for example, because of restrictions on marketing expenditure by the government (Pharmaceutical Price Regulation Scheme), several companies had to withdraw all support for a number of products whenever they launched a new product in the market. In India, Searle was seen to divest many products.

In reality, firms adopt a hybrid of strategies depending upon their size, diversity, position in the market, rate and type of external change, resource commitments, and management attitudes towards concepts and database. It has been observed that all these strategies do not yield results if the firm does not try to understand the customer and end-user—the physician and patient, in our case.

CASE

Cifran—The Story of a Brand[1]

Before we were getting ready to market our brand Cifran, our Product Management Group wanted to know what exactly we were planning to achieve and how. Were we to establish a new and superior line of treatment for infections or were we to aim beyond that? We knew we had a very powerful product on hand but to make it a powerful brand we undertook an elaborate exercise to figure out what we must do and, more importantly, in what priority.

This, I presume, is the situation with every major product that a company is about to launch. While a wealth of medical information was to be sifted, the germane issues were the relevance and the criticality of the information that we would have to take to the medical profession.

There were many new and exciting things to talk about in the case of a new product like Cifran. We had to research and find the gaps in the anti-bacterial therapy that a specialist or a GP faced at that point of time. This brought out interesting facts: Many doctors thought that while the spread of the spectrum was important, the killing power of anti-bacterial, particularly in terms of recurrence of the same infection, was far more engaging. We also found that the importance of the commonly talked about 'blood level' was secondary to that of 'tissue levels'.

In retrospect, I believe, one reason for Cifran's success was the strategy for our communication to the selected groups of doctors. Our field force was given the right pitch and the right sequence in which the story was to be unfolded. We believed in the simplicity of what we said and how we said it. If messages are long-winded they lose transparency. When our field force saw the whole presentation, down to the last detail, they were enthusiastic. They made Cifran a major brand.

When one is keen to innovate, there is always scope. If Cifran was an outstanding product with a successful brand name, its packaging and dosage elegance had also to rise above the ordinary. Cifran's packaging design, graphics and colour were simple but attractive. Each tablet was

---

[1]*This case has been contributed by Mr. S.K. Chakraborty, Vice President—Marketing, Ranbaxy, New Delhi.*

given a shape and an embossed logo that stood out. These were necessary.

For sustaining quality there has to be a price benchmarking. This was not an easy task, particularly in our environment. But we did it successfully to ensure value for money on a sustained basis.

When a brand like Cifran is marketed, the whole organization has to be on drill. Coordinating the activities of the product and packaging development, marketing, manufacturing, medical, regulatory, finance and distribution divisions assumes critical importance.

One delay can upset the entire chain of events. The process has its difficulties, disappointments, and joys. Unless everyone takes part in it, creating a brand becomes difficult. I remember that after Cifran was launched, everyone in the organization was eager to know how we were progressing. At every level there was the feeling that we must do well and for that no task, however hard, was unwelcome.

LEARNINGS

Successful Strategic Stance

- It is essential to grow intelligently and emotionally to have a successful strategic stance. The firm should balance its risk and resources as they are related to market behavior, and capacities and capabilities as they are related to the firm's own commitment to service markets.

- Formulation of a strategic stance is crucial before proceeding further. Strategic stance at the corporate level is more demanding in the existing environment than that at the marketing level. If the firm cannot allocate resources to marketing, the formulated strategic edge remains only on paper.

- There are *fourteen* different options for any firm relevant to the existing and forthcoming environment. These options could be classified in three major areas:
    1. International and national environment related.
    2. Firm related
    3. Markets related

- A firm needs to decide its strategic stance and then allocate resources to the direction which it wants to give to markets and products as they need to match from the business point of view.

Strategic Marketing Options and Methodologies

- There is a range of options open for product-market matching. A few of them are related to products and their attributes, and a few are related to markets. Other product-mix options are available in the context of profitability.

- Often, those who take a strategic marketing stance need to look at the options of available concepts. All marketing concepts, starting from that of the product like-cycle to Porter's concept of competitive marketing, need to be integrated to create powerful stances for products.

- As a strategy, you can consider the options of expansion, maintenance, milking and divesting.

- Constraints which were imposed on the pharmaceutical industry and marketing are getting diluted, and many options have now become available for everybody. Now is the time to cope with borderless markets.

CHAPTER **5**

Evolution and Change of Gear

After one long hot European summer, the price of potatoes rose steeply in the shops. One Saturday, Alan went shopping with his friend Percy, a successful ship broker. Alan was one of those men who was clearly very wealthy but always needed to borrow money. They were shocked by the staggering price of potatoes, and walked out of the store refusing to buy any.

Two weeks later, Alan saw Percy again. 'Remember those potatoes, Percy said, 'What did you do about them?'

'I went home and decided to buy rice instead.' Alan replied, 'Why, didn't you?'

'Oh no, I rang up a contact in Kolkata, ordered 2000 tons of Indian potatoes at £ 100 per ton, arranged freight and insurance for £ 30 per ton, and sold them in advance to a London merchant I knew for £ 230 per ton.'

'But Percy' Alan said, 'that's £ 100 per ton profit...and on 2000 tons...!'

Alan switched to rice . . . Percy made a neat packet of nearly £ 200,000.

Percy maintained an extensive network. He had ready information on his fingertips. Alan wouldn't have known who to ring, how to import, at what rate to buy and what rate to sell, whom to approach, whom to promote to, how to get the money! Percy knew.

People like Percy who understand their customers and their needs, and maintain a good database of their customers and suppliers can seize an opportunity when it presents itself. Then they can make profits in no time.

For succeeding in the pharmaceutical industry, understanding the evolution of its customers is an important prerequisite. Let us attempt this here, and see how we can thus, add value to our marketing efforts.

PHYSICIANS, PATIENTS AND THERAPIES

Every business is characterized by the contribution it makes or the value it provides to the customer. The pharmaceutical business basically contributes to two primary segments: the sick and the healthy. The most obvious contribution so far of the pharmaceutical industry to health-care has been through safe and effective medicines using systematic diagnostic procedures and effective therapeutic agents. This indirect contribution gets directed through physicians with the help of therapies, and medicines help patients remain healthy.

Thus, the pharmaceutical business has been built around three equally important variables: the physician, the patient, and the therapy. Awareness, credibility and reliability of a particular therapy determine whether or not the physician will choose it for the patient to provide him relief. It is therefore important to build the physician's confidence in the therapy.

During the last few decades considerable evolution has taken place in the physician-patient-therapy interactional patterns owing to the altered values, beliefs and paradigms of doctors and patients the world over. Socioeconomic aspects along with revolutionized therapies have been responsible for these evolutionary changes.

The role of a physician in managing the health of his patients is dependent on several factors. Changes in society from the combined family to the unit family system has meant that physicians have to now respond to even elementary ailments like cough and the common cold. Earlier, these symptoms were treated by grandmothers. Economic changes have also necessitated health be given a priority status. Similarly, political changes lead to tension, terrorism, and war. Their manifestations affect patients physically and psychologically and their after-effects lead to many new complications to which physicians have to respond to by using deductive logic.

Those physicians who try to respond to these new situations have to adapt themselves and change their beliefs, attitudes, paradigms, behavior and ultimately their roles while treating patients.

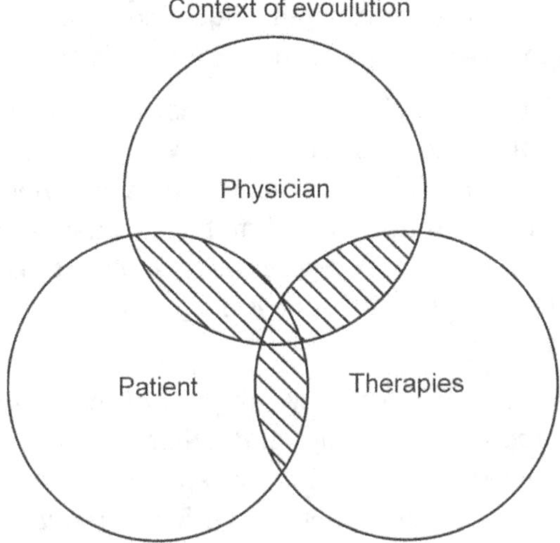

Figure 5.1 The physician-patient-therapy interaction

EVOLVING ATTITUDES OF PHYSICIANS

Ancient Indian, Chinese, and Persian systems used the 'holistic' approach as opposed to the present-day scientific or reductionist approach. Hence, those who healed many were regarded as 'miracle-generating' humans and their cures were thought to be out of the realm of scientific reasoning.

Ayurveda, meaning 'the science of life'—and ancient Indian system of medicine—even today believes in a synergy of mental, physical and spiritual factors. A crucial difference between the scientific approach and the holistic Ayurvedic approach lies in the fact that in the former approach the physician 'attacks' the disease or ailment, while in the latter the vaidya (physician) develops strength in the host (patient) and builds up his immunity to fight the disease or ailment. This is basically achieved through a combination of different herbs, which counterbalance each other's toxic effects along with proper regulation of diet and sleep pattern, and self-control.

On the other hand, in the reductionist approach, the active ingredient from natural herbs is extracted, using only of the many benefits of the herb; and it is then used for relief of a specific ailment. Liquorice is one of the famous roots in India. This root was extracted and a molecule of 'deglycerizinated liquorice' was prepared and recommended to provide relief for peptic ulcer patients.

You will find it surprising but it is true that Ayurveda operates on the same definition of health as is accepted by W.H.O. which states: 'Health is the state of complete physical, mental and social well-being and not merely the absence of disease or infirmity.' This definition then widens the role of the physician today. Successful therapy often depends on the physician's ability to restore the physiological conditions which favour natural resistance.

In the seventeenth century, the progress of medical science closely followed the progress of biology and other natural sciences. It was Descartes who introduced the theory of separation of 'mind' and 'body'. In fact, the Cartesian view is well known for its reductionist approach, which regarded the human body as a machine and in which disease was seen as a malfunction of the biological mechanism. The Cartesian paradigm has greatly influenced even today's medical thought.

In the eighteenth century, medical science progressed towards cellular and structural changes. Rudolf Virchow postulated that all illnesses involved structural changes at the cellular level. At about the same time, Louis Pasteur, working on microorganisms, demonstrated the relationship between bacteria and disease. The focus of the physician for the first time moved from the individual organ to mechanical and biological interventions. It then moved further to the structural aspects of cells, and finally it focused on the control of invading bacteria.

With this change a major shift in the direction of treatment and therapy took place, with physicians aiming to 'kill' bacteria to provide relief to patients.

In the nineteenth century, while Pasteur continued his work on bacteria, Bernard studied the environmental factors related to disease. But the concept of a specific etiology for disease was formed by Robert Koch. At the same time, medical technology was also upgraded and stethoscopes, blood-pressure instruments, and other surgical instruments were invented. Pathologists helped physicians to locate, diagnose, and label diseases. Hospitals were transformed from 'houses of mercy' to 'centres for diagnosis, therapy and teaching'. The availability of diagnosing tools and the gradual shift in focus from the 'patient' to the 'disease' led to specialization, with separate roles for general practitioners and specialists.

The twentieth century witnessed progress towards a more specific understanding of biological phenomena and invention of newer medicines. The first major advance was the development of vaccines for typhoid, tetanus and diphtheria. Invention of other vaccines led to virtually a conquest of the three major tropical diseases—malaria, yellow fever, and leprosy.

In 1928, the invention of penicillin ushered in the era of antibiotics. By 1950 many antibiotics had been invented. At the same time, another broad range of psycholeptic drugs such as tranquilizers and anti-depressants were also invented.

The biomedical model now began working in a different direction. Physicians started facing the side-effects of the medicine prescribed by them. The existing medicines were not strong enough to induce 'rest' to the patient, and the role of tranquilizers became important, along with curative medicines. This brought about a change in the attitude of physicians. On the one hand, they began 'attacking' the bacteria like *Mycobacterium tuberculosis* with stronger drugs, and on the other, prescribed rest while making use of tranquilizers to provide relief from continuous coughs at nights, preventing sleep and disallowing rest. The effects and side-effects of these different medicines were analyzed, and physicians gradually adopted the use of different therapies to provide complete treatment inclusive of treating the psyche.

EMERGING ROLE OF THE SURGEON

While physicians improved their skills and changed their attitudes on the basis of increased knowledge, surgeons acquired detailed knowledge at the cellular and molecular levels. To begin with, blood groups were discovered, which made blood transfusions possible. Substances to prevent blood clotting were discovered and anesthesia was invented. Surgeons could thus perform 'miracles'. Newer medical technologies allowed them to maintain normal physiological processes even during prolonged surgical intervention. Thus, a new specialization of 'surgeons' came to the forefront.

The speciality further went in to 'super-specializations', and in 1960, Dr. Christian Bernard transplanted a human heart. With this successful experiment, surgery became all-pervasive in modern medical care.

Thus, a general physician slowly transformed into a specialist and then into a surgeon with the formation of the three separate entities— the general practitioner, the specialist, and the surgeon. There was a sharp decline in infectious diseases all over the world. However, this did not happen to that extent in India as ecological conditions and hygiene were still below acceptable levels in the late nineteenth and early twentieth centuries.

THE SIMMENTONIAN APPROACH AND NEW TECHNOLOGIES

Carl Simmenton's approach to cancer is the most recent, and it is likely to further change the pattern of treatment, care, and the attitude of physicians. Today, patients are treated through chemotherapy, radiation, surgery, or a combination of these. In fact, such treatment is drastic, negative and causes further injury to the body. The Simmentonian approach affirms that the development of cancer involves a number of interdependent psychological and biological processes; it views the problem as involving the whole person and does not view the tumour in isolation.

Simmenton has developed a fully consistent view of health and healing. It has been observed that cancer cells are not strong and powerful and that they do not invade, attack, or destroy; they have a dangerous effect because they overproduce. A cancer cell begins with a cell that contains incorrect genetic information because it has been damaged by harmful substances or other environmental influences, or simply because the organism itself occasionally produces imperfect cells. This prevents normal functioning of the cell. If this cell reproduces other faculty cells, they overgrow.

This suggests two approaches—one, to tackle the cause of formation of such cells, and the second, to strengthen the immune system of the body. The disease or malfunctioning suppresses the body's immune system, and at the same time, leads to hormonal imbalances that result in an increased production of abnormal cells. This encompasses both psychological and biological processes.

Simmenton's approach and other similar techniques brought about the concept of 'energy medicine.' Bioenergy, according to Wilhelm Reich, flows in wave movements and its basic dynamic characteristic is pulsation. This concept comes very close to the Indian concept of *Nadi* and the Chinese concept of *Chi*. The basic premise is that the human body consists of chemicals, bones, muscles, and also 'waves'. 'Waves' were regarded as the scientific form of 'spirit' to complete the whole—mind, body and spirit. Such new revolutionary concepts in scientific thinking can surely have a powerful influence on the attitudes of physicians, and the social structure and belief systems of patients.

You will thus, observe that over time there has been a paradigm shift in the attitudes of physicians. Though a process of constant re-examining of their contributions, they have now adopted a more holistic approach.

IMPACT OF CHANGING BELIEFS OF PATIENTS

Over the last three centuries, changes in the social structure, and increased knowledge of new situations have also led to considerable changes in the belief systems of patients. Consequently, their expectations from the physician in terms of effective therapies have steadily increased. The patient who once had complete blind faith in his physician or 'healer' has evolved into a doubting Thomas. And today, the prime criterion with which he judges the efficacy of treatment is the speed and extent to which he gets complete relief. As a result, the physician too has had to change his response towards his patients.

In many societies even now the belief systems of patients vacillate between, or sometimes go hand in hand with, traditional and modern approaches to medicine and therapy. The wisdom and sophistication of traditional systems were based on two schools: The Eastern ayurvedic system, and the Western belief with Hippocratic medicine lying at its root. Hippocratic medicine believes that illness is not caused by demons or other supernatural powers, but is a natural phenomenon which can be studied scientifically. In fact, the well-known Hippocratic Oath was established by Hippocrates and the code of medical ethics has still remained the ideal of the present-day physician.

It was the German physician, Samuel Hahnemann, who founded the formal therapeutic system in the eighteenth century. Earlier, patients believed healing to be an art or skill, and hence placed their faith in skillful physicians irrespective of their approach. Owing to the lack of any scientific explanation, homeopathy and ayurveda remained controversial healing arts.

India is one country where perhaps one of the largest variety of belief systems co-exist, keeping different therapeutic approaches alive. Besides the modern allopathic physicians, surgeons, and super-specialists, we have the practitioners of homeopathy, ayurveda, naturopathy, chiropathy, yoga and even therapies based on superstition and blind faith such as the shamanistic therapy. A 'shaman' is a person who is believed to have the power to enter into a non-ordinary state of consciousness and make contact with the spiritual world. The belief is that all humans are integral parts of an ordered system and all illnesses are caused by some disharmony with the cosmic order.

In India, you can observe a variety of belief systems among different social strata in different parts of the country. Thus, you can find an exceptionally modern and scientific approach being used in one area, while a traditional approach may be being used at another place. On the other hand, gulping a 'tiny fish' is the advice given to patients at some places in Hyderabad to get relief from asthma. Above all, yoga is advocated for building capacity to breathe.

IMPACT OF CHANGING SOCIAL STRUCTURE AND INDUSTRIALIZATION

In the twentieth century, as we have seen, the existing social structure was dramatically eroded with increased incidence of alcoholism, drug abuse, terrorism, accidents, suicides, and chronic and degenerative diseases. This was of concern to the medical profession.

Thomas McKeown studied infections and found that poor nutrition, hygiene, sanitation, poverty, and filth are the basic causes of increased infection.

Industrialization added to the complexities of such diseases with erosion of the rural base that changed the demographics and lifestyles of patients and physicians. The challenges of today, then, are largely due to an imbalance in the social structure, industrialization and the degenerative nature of diseases.

Factors such as lifestyle, nutrition, hygiene habits, sanitation facilities, literacy, availability of resources, economic conditions, and so on, also have a direct bearing on the belief of patients and disease patterns. Quite often, owing to poverty or ignorance, patients avoid going to proper physicians to be cured of their ailments, and resort to cheaper or unscientific therapies. This not only lands them into trouble but in the end they lose faith in the therapy itself.

Population density is another factor responsible for 'localized' illnesses, especially in cities like Mumbai or Kolkata. In these mega cities horizontal expansion has not kept pace with increases in population. It is estimated that by 2020 the population of India would be 1.38 billion and that the total healthcare spending in local currency terms would be USD 195.7 billion by 2020.

Other environmental factors have caused major manifestations, like asthma in Bengaluru, eosinophilia and tuberculosis in Mumbai and Kolkata, and peptic ulcer in Jammu & Kashmir and Andhra Pradesh.

An appreciation of the various factors that have led to changes in the belief systems of patients about therapies, medicine systems, and physicians is therefore essential to our understanding of the pharma marketing environment.

EVOLUTIONARY FACTORS

There have been four major factors that have contributed towards the evolution of physicians in the world:

1. Development of the biomedical model
2. Shift from the segmented to the holistic approach
3. Improvement of technology and skills in surgery
4. Initiation of the health concept

Through the centuries physicians have changed their ways of treating patients on the basis of biomedical inventions, therapies, and belief systems of patients. New ways to look at diseases have led to new therapies and new chemical entities. And their clinical success has been largely dependent on the patient-belief system. This has evolutionalized the entire philosophy of physician-patient-therapy interactions.

What is required for today's general physician, specialist, or surgeon is to understand the environment and belief system of patients, and evolve new therapies in a holistic way. He would then be able to perform his role in such a way that he contributes to the 'total health' of a patient.

In the last century considerable attention has been paid to those who are healthy. Consciousness about health has also been greater. Tailor-made information is now available on how to remain healthy and fit. The value of proper nutrition, dietary habits, and exercise has been recognized by those who are healthy.

Besides this awareness, people now tend to take prophylactic action to ensure good health. Unusual symptoms are detected early and acted upon in time. People have learned to be proactive and responsive.

In India, this has, statistically speaking, brought down the infant mortality rate from 80/1000 births in 1991—92 to 38/1000 births in 2015. The death rate has also been brought down from 9.8/1000 in 1991—92 to 7.3/1000 in 2015. The birth rate reduced from 29.3/1000 in 1991—92 to 19.8/1000 in 2015. At the same time, life expectancy improved from 59.9 years in 1991—92 to 67.3 years for males and 69.6 years for females between 2011-15. All this has been possible because of education and greater awareness. But plenty more needs to be done for the health of individuals.

The medical profession, pharmaceutical industry, health ministry, government, social organizations and other industries together have to accept the challenge to make life enjoyable. The pharmaceutical industry, especially, must play a major contributory role.

MARKET DYNAMICS

Continual changes have evidently transformed physicians, patients, and therapies. Pharmaceutical marketing is dependent on understanding the dynamics of this changing market. There are *three* major variables in any market which interact with each other:

1. The size of the present and future member of physicians, retailers, and patients
2. Observable prescribing or stocking behavior
3. Their capacity to prescribe and stock as well as consume

Market dynamics comes into play when these three variables start interacting with each other. For instance, take the case of a disease like breast cancer. Here you need to identify the number of breast cancer patients, oncologists and special hospitals where the products are stocked. Also, you will have to study their behavior and capacity to stock or prescribe anti-cancer products. This study can help focus your attention to persuading the oncologists to prescribe or use your brands.

MARKET SIZE

In India physicians have proliferated greatly, with over 9.6 lakh registered medical practitioners spread all over the country and 381 medical colleges churning out at least 50,000 medical practitioners every year. In addition, 2827 ayurvedic hospitals add more than 3.9 lakh ayurvedic physicians every year. Add to this, another 30,000-50,000 government hospitals, civil hospitals, ayurvedic hospitals, ESI (Employees State Insurance) and ayurvedic centres, dispensaries, primary health centres, etc. who employ physicians on full-time or part-time basis. These dispensaries and nursing homes have at least 1:3 ratio of doctors to patients. There are around 25,308 primary health centres and 1,53,655 sub-centres. A paramedical population with around 16,73,338 registered nurses and mid-wives completes the total picture. (The statistics given here are as of 2015).

This complete population is spread over tribal, rural, semi-rural, and urban areas in India. The major facilities are located at urban areas which compel patients to travel to these areas for the treatment of complex and chronic diseases.

From such statistics it is quite evident that there has been a proliferation of physicians and paramedics in India. However, this is not a cohesive mass. And although there are more than 9 lakh registered practitioners existing, specialists like gastroenterologists number not more than 1000! The clusters of specialized physicians are quite dense, unique, and as a result, powerful.

Since the last two decades more than 8 lakh traders and chemists have also emerged as an important force in the marketing of pharmaceutical products. Today, the power of generating and encashing prescriptions has been bifurcated. Physicians retain the power to generate prescriptions but traders and retailers have gained the power of encashing these prescriptions.

Hardware technology, medical instruments, equipments, and diagnostics have aided the formation of other clusters in India. For instance, in Kerala, small nursing homes attended by technicians have changed the homogeneity and complexion of medical practice in the state in the last two decades. Polyclinics formed by groups of physicians have sprung up. There has been a proliferation of small, medium and large hospitals with diagnostic facilities and proper infrastructure. Besides this, there are other clinics where yogic, ayurvedic and homeopathic treatments are administered.

Thus, we can classify the customer group in India into the following categories:

- Physicians
- Physician-cum-dispensing chemists
- Retailers/traders/chemists
- Nursing homes with technicians
- Nursing (maternity) homes with attached beds
- Polyclinics
- Small, middle and large hospitals with ready availability of medicines and drugs
- Nature cure clinics
- Yoga institutes
- Diagnostic centers
- Rehabilitation centers
- Clinical and pathological laboratories
- Others

With such a large variety and size of the customer group, the task of identifying the right customers can indeed become difficult. At this point, it would perhaps be pertinent to ask a few questions:

- Do we identify and assess the potential of physicians and other customers for available medicines and therapies?
- Do we study demographics (such as age, education, income) and psychographics (prescription habits) to identify their prescription behavior?
- Do we correlate other factors (such as corporate image price) which are relevant in the assessment of prescription behavior?
- Do we segregate prescribing and dispensing customers for better individual products and brands?

- Do we identify the role of influencers and opinion-makers in the prescribing habits of general practitioners, who constitute about 70% of the medical force?
- Do we identify the role of decision makers in institutional buying in the private sector?
- Do we identify the role of other panel members in industrial organizations for buying medicines?
- Do we identify the role of decision makers in government and public sector institutions?
- Finally, what weightage do we give to select the appropriate customer base for effective marketing?

Answers to these and related questions can help us develop the right customer base, which we now turn to.

DEVELOPING A DATABASE

There are several methods that can help you identify the right customer base.

1. **Retail Chemists Prescription Audit (RCPA)**

   RCPA basically focuses on identifying the major competitive prescribers of a locality, and the quantum of prescriptions of such doctors for a chosen therapeutic group. It does not deal with finding out the share of a company's product from the retailer. This way identification and assessment of a physician is quickly done from A class retailers. (The A, B, C classification of retailers is dependent on the daily sale of the retail outlet). This data may not be very accurate but can give you a 'trend' which can be cross-checked from other retailers. Clusters of retailers are surveyed continually, to provide accurate identification of physicians-customers.

2. **Continuous Prescription Audit (CPA)**

   The continuous prescription audit (CPA) is based on the scrutiny of actual prescriptions. Every month, a decided number of prescriptions are scrutinized and the data is analyzed to identify the customer base.

3. **Speciality Survey (SS)**

   Almost all organizations are dependent on a few specialists. The product mix of most organizations is skewed towards one, two or more specialities. For instance, the product mix of GSK is skewed towards general practitioners and physicians, and Torrent towards psychiatrists and cardiologists. Each speciality exhibits different behavior. It is also easy to obtain the names and addresses of such specialists, and study their behavior. For instance, for a peptic ulcer product, it is easy to get a list of the most potential 300 gastroenterologists in the country. Selective samples can be identified and a survey conducted to understand the prescription behavior of such specialists.

You can classify this survey into two categories: (i) exploratory and anticipatory, and (ii) fact-based. Both can be carried out to enhance the scope of qualitative research as there are specialists who have different opinions from others.

4. **Stockists Continuous Audit (SCS)**

   Usually stockists are responsible for the availability of products at the retail level. Hence, it is important to make a continuous audit to arrive at the 'availability' to corroborate the accuracy of the information received from RCPA. Present and potential territorial clusters can be identified on the basis of continuous availability of specific products. These clusters can be further explored for those specific products.

5. **Continuous Institutional Audit (CIA)**

   CIA gives the 'profile' of a particular institution. The decision-makers, influencers and products available in institutions keep changing. Similarly, funds and grants allotted also vary. Since the potential and profile of each institution keeps changing, continuous audit is needed.

   These are then the different options open to all pharmaceutical companies before they build up a customer base and keep it continuously updated for their own benefit.

FORMATION OF CLUSTERS

All types of physicians can be clubbed into *three* major clusters:
1. General practitioners
2. Specialists
3. Full-time, hospital-attached practicing and teaching staff

The last category includes state or central government schemes, public sector hospitals, private sector hospitals, and schools/colleges/teaching institutes along with industrial institutions. All three groups can be further classified into individual and group practices. Depending on the therapies and type of patient profiles, an organization can work on its own customer identification process.

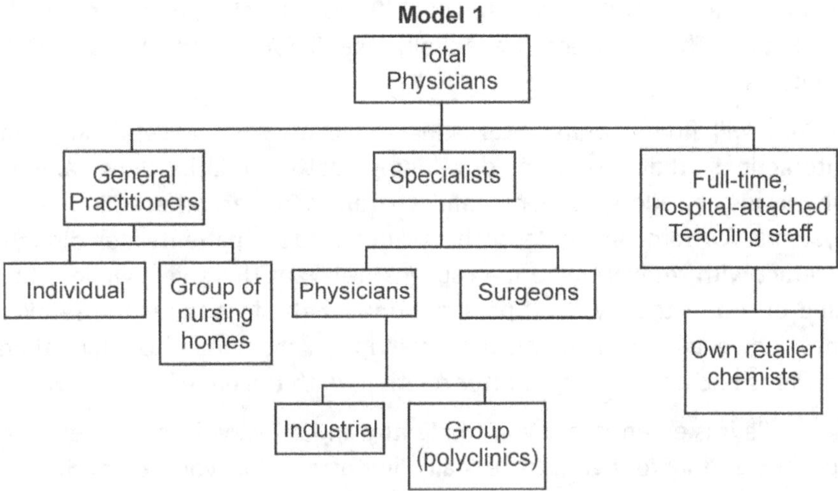

Figure 5.2 Model 1- cluster of physicians

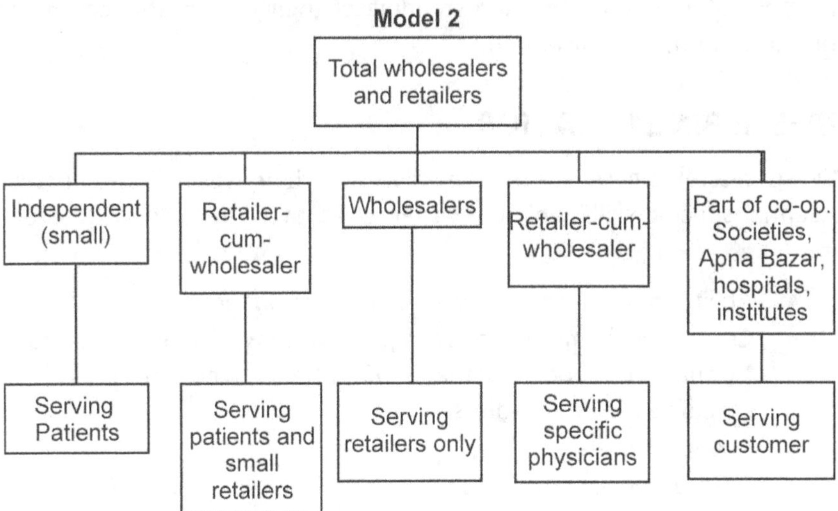

Figure 5.3 Model 2- range of retailers

As we have classified physicians into three clusters, you can also classify retailers—your second customer.

You can classify retailers into A, B and C categories and arrive at the potential of each retailer depending on the counter sale of each day. Similarly, the role of the wholesaler and retailer attached to the doctor as well as a retailer attached to a hospital is very crucial for a few brands. Each brand may need a different retail mix for effective marketing. These outlets are equally useful for health-care and OTC products.

You will find it quite interesting to observe the several different interactions that go into developing better relationships among physicians, retailers, patients and therapies under different type of systems. For some ailments, such as skin disorders, patients may directly interact with retailers who may suggest relevant therapies, while other kind of products may need prescriptions for the first time. The retailer may, however, not insist on the prescription the second or third time onwards once he develops better relations with the patient.

While it is essential for you to identify and select your customer base for better marketing, it is equally important for you to study the behavior of physicians and retailers as they form your customer groups. While the physicians generate prescriptions, retailers give 'orders' and maintain 'shelf stock'. An understanding of their relationship can make for better brand establishment.

PRESCRIBING BEHAVIOR

All successful physicians irrespective of their specialities possess essential specific skills which get sharpened over time. Some of these are:

- Ability to probe to get more out of their patients
- Creative listening—a knack to go beyond words and understand through the body language of patients who are unable to verbalize their complaints
- Analytical skills
- Differential diagnostic abilities
- Regularity of follow-up
- Interpersonal skills

- Communication skills
- Ability to make good presentations
- Assertiveness
- Commercial acumen

A majority of these skills are used to find out 'what is wrong with the patient'. Hence their day-to-day practice gives them enough opportunities to sharpen these skills. And over a period of time they develop good 'reflexes' to carry out their routine efficiently. The degree of sharpness of these skills is dependent on the size and complexity of the practice, and of course, the individual ability, sensitivity and competence of the physician.

But ultimately prescription becomes a motor reflex of the physician's mind. Once a brand acquires a place in the physician's mind, his reflex to prescribe the brand can be developed slowly. It is the brand's effectiveness and the physician's experience with the brand that can provide an impetus to or hinder prescriptions.

You will need to do a lot in the area of personal communication, if you want to develop such reflexes speedily. The physician needs to be convinced and helped to associate the brand with the stimuli he receives while prescribing the same brand for his patients. Once the reflex is transferred onto paper, it takes the shape of a prescription. Usually it is observed that physicians do not think while prescribing. It is almost entirely a reflex.

While cultivating this reflex is vital, it is equally important to follow up with the retailers to see that the brand is well stocked because it is up to the retailer to honor the doctor's prescription. If a retailer has adequate stocks of the product, he will honor the prescription. However, if the retailer has stocked other competing brands, or is likely to earn more profit by selling other brands, he may substitute the product or try to convince the patient that the competitive brand is equally good if not better. Very often, such substitution or advice takes place when the prescribed brand is not adequately stocked or make available. Hence sufficient shelf stock of the brand is very important for better market dynamics.

You can gain an indepth understanding of the physician's behavior by following the classification table given below.

S. No.	Physician's name	Physician's age	Education	Type of practice profiles of patients	No. of patients seen each day	Relative income	Location

Figure 5.4 Physician's behavior format

CLASSIFICATION OF PHYSICIANS

Physicians can be categorized into *six* different classes depending on their prescription behavior. Two distinct patterns emerge: loyalty patterns, and adoption patterns.

1. Loyalty Patterns

(a) ***Corporate loyals:*** It has been observed that doctors exhibit loyalty patterns. Those who prescribe more than three brands from a company consistently are called corporate loyal. They prescribe because of a company's influence and its special characteristics, which they value. These doctors can be general practitioners, specialists, or hospital-attached. They are proud of their choice and decision. And, if need be, they exert their influence on other colleagues and justify their actions of prescribing these many brands from one company.

In the eastern sector of India, you will find a majority of doctors who have a faithful allegiance to a few companies like Alkem. As a result, more than 50% of the contribution in sales of this multimillion rupee company comes from the East alone. Each of these physicians, are capable of influencing at least ten other practitioners, and thus are able to set the trend of prescriptions.

(b) ***Brand loyals:*** Hard-core loyals are those who prescribe one particular brand all the time. Thus a prescription pattern represents an undivided loyalty to the brand. Soft-core loyals prescribe more than two brands, but the loyalty is divided between only these two. Erythromycin was one brand that found loyal prescribers in Bihar especially in Muzaffarpur. However, as competition is increasing, a few loyals have divided their loyalty between the two major brands. This trend is observed in case of vitamins and protein products also.

(c) ***Brand shifters:*** Some doctors shift their loyalties from one brand to another since they do not find any difference between a few brands. As the competition is steep, and communication aggressive, seemingly many brands of a molecule look alike. When such a belief sets in, doctors behave in this fashion and shift their loyalties. A majority of doctors today behave in this manner.

2. Adoption Patterns

(a) ***Early adopters:*** About 8 to 10% of the total physician population in India exhibits such a pattern while adopting any new product. Irrespective of speciality, these traits are found in some doctors since they like to 'try' new things ahead of others. They are usually curious to try out new therapies, new technologies. They are experimental in nature. This class is useful for any new product for a short while at the initial phase of launch.

(b) ***Late adopters:*** This category of doctors waits for reinforcement. Many general practitioners act in this way. Once they observe their reference doctor-consultants, they gain confidence to use and prescribe those product/brands. These doctors do not wish to take a risk with patients and themselves. They exhibit cautious behavior.

They do not wish to experiment at all, and find it difficult to cope with the plethora of new products. They usually are 'yesterday's' doctors.

We have seen above the loyalty and adoption patterns of doctors representing six types. If you divide the territories of your MRs in these six groups, you can direct them to adopt certain specific practices to deal with them at the individual level.

CLASSIFICATION OF RETAILERS

Retailers can be classified into *three* categories:

1. **Image-oriented:** Such retailers are conscious about their image in the industry, and are ready to cooperate to enhance their image. They were willing to spend on displays, merchandising, and shelf-space, and also like to keep a range of products. They have a steady clientele, and advise patients freely.

2. **Cash-oriented:** This category is usually 'trade-minded', and weigh their decisions on pure commercial terms. They are more influenced by margins, discounts, free-bonus offers, and other monetary benefits. They invest proportionate to their returns, and may even overstock a few brands if they see a potential fortune.

3. **Efficiency-oriented:** This category develops its own style in servicing their patients. They may stock their brands in convenient patterns like all ointments at one place to provide quick service to customers. They act quickly and work energetically at the counter.

   You may need to deal with each category differently. It is also possible that you might get all characteristics in different degrees with just one retailer.

   If you can gather this kind of information for at least those physicians who matter, you can calculate the individual potential of a particular doctor for your company. If you know some of these parameters, you can even anticipate the behavior of a physician in advance while calling on him. For instance, consider a registered medical practitioner, age 55, having a majority practice dealing with children, and handling about 50 patients per day. Suppose he is located in one of the rural parts of India, and charges around Rs.50 per patient. It may be worth your while to spend considerable amount of time with him, detailing your brand. And then it all depends on you and your communication skills to cultivate in his mind a reflex for your brand.

   On the other hand, take another case of a young doctor, say an FRCS or a specialist, who maintains an extremely busy schedule with his patients. Based in a city like Mumbai, his relative income may be quite high. You can very well imagine how disinterested he may be in your detailing.

Thus, a more detailed study of these parameters can provide useful tips for field staff.

IMPORTANCE AND IMPACT OF A CUSTOMER BASE

It is really futile to market any brand unless you have properly studied your customers. It is therefore important to identify your customer base, study its characteristics and then decide to market. This information must be based on facts, and not on feelings and experience alone. Experience and feeling can certainly help analyze the facts, but cannot substitute them.

The Impact

As soon as an organization starts relying more on facts and develops its customer database, you can immediately feel the impact, which can be seen through:

- More accurate objectives and fulfillment of objectives
- Focused, concentrated efforts
- Proper allocation of cost of inputs
- Maximization of each call since the potential is known
- Minimization of wastage
- More quantifiable results
- Propensity to implement a specific strategy
- Greater job satisfaction among field staff

The Process

Comprehensive data often conceals the comparatively rapid competitive shifts which represents many local markets. You need to closely examine individual markets on a continual basis to identify such shifts.

This process can be initiated in the following sequence:

1. Analysis of industry trends and other indications of therapeutic groups and territories—secondary data should be studied and collated

2. Identification of the parameters required to be studied for an organization to establish a customer base
3. Assessment of these parameters to evolve an accurate and updated database
4. Determination of a methodology to carry out the survey on a continuous basis
5. Design of the data collection forms
6. Starting of data collection, and developing clusters on the basis of potential
7. Use of the data

The prime value of the creating of a customer base will become obvious when you inherently begin to recognize that each and every territory is different. This base provides sufficient perspective of the present and potential prescription behavior of physicians, and their in-clinic behavior. It also gives the representatives a mechanism to calculate the ROTI (return on time invested) and thereby the market share. It also provides information about shifts in customer behavior in each territory. Managers thus become capable of understanding market shifts, and can qualitatively contribute to the short-term and long-term definitions of the markets for tomorrow.

Markets are usually defined as a group of present and potential customers, who have a desire to prescribe, stock or dispense brands, and those who have prescription, dispensing or stocking power. Every territory is a part of this market. It is therefore essential for you to qualify each market and analyze it in quantitative terms before you start any marketing exercise.

CASE

Database Marketing of Cipla[1]

Multimedia marketing in Cipla was launched in June 1991. It was then called direct marketing.

Preparation

The computer program was prepared by mid-July 1991, and the software and hardware were readied to create a database of doctors.

---

[1]*This case has been contributed by Interlink Marketing Consultancy Pvt. Ltd., Mumbai.*

Initially, the categorization was done on the basis of available information, about doctors. To procure the correct address of each doctor, Cipla mailed out reply-paid postcards to get the basic details—where the doctor wanted to receive his precious mail (either at his clinic or his residence), his complete address date of birth, telephone number, wedding anniversary date, hobbies, etc.—on one side. On the flip side, he was asked to mention what information and services he wanted from Cipla. When Cipla received these cards back, the addresses were immediately corrected on the existing list and the telephone numbers were entered. Any other request mentioned in the card by the doctor was also attended to immediately.

These doctors were then classified into A+, A, and B categories depending on the speciality of doctors.

The data file system and mail-merging were meticulously developed. Stickers with the doctors' addresses were taken in two sets: one, for the outer cover, and another for the envelope containing the 'Dear doctor' letter. The immediate task was to develop a computer program that could reduce the burden of creating a mail list and increase the dispatches. It was decided to send at least one parcel to every doctor every month. A controlling courier system was also evolved.

Implementation

The first phase started with sending samples and literatures to the doctors. The contents of each parcel were dependent on the speciality of the doctor and his classification (A+, A or B).

Feedback system for the unaccepted parcels was elaborately formulated. Necessary actions were also designed to take care of those doctors.

Activity in the second phase was also planned with the addition of newsletters and reports. So there were Lomac newsletters, gynae booklets, 'Medical Flash' series for the anti-hypertensive, anti-asthamatic, anti-arthritic, anthelmintic and anti-bacterial ranges, latest reports on the Cipla-Protec range, and so on. These special letters were sent in between the parcels containing samples and literature. A calendar of events for the year was also planned.

All doctors were informed that any product of Cipla for their personal use would be sent to them if they wrote to Cipla or even called over on the phone.

This really popularized Cipla among doctors. In the absence of the samples sales stock was sent by courier/registered post with a letter requesting support for the brand. In these operations Cipla and Protec were one. Each and every response was looked after by the administrative staff.

New Product Launch

Cipla launched Ciplox Eye Drops with this database approach. Letters to the chemists were also sent after the product was sent to all selected database doctors. A special gift pack was sent with four samples and a digital clock to the ophthalmologists. The product clicked immediately. The same pattern was followed for the introduction of all new products. In Chennai, coincidently, there was an outbreak of the 'Madras eye' at about the same time. This epidemic gave a boost to the sales in that region.

Reminders (Value-Added)

As reminders a system of using Doctor Mailing Cards (DMCs) was conceived. These cards had the product message on one side and visuals of the disease/disorder or new techniques, etc. (with retention value) on the other side. They were sent with the parcels. Charts on asthma and on recuperative exercises were prepared and sent to the doctors. The Novaclox poster was admired by all doctors as they were directly sent. Terfed posers were used in the meetings of doctors and then they were distributed to them. Patient tear-offs on various disorders, do's and don'ts, checklists, etc. were also evolved for increasing the involvement of doctors. Wherever possible, they were handed over personally.

Reasons for Success

These innovative campaigns were possible to implement as Cipla invested in creating a database of doctors. The firm conviction with which Cipla went about using this database made these campaigns successful. It involved a lot of hard work and dedication but it paid off. It took an investment of about Rs.25 lakh to generate the active database.

LEARNINGS

Physician-Patient-Therapy Dynamics

Health-care has two fundamental dimensions: It addresses to the sick and the healthy. Its up to you as an organization to decide whether you would like to address one of these two dimensions or both of them.

When addressing patients, it is important for you to understand the physician-patient-therapy interaction pattern. This will give you a bird's eye view of the total picture. You can then exercise your choice and select the physicians, patients and therapies you would like to work with.

Market Dynamics

Before identifying the business and marketing parameters, it is essential for you to gain an overview of the market. You can do this by studying *three* major factors:

1. Size and potential of the present and potential customer/end-user/retailer
2. Their prescription, stocking and consuming patterns
3. Their willingness to promote and invest in your selected therapies

Developing a database is useful for understanding the inter relationship of physicians, patients and therapies in the complex market situation.

If this fundamental database approach is missing, firms will find it difficult to create added value and build brands in a competitive market like India. And marketing efforts will be divided between selling and trading principles.

CHAPTER **6**

Strategic Plus

In the epic *Mahabharata,* Lord Krishna proved to be the greatest asset for the Pandavas in the war fought at Kurukshetra. Besides being very knowledgeable, he was an excellent diplomat and strategist. Even with all the capabilities to win at their command, the Pandavas would have lost the battle, had it not been for Lord Krishna's advice at every stage. It was indeed Lord Krishna's role in the war that gave the Pandavas a strategic competitive advantage.

The turning point of the war was the grand fight between Arjuna and Karna—the anchor of the Kauravas, the right-hand man of Duryodhana. It was only Lord Krishna who knew that Karna was the sixth Pandava, the eldest one. By letting Karna know of this secret, he was able to ensure that Karna promise his mother, Kunti, that in all circumstances, 'five' Pandavas would remain alive. This implied that Karna would only fight Arjuna and none of the other four brothers. He also strategically took away Karna's God-given shield with the help of Lord Indra before the day of the battle. He thus, ensured that Karna was both *physically* and morally affected even before he battled with Arjuna. Except physical capability on a one-to-one basis, Karna was not left with any special advantage while fighting with Arjuna. In terms of might and skill, the two rivals were almost equal, and a lot depended on the situation at a given moment.

During the grand fight, Karna fought Arjuna valiantly, but his chariot wheel got stuck in the ground, making it difficult for him to move. The battlefield conditions suddenly went against him, and under instructions of Lord Krishna. Arjuna killed Karna when he was trying to move the wheel of this chariot. The right 'moment' was found by Lord Krishna who ensured that the same moment was exploited by Arjuna. Many such incidents during the war clearly indicate that the presence of Lord Krishna itself gave a competitive strategic advantage to the Pandavas.

If you examine this, you will agree that victory or defeat in war is dependent on the quality of the strategy, diplomacy, knowledge, and on whether you have competitive advantage.

The episode also throws light on the *five* components of strategy in war, which is equally applicable in pharmaceutical marketing. Suppose a firm has researched a new chemical entity in the anti-ulcer market. The *qualities* the firm exhibits are different from the qualities of those who may follow it in the market. It therefore has enough *moral* strength to launch its products. With 500 MRs to cover India, it has *physical* power. Simultaneously, it has designed its distribution in such a way that *mathematically* it can grab a 60% distribution width within the first four months. It has also observed that Jammu & Kashmir, Andhra, part of Kerala, and all the metro cities provide *geographical* advantage as these markets command maximum share of the total market in India. Finally, it has decided to monitor the inputs and output *statistically*. The firm has thus woven together all the five basic elements for achieving strategic advantage: *moral, physical, mathematical, geographical, and statistical.* You should never segregate these elements since you can gain a *strategic edge* from integrating the five elements and not from their summation. The competition factor is built into these five elements as they are all relative to competition or competitors.

THE PROCESS OF COMPETITION ANALYSIS

To understand the competitive threats and opportunities, you need to (i) analyze the competing marketing forces and (ii) the performance abilities of your competitors. This gives rise to *five* crucial issues:

Identification of competitors

1. Competitors' ability to take risks and invest resources
2. Competitors' capabilities (reflexes)
3. Competitors' performance
4. Competitors' motivation and marketability

The competitive analysis process is depicted in the following box.

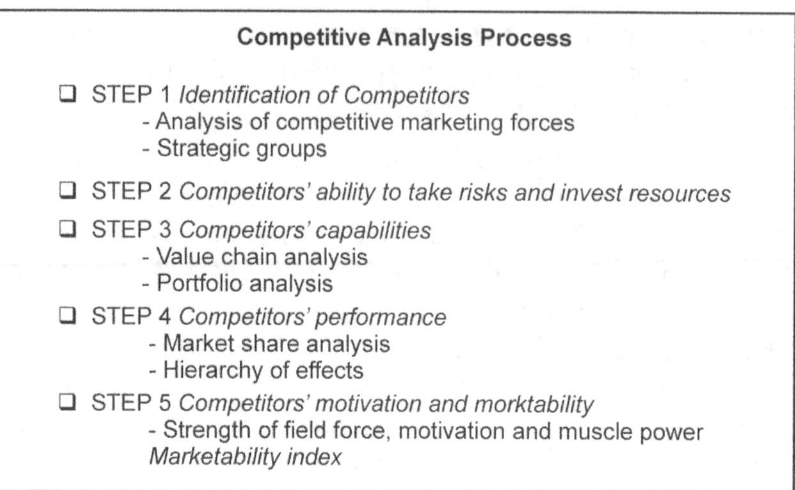

Figure 6.1 Competitive analysis process

Competitive Marketing Forces

(i) ***Identification of competitors:*** A key problem in the identification of competitors is the prevailing feeling among marketing professionals that they know their competitors, their strengths and weaknesses, their people and their strategies. The fact, however, is that they on most occasions rely on rather partial statistics based on information which is often limited to their own experience. Often, the management's understanding of competition is casual, clumsy, and inaccurate.

Systematic, appropriately organized, and objective information is the key to rigorous competition analysis. Competitive force analysis is based on market segmentation, product positioning, and analysis of R&D capabilities. Target-market and positioning analyses are useful approaches to identify the key players in the marketplace. By studying the target-market segments of competitors and their perceived positioning in the eyes of the targeted customers, it should be possible for you to conveniently pinpoint direct competitors. Alternatively, you could go directly to the prescribers and ask them which drugs they would consider prescribing for a specific disease. The available research capabilities of the existing and potential competitors can further expand the previously identified competitors.

Strategic groups as stated by McGee & Thomas (1986) are basically groups of competitors in an industry pursuing similar strategies and having certain common characteristics (e.g. size, commitment to the ethical drug business, R&D intensity, etc.) (McGee and Thomas, 1986). These strategic groups are useful tools to segregate homogeneous competitors into heterogeneous markets.

(ii) ***The emergence of new customer groups:*** Considering the state of development of each country in terms of priorities in healthcare, new customer groups will emerge. These new groups will be subdivisions of existing groups or new customers who would be more literate, demanding, agile, and active.

These new groups would act as a regulator force (in addition to the government) as they are already doing in more developed countries. Their needs and demands have to be studied before marketing products. Physicians have to undergo changes in attitudes to serve patients better, and will demand better service from pharmaceutical companies.

(iii) ***Globalization:*** In the next decade, the explosion in economic growth in pharmerging countries will probably mean an increase in pharmaceutical sales with fierce global competition. As a percentage of total healthcare spending, the USA spends only about 11.9% on pharmaceuticals in comparison to Italy and Germany, who spend up to 14-18%. Japan is the second-highest after USA, spending about 10% on pharmaceuticals. On the other hand, India spends only about 6% on pharmaceuticals.

(iv) ***Impact of european union (EU):*** With the EU approach becoming more market based and the FDA system becoming stricter with emphasis on the prevention and cure of public health, there will be a change in regulatory philosophy. This may lead to more line extensions of patented and innovative drugs. As a result of liberalization in the licensing policy, more synchronized launches and many molecules throughout the world will be the order of the day, with more intense competition.

(v) ***Faster approaches of new molecules:*** In 2015, 45 new molecular entities were approved by the US FDA's Center for Drug Evaluation and Research (CDER). They reflect several important industry trends. CDER identified 16 of the 45 novel drugs in 2015 (36%) as first-in-class drugs, one indicator of the innovative nature of a drug.

About 47% of the novel drugs approved in 2015 (21 out of 45) were approved to treat rare or orphan diseases. 14 of the 45 novel drugs (31%) were designated as Fast Track, meaning drugs with the potential to address unmet needs. CDER designated 10 of the 45 novel drugs (22%) as Breakthrough Therapies. 24 of the 45 novel drugs (53%) were designated as Priority Review. Additionally, CDER designated 6 of the 45 novel drugs (13%) under FDA's Accelerated Approval Program, which allows early approval of a drug for a serious or life-threatening illness that offers a benefit over current treatments. From 2006 through 2016, CDER averaged about 28 novel drug approvals per year.

(vi) ***Pricing and IPR impact:*** The downward pressure on pharmaceutical prices will reduce the potential profit required profit required to support R&D investment. Thus pricing strategy needs to be investigated, and properly adjusted. Positive changes in 'pricing policies' are bound to take place sooner or later the world over.

(vii) ***Limitations on resources***: There is always pressure on existing resources. As a result of the overall emphasis on value-for-money (VFM) and not on cost alone, it is important to make the best use of limited resources.

(viii) ***Positive trends:*** The creation of an aging customer group of relatively wealthy and sophisticated consumers in developed countries, and the continued economic development of the Third World, have led to a demand for quality, branded drugs. There are large gaps in therapy for genetic disorders. Low-cost drugs with high therapeutic benefits will benefit from more favorable regulatory procedures.

(ix) ***Market growth:*** Although there has been a growth rate of 95% over the last five to ten years, the unit growth of these therapeutic categories has been flat in eight developed countries, namely Japan, German, France, Italy, UK, Canada, and Spain, which account for over 70% of the world-volume product replacement. Unit growth will account for 2% (compared with new products 5%, and price 1%). The rest of the world is at different stages of developing health-care. Hence, most of the growth is likely to come from outside there eight key markets.

(x) ***Generic competition:*** Lack of brand awareness and cheaper generic availability will force generic competition to take 25% of the market share in the coming years. Integrated supply chains, comprising manufacturing, whole-selling and retailing, pose a strong threat to the industry. They will use their labels for generic products, and discretionary substitution in pharmacies could badly affect brand manufacturers. The wholesaler's ability to make profitable arrangements with manufacturers will also squeeze the margins of manufacturers of branded products. In this environment a switch from prescription to OTC products will be witnessed.

(xi) ***Cost of innovation in promotion:*** The widely accepted promotional approaches based on convincing physicians of the uniqueness and scientific benefits of a product may prove inadequate. On the other hand, cost will increase with inflation and companies will have to be innovative.

(xii) ***New technology:*** Access to new technology and its utility has caused a few problems. To suit the culture of a particular country, companies may have to identify appropriate technologies to take advantage of the available infrastructure. Sodium nitroprusside was launched by a small company of Gujarat in competition with Roche. It was essential to pack this product in aluminium foil since it was a blood pressure monitoring agent during surgery. It could not take advantage of the situation due to lack of technology and infrastructure.

(xiii) ***Changing structures:*** Increased competition and greater access to technology will lead to dissolution of the existing industry structure. To survive, multinational firms will have to become therapeutic or regional specialists.

To summarize, there have been far-reaching effects on the environment, markets, and organizations. These changes will drive out weak, marginal players, such as family-owned companies, and survival will be virtually impossible for start-up companies. There will have to be a focus on size—the organization size will have to be optimum if it is to compete successfully at both the national and global levels.

(xiv) ***Customers:*** Prescribers, retailers, health-maintenance organizations, hospitals and the Consumer Guidance Society will progressively put more pressure on drug companies to develop genuinely 'new, effective, and efficient' drugs, and to inform customers better about the value of available drugs. Furthermore, the concentration in the prescriber population will have to be considered. More specifically, pharmaceutical companies will be competing for fewer core clients. Pharmaceutical companies will also have to rethink their size and the role of their expensive sales forces in the light of the more concentrated prescribers' market.

The role of wholesalers varies dramatically from country to country. In Germany, for example, a highly concentrated wholesale sector has strong bargaining power both with drug manufacturers and pharmacists. In Belgium, a fragmented whole-selling industry has no power at all. In the USA, the growth and greater efficiency of retail chains and wholesalers through mergers and the formation of buying cooperatives has increased the distributors' leverage with manufacturers. In Japan, most of the major pharmaceutical companies have direct interests (and investments) in the wholesale distribution sector. In India, AIOCD (All Indian Organization of Chemists & Druggists) has enough regulatory power and negotiate and bargain with companies. They can also regulate the quality of drugs and come in the way of launching any new products if not taken care of.

Institutional customers, such as hospitals, constitute another force in the market with a strong bargaining power with drug manufacturers. In India, government and non-government buyers can be segregated. Able to place large orders and regarded as opinion makers by some prescribers, hospitals are powerful negotiators in the drug industry.

(xv) ***Rivalry at the industry level***: An oft-cited summary measure of the market power of firms in an industry is the concentration ratio. The usual way of constructing this measure is to compare the sales of the top four or eight manufacturers with the overall market volume. These ratios are referred to as the C4 and C8 indices respectively.

These concentration ratios can be computed at a number of different levels. For the drug industry these levels could be the total market, the therapeutic class, and the product level. Such a computation for the total market size of the first ten companies may, for instance, reveal that these top ten companies have covered 30% of the total market. In other words, there is a huge possibility to top and exploit the remaining 70% of the market.

After studying the strengths and weaknesses of the product mix of these ten companies, each company can develop strategies for itself to gain competitive advantage. Thus, such computation can lead to internal competition.

Analysis of Competitor's Ability to Perform

(i) ***Competitor's ability to take risks and invest resources:*** It is important to figure out whether the competitor is ready to invest money and time, and to focus on the product in competition.

(ii) ***Competitors' capabilities (Reflexes):*** It is difficult to anticipate what the competition will do next. Nevertheless, it is crucial to try to figure out explicitly what strategies the competition might pursue in the future. To improve the understanding of what competition will or could do, we can look at their past reflexes and arrive at reasonably defined attributes. Unless major changes in policies, values and management have taken place, we can assume that capabilities exist. The R&D, registrations, manufacturing, marketing and distribution of competitors should be analyzed. Analysis of how each of these five functions is performed by the competitors could provide a deeper understanding of the competitive advantage and the likely future moves of competitors. This business system analysis identifies the strengths and weaknesses of the competition, and therefore, indicates where the competition will be aggressive and where vulnerable. This analysis is a useful tool to get a better understanding of the capabilities and sources of the competitors' strengths and weaknesses.

(iii) ***Competitors' performance:*** Indicators of performance are usually market share, sales growth and profitability. Information about changes in these indicators over time is essential for an accurate assessment of competitors' performance.

(iv) ***Competitors' motivation and marketability index:*** It is important to grasp the competitors muscle power and philosophy and the way they perceive themselves and their competitors' to anticipate their future moves. Do they perceive themselves as the clear leaders for tomorrow in the market or simply as followers? How are they and how do they want to be perceived: aggressive, defensive, or conservative? Does their organization allow them to act and react quickly to their opponents' moves? Do they provide substantial autonomy to their subsidiaries? For example, everything else being the same, Swiss companies have the reputation of being slower and more conservative than their American and Japanese counterparts. Japanese companies are perceived as centralized and managed from the company's headquarters in Japan (Bartlett and Ghoshal, 1989).

The point is that when you predict a competitor's strategy, you should try to think as they would, and not think in terms of what your company would do in the given circumstances. Another danger in this context is to become deceived by some existing 'halo' effects in the market about certain competitors. These company stigmas could be rather inappropriate generalizations, and not hold good in particular market situations.

How do they really react? Is their field staff really motivated?

STRATEGIC COMPETITIVE ADVANTAGE

Sources of Competitive Advantage

A distinctive capability of any organization becomes its competitive advantage, when it is *applied in an industry and brought to the market.*

There are *three* distinctive capabilities which help an organization to review its status of competitive advantage.

1. Structure and culture
2. Reputation
3. Innovation

(i) ***Structure and culture:*** Although IBM's products and its achievements in the marketplace are universally admired, its culture is not to everybody's taste. Employees are fiercely loyal and those who find the organization uncongenial leave. Similarly, over a period of time, each company establishes a structure, a style, a set of routines, which operates to get the best out of relatively ordinary employees. Such routines have been known to produce exceptional corporate results over many years and through many changes in the economic environment. The power of shared knowledge through commercial relationships benefits every organization.

The competitive advantage typically arises through the acquisition of organizational knowledge, the establishment of organizational routines, and the development of cooperative ethic.

This allows flexible structure and response, the culture of sharing of information, and process in which monitoring of quality becomes second nature to the organization.

In such an organization, the driving force is usually the one who directs the company and pushes it towards acquiring its distinctive capabilities. A few people are suited to playing such a role; many aren't. Only a few companies in India have been able to acquire distinctive capabilities. GSK, Sanofi, and Pfizer among MNCs, and Ranbaxy, Wockhardt, Alembic and Cadila among NCs have this capability. Other similar companies simply cannot emulate the structure and culture of these organizations.

(ii) *Reputation:* Good reputation is always a commercial benefit. Reputation can be a substantial and sustaining competitive advantage. In the long run, it can only be earned by providing high quality consistently. For instance, GSK's or Ranbaxy's competitive advantage was based on the reputation of Zinetac and Cifran.

(iii) *Innovation:* Costs and uncertainties are always associated with innovations. Sony is an excellent example of innovation, and so is Dr Reddy's Laboratories. However, if you consider innovation in isolation, these organizations may not have competitive advantage. As a matter of fact, these organizations have achieved a distinct reputation owing to their structure and culture fostering continuous innovation. Dr Reddy's Laboratories and Sun Pharma are examples of organizations which have all these three distinct capabilities to develop competitive advantage.

If these distinctive capabilities are properly applied to markets, they create competitive advantage. Natco has the distinctive capability of producing a slow-release form for any molecule. If this capability is used in the market by defining demand, physicians' needs, and appropriate price, it will create a competitive advantage.

Strategic Group and Strategic Market

The strategic group and strategic market together define the competitive battlefield. The strategic group is determined by classifying together companies with similar strategies. Eskayef and USV have similar capabilities to produce time, release products. So these two companies form a strategic group. Many companies are getting their SR (slow-release) formulations manufactured by Natco. They also form part of a strategic group.

The strategic market needs to be properly identified and deployed. In the case of Natco, the market could be those companies manufacturing their SR products. Natco then becomes a supplier to pharmaceutical companies. It is also possible for Natco to focus on physicians prescribing SR molecules for asthma.

So Natco has to identify its 'core market'. Once this is done, the market needs to be deployed fully with the help of distinctive capabilities. As we have already said, Natco has a choice. It is also possible that it will work on both options.

Mergers

Mergers can add value. It is often profitable to use the distinctive capabilities of more than one party in combination. The mergers of Warner Lambert and Parke-Davis took such a long time that the distinctive capabilities of Parke-Davis in ethical pharmaceutical markets could not be exploited at all. The reputation of Parke-Davis was so distinctive that Warmer Lambert should have capitalized on it. But the organization chose the different options of exploiting Waterbury's, Halls, and Chiclets. The effect of this merger is yet to be studied.

Joint ventures and strategic alliance are other methods to gain competitive advantage. Nova started manufacturing and marketing Human Insulin with Torrent. Nova's products were manufactured by Torrent but sold by Boots.

Divestments and takeovers are not observed so often in pharma as in other industries. GSK divested its other businesses and chose to concentrate on pharma, showing that it is also possible to gain competitive advantage by consolidating resources.

Developing Strategic Competitive Advantage

Can a company develop strategic advantage? The answer is clearly yes. You can develop this advantage if you build up an ability to do something better than your competition consistently due to your innate or acquired strength.

One or more big advantages or a number of small advantages adding up to a big one can give you the strength of a 'moral' backing which you require to sustain this advantage. A new chemical entity researched by you and licensed to a franchisee might give you one or more advantage; while generic products could give you a number of small advantages in terms of quality, price, less side-effects, efficiency, and availability, adding up to a margin advantage. If no advantage is perceived, you may have to work towards:

- Greater customer orientation and convenience
- More integrated structure of marketing and manufacturing to offer price differential
- Concentrated market focus by deploying a niche or core group
- Accepting the realities of competition and taking a stance for your brand
- Investing in R&D to develop an advantage through break-through of technology

You may use the above criteria for analyzing your brand and its perceived advantages in the context of the Indian scenario.

The strategic advantage has to be backed by power of field force and implementation, together with promotional tactics.

CASE

Strategic Advantages of the World's Best Three Companies in the 1990s[1]

Merck and Co.

- ***Winner in prescription support for more brands:*** Merck & Co. had been a winner in prescription trend analysis in three fastest growing major therapeutic groups. They were leading as a result of the maturity of these products in the market. Five of their brands were among the first 50 top brands.

---

[1] *This case has been contributed by Interlink Marketing Consultancy Pvt. Ltd., Mumbai.*

- ***New product strategy***: Of the top 40 companies, Merck & Co. had 98 R&D drugs, 75 own drugs, and 23 under license then. This provided a high leverage for the existing and mature product mix. Their method of introducing new products also gave a fresh leverage.

- ***Image building***: Merck's image had also been responsible for its momentum and success in each area. Image building takes up large proportion of investment, which then pays off in areas like selection of quality personnel, quality products, and goodwill.

GSK

- ***Market-driven strategic base***: Considering the critical success factors, GSK was heading for the numerouno position as a result of a market-driven strategic base. It was supported by continuous management development, size and quality of sales force, its aggressive attitude of outstripping competition, concentrated focus on markets and products, priority investment in advertising, quick response to potential market needs, and market-driven policies.

- ***Speedy commercialization of R&D efforts***: GSK invested around US $ 400 million in R&D then. Its philosophy of developing 'research satellites' yielded nine fully developed, sixteen exploratory, and seven new compounds. Among the 40 top companies then, GSK had 40 R&D drugs, 21 own drugs, and 19 under licensing. Speed and efficiency in registering dossiers and pushing products from the development to the commercial stage in minimum time contributed to its success.

- ***Business growth through products and market***: Of the leading 50 brands then, three came from GSK. For the next five years. GSK capitalized on existing products, expecting two-thirds of its business growth through today's products, of which one-third was from Zinetac and one-third from new products. It relied heavily on the quality of its products.

- ***Image-building activities***: A few activities like constructing a pharmacy building and other specific events showed they would like to be no. 2 in image creating after Merck & Co.

- ***Focus on profits-bottomline increase***: Profits in 1989 were better than those of Merck & Co., i.e. US $1229 million as against Merck's US $749 million.

Takeda

- *Focus on improvement:* The critical success factor of Takeda was smartly hidden in its orientation towards improvement of products. In 1988 alone, four products were improved by Takeda.

- *Reliance on R&D base*: R&D expenditure represented 6.6% of total sales and there was a move to strengthen it by a further investment of Yen 30,000. Among the top 40 companies then, Takeda had 46 R&D, drugs, 42 of its own drugs, and four drugs under licensing.

- *Better management*: Takeda streamlined its organization in an effort to reinforce effective interaction, cooperation and communication at all levels to ensure effective planning of business activity. Although the sixth or seventh largest company and having one brand in the top 50, Takeda wanted to play it safe, relying on joint ventures rather than mergers.

- *Insufficient capital*: Their capital was insufficient to make waves in markets overseas.

LEARNINGS

While building competitive advantage, we must analyze the competition and competitors. This is a two-step process involving:

- Analysis of competitive marketing forces
- Analysis of competitors' abilities to perform

On the basis of this analysis, any firm can exercise its choice of a group of competitors to deal with in future.

Competitive advantage then helps the firm have an edge over chosen competitors. This advantage is dependent on:

- Distinctive capabilities of the firm
- Application of these capabilities to the market

It has been observed that those who have created an advantage for themselves have led the industry and maintained their position irrespective of environmental changes.

CHAPTER **7**

Force of Segmentation

Shivaji, the great Maratha ruler, always formulated his battle strategies based on information about the strengths and weaknesses of his enemy. On several occasions, he attacked the enemy unexpectedly. On one occasion, he surprised Shahiste Khan, the Mughal general, at LalMahal, Pune, at midnight, who not only had to yield to him but lost four of his fingers in the bargain. At another time, Shivaji killed Afzal Khan, another Mughal general, in his own tent. Shivaji on this occasion feigned that he was surrendering.

Shivaji never took on the Mughal force in a frontal attack, as the size of his own army was very small in comparison. He instead adopted another strategy to fight the Mughals; he always attacked it in segments. Each segment was chosen on the basis of its relative strengths and weaknesses. Shivaji was able to learn of the plan of attack of the enemy segment in advance through his spies. He and his soldiers knew the entire Deccan like the lines on their palms. They could wait around valleys or hide their force till the segment of the Mughal force arrived on the scene. No sooner would the Mughal segment approach them, they would attack them from all sides. The attack was unexpected, powerful, and concentrated. The strategy ensured that not a single enemy survived.

Like Shivaji's war strategies, the power of strategic marketing also lies in attacking markets in segments.

In the Indian pharmaceutical environment, there are some popular misconceptions about segmentation. Some of us tend to believe that if every medical representative in his territory selects about 20-25 class A physicians from a given speciality and then concentrates on them as the 'core segment', he would have more or less the entire territory taken care of. The case is similar to that of a person whose head is in ice and legs on fire, and we therefore were to conclude that he would be comfortable because his average body temperature is at the comfort level.

The marketer who develops strategies and tactics for the core customers considering the comfort level is usually on the path of disaster. Over a period of time, the same 20 to 25 physicians in each MR's area are concentrated upon by practically all manufacturers in that speciality. Due to the competition, the core segment of a company gets overcrowded. Concentrating on the same segment no longer works.

At the other end of the spectrum is another group who reach the conclusion that no segmentation can work. They feel that you can get something out of every physician. Hence, they look at each physician as the average. Now, this is similar to the case of the statistician who waded through a river with an average depth of one meter and drowned. Only as an exception does the MR identify and select a few physicians for giving special emphasis and treatment. As the physicians in number are usually more, they get average inputs, and the MR at times does not even produce average results.

How do you differentiate the practices described above from a good segmentation scheme? A good segmentation scheme is one that identifies segments which are homogeneous within the segment, and heterogeneous across segments.

The purpose of segmenting should be subgrouping. It should be done in such a way that the product manager or marketing manager is able to design a marketing mix which matches the needs of individuals in a selected segment more precisely.

PROBLEMS IN MARKET SEGMENTATION

Even today many pharmaceutical companies have not adopted market segmentation as part of their overall philosophy. The reasons for this are not difficult to identify. It requires an understanding of certain key issues:

Lack of Faith in a Focused Approach

First, market segmentation requires a focused approach. You should be ready to put all your eggs in one basket. Risky? Yes, but the returns are really maximized if it works well. If you are sure of yourself and are able to clearly identify your target and concentrate on this focused group of doctors or retailers, you have got it made. But you should be confident of doing it consistently right and producing the results. There are some who are not willing to take such a risk. A few marketers believe that all products can be prescribed by all doctors. They insist on exposing all the products to all doctors. GSK did it successfully. However, the same approach was used in Sandoz; it just did not work. It depends on the maturity of the market and the product-mix utilities.

Companies who do not have a well-trained field force and have less capabilities in target selection, sometimes adopt a kind of 'hit-and-miss' approach based on random selection.

Strategic Vision and Resourcefulness

Markets do not always develop smoothly. You need to develop a 'strategic vision' to continuously update the core group of doctors. They are usually the same for all competitors. It then becomes difficult to keep them motivated. And this requires a lot of resources as all of them understand that they are being picked up by everyone. The commitment level of doctors to a particular company goes down. The whole issue of core segmentation gets vitiated. As a result, more and more resources are spent on the same core doctors.

Strategic vision in terms of developing a second 'line of defense' among core doctors is very important. So you must develop a relationship between the core and a second larger group of 'would-be-core' doctors simultaneously. Those companies who do not have any strategic focus find it difficult to segment today's and tomorrow doctors.

Take the instance of the chief of a cardiothoracic surgical ward who was so eminent that every company was attending to him. There was a registrar who assisted him. But all companies ignored the registrar. After a period of just five years, the registrar became chief surgeon in another hospital. It was then too late for those companies who had ignored him earlier. Identifying such core and would-be-core doctors is very crucial for success. What is needed is foresight and vision. But many find it tedious to give such careful attention to the territorial selection process.

Specificity and Practicability

There are no water-tight compartments for different categories of customers. There can be none; they are bound to overlap each other. However, for developing a perfect segmentation scheme, 'specificity' is essential. Consider a segment of corporate loyal doctors. Some of them may have more followers than others. Where do you draw the line? Here, there is a need to specify the 'range' of followers to make the segment work properly. For instance, a corporate loyal doctor, to begin with, may be prescribing a brand, but as time passes his brand loyalty changes to corporate loyalty.

Sometimes there is a problem of the sheer presence of specialists whom you may like to make corporate loyal. Suppose you require 20 gynecologists in a territory to make up a target group, and you find there are only 15 specialist gynecologistsin a specific given territory. What do you do? Do you then add GPs who also handle gynecology cases? Do you then add those GPs who have a predominant female practice? Do you dilute the target group or do you not? And can you then expect the same results from this territory?

Such practices take away the major spirit of strategy and segmentation at the level of implementation.

Micro and Macro Disparity

In countries with wide disparities like India, macro-level policies do not always percolate or get implemented at the micro level, especially in the villages. This phenomenon is of course not exclusive to marketing. Therefore, at the village level, the segmentation strategy needs to be fine-tuned and adjusted locally to suit local situations. At the same time, it should not happen that the strategy is so totally submerged by the local conditions that the segmentation system is forgotten. The system must be amended for better implementation and not for segmentation. The original concept must remain. The modified system can then be communicated to the sales management to execute. However, in practice, restraints and constraints overtake the concept. And these difficulties defeat the purpose of segmentation.

In many organizations, there is little control on implementation. Hence, the results from such segment-oriented strategies are bound to be less.

Commitment of the Field Force

In the final analysis, the success of any segmentation system or target-market selection is largely dependent on the commitment of the field force. It is often heard that this commitment is lacking. The field force fear loss of their freedom and feel they will get straight-jacketed. They take it as an unwarranted interference in their functioning.

They instead defend their own line of action, and argue that they are in fact implementing a far superior segmentation strategy based on individual relations. Moreover, each MR has his favorite set of doctors with whom he has a special relationship. They are unable to sometimes evolve a proper equation with those whom they do not know but are potential for the company. In this process the range of supplementation gets diluted. Therefore, much depends on the degree of relationship of an MR with his group of doctors.

Apprehension Regarding Ability and Skills of the Field Force

The sales force sometimes needs to acquire new skills to work on innovative campaigns. You should not underestimate the MRs' willingness and ability to learn and adopt new ideas. We have seen that a small proportion of physicians adopt a new product early; similarly, there is a small percentage of pharmaceutical MRs who adopt new approaches early. This requires skill on the part of the sales force to implement new ideas. These approaches and skills need to be developed and nurtured so that the MRs get accustomed to deploy new ideas and are proud to do so.

It is equally important to develop skills to cope with new challenges. Such a transition requires new skills in analyzing the markets, developing marketing strategies, and organizing the sales force.

Segmentation also requires the availability of additional, and often costly, data to provide insights into the market. Feedback is required to check the appropriateness of the segmentation approach and the performance within the chosen segments. Only standardized syndicated data is not the best basis for segmenting markets. You may have to conduct tailor-made database research. Many companies are not sure whether all these things yield results, and are possible or not, in the present environment.

Dilemma of Positioning and Segmentation

Many companies also feel that once they select a specific 'indications related' positioning, they do not require to further look at segmentation.

They make the error of thinking that there is no difference in segmentation and positioning in pharma marketing.

This fallacy often prevents managers from thinking of markets, which is crucial for success. Baralgan was positioned to provide speedy smooth muscle spasm relief as it was an important indication. But it was further targeted to those heterogeneous groups of doctors who wanted to use pain relievers along with every anti-diarrhoeal preparation as their patients were suffering from gastroenterologists; it consists of 'co-prescribers'. Although the difference is subtle, it is evident.

Let us now take a look at the different segmentation methods.

METHODS OF SEGMENTATION

Having understood the problems of segmentation, let us see the different methods to segment the markets and develop target markets. The basis of segmentation is dependent on:

1. Sensitivity of physicians
2. Demographics
3. Geographic
4. Socioeconomics
5. Psychographics
6. Prescriber and retailer behavior
7. Brand relationships with 'inner circle' doctors

Based on the above factors, seven different methods emerge.

1. Sensitivity of Physicians

It has been observed that in India, the response of a physician to prescribe or dispense sometimes depends or his relative sensitivity to a variety of promotional tools and the attributes or galenical forms of a product. We can identify physicians on the basis of their responses and club them in different segments.

When we talk about homogeneity within a segment, we mean that the members of a segment have similar needs or manifested behaviors or habits. Based on this criterion, the best segmentation scheme would be at the level of implementation where you identify each individual physician as a segment.

Although this is not viable in totality, it does work when an MR wishes to sell a product in bulk and he identifies a dispensing GP who has the capacity to dispense. It works when we manage each territory separately.

For purposes of our study, we have identified below six major sensitivities that can help you as a marketer to observe the relative response of physicians and develop segments. They are as follows:

- (i)   Sensitivity to sampling and galenical forms
- (ii)   Sensitivity to special prices and galenical forms
- (iii)   Sensitivity to price and dosage of a product
- (iv)   Sensitivity to extensive use and availability of all galenical forms
- (v)   Sensitivity to medical information and side-effects, contra indications, and drug interactions

(i)   ***Sensitivity to sampling and galenical forms:*** Some injectables have a relatively high degree of sensitivity to sampling in comparison to tablets. One multidose vial can be injected to a patient regularly. The patient also has to pay for these injections. Thus, sampling assumes high relevance in such products.

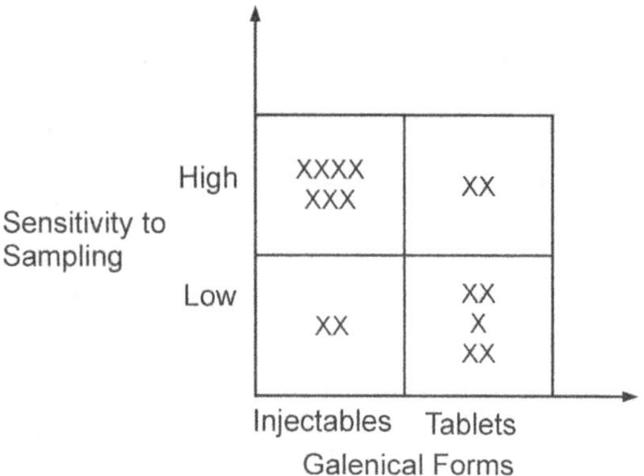

Those who prescribe may look for speed and onset of action of the galenical form.

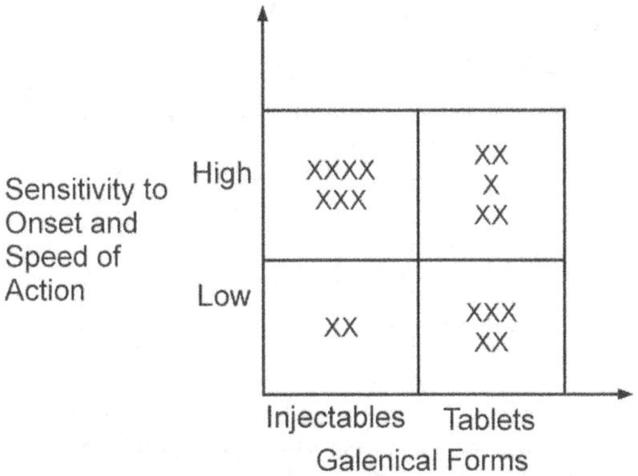

(ii) ***Sensitivity to special prices and galenical forms:*** Bulk packs of tablets as well as liquid preparations are bought by many physicians in rural India. As they buy and dispense in divided doses to their patients, they look for special prices or discounts. Their sensitivity to special prices is relatively high when they decide to buy.

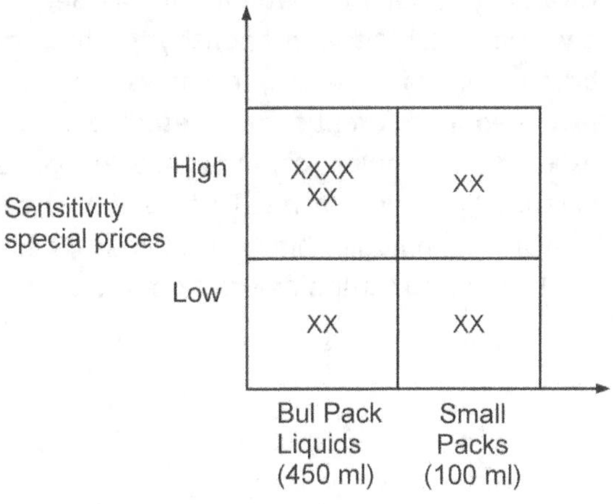

(iii) ***Sensitivity to price and dosage of a product:*** Sensitivity to price is observed in the case of single-dose and multi-dose therapy. For instance, a physician will look for economy of the therapy in the case of a condition that needs continuous treatment for longer periods of time. His sensitivity to use an economic brand will thus, be relatively high.

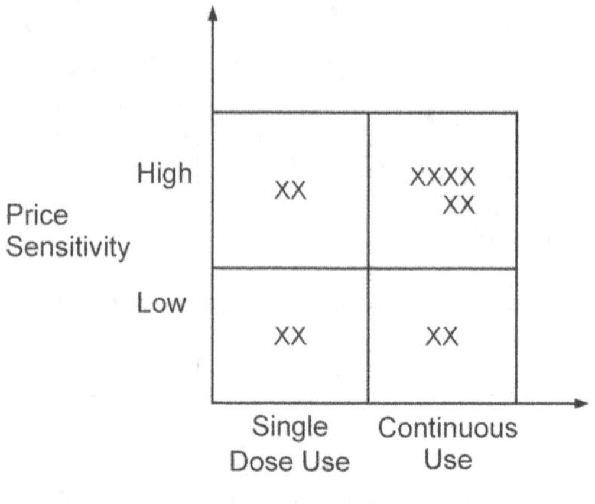

(iv) ***Sensitivity to wider usage or prescription and availability of forms of a product***: A brand gets its widest usage when it is available in all forms like tablets, capsules, injectables, syrups, and suspensions. Physicians can then prescribe it to all age groups of patients. It has been observed that physicians exhibit a propensity to prescribe the same brand more often when he knows that the brand is well extended in different forms. Betadine and Wockadine are excellent examples of increased usage due to more extended galenical forms. To extend its usage, Wockadine is available in liquid, ointment, gargles, pessaries, mouth-wash, and also scrubbing solution.

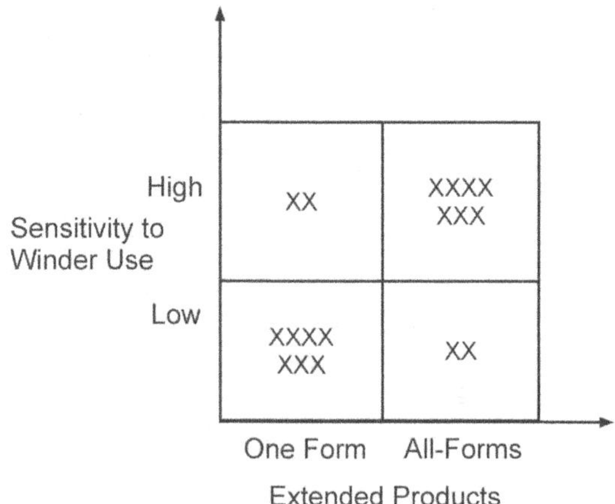

(v) ***Sensitivity to medical information regarding side-effects:*** Physicians need more information when they are apprehensive about the side effects, contraindications or drug interactions of a particular product. It has been observed that while adding any multivitamin or fat solution to infusion, physicians insist on the compatibility data as the patient's life can be endangered. So sensitivity to more medical information is very high in such situations.

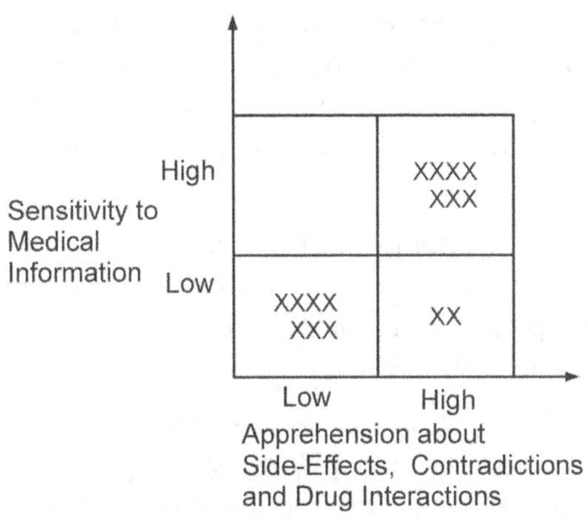

2. Demographic Segmentation

The method of segmentation involves dividing the market into different groups of prescribers as the basis of age, sex, education, size of practice, location, and specialization. The size of practice and specialization of the physicians can be especially useful segmentation variables. Doctors with large practices can be interesting targets because of the obvious potential of specialized drugs which are only prescribed by specialists. Often, however, it is necessary to segment these demographic segments further with other psycho-graphic criteria.

Take the case of gynecologist in Tamil Nadu, age 50, who is visited by at least 10 female patients per day. She does not believe in Sustained Release (SR) therapy and so does not prescribe it. She is rude to the field staff who tries to push such products. You can gather many clues from this case on the basis of demographics.

The demographics of a particular area also help us in ascertaining the capacity of doctors in terms of prescription or dispensing power. Information on age, education and number of patients a doctor treats per day provides us the relative potential of two equally good doctors who may behave in a similar fashion. Two similar types of doctors may have more or less the same capacity to prescribe, but one may be treating more than 100 patients a day, the other just 25. Again, you can judge their relative potential.

There is one more dimension to this—location. A doctor in a rural town such as Gadchiroli in Maharasthra may differ in prescribing potential from one in a city like Mumbai or Pune though the number of patients he treats in a day may be the same.

Finally, the income level of the patient also plays an important role. If the buying or paying capacity of the patient is limited, he naturally prefers to go to a doctor whose fees are low and who prescribes cheaper drugs.

Conceptually, all these factors—age, education, number of patients, location, and buying capacity—have to be carefully considered while selecting the target market. In practice, it is difficult to justify the selection of a segment taking all these factors into account. But the exercise can give you a fairly good idea of the potential of the chosen segment.

3. Geographic Segmentation

Geographic segmentation, as the name implies, entails subdividing the market into regions, cities, districts, and villages.

The urban-suburban-rural criteria can be useful in characterizing target markets since the ailments demand specific facilities like SGOT, SGPT in liver disorders and T1, T2, T3 in thyroid investigations. The availability of specialized investigation facilities help physicians prescribe related products. In the absence of such facilities, they may give up, and shift the patient to urban areas. Thus, since the needs for such doctors in areas differing geographically are different, it is possible to segment markets on the basis of geographical location.

Target marketing is an efficient way of using scarce resources. For example, if the available size of the registered physician population is in range of 9-10 lakh you will find it impossible to reach all of them even with the help of a large field force. Hence, marketing efforts are inevitably concentrated on representative-stratified samples of target doctors who are likely to yield higher prescriptions and profits. Geographically, these markets can be clubbed together depending on their rural or urban criteria.

By selecting such specific target markets, you can ensure concentrated efforts. It has been observed by many companies that they make a base town on the basis of target-market segmentation. Over a period of one or two years, that market starts yielding results. The moment competition notices this, they start appointing their MRs in the same market. As a result, the market gets overcrowded irrespective of its potential. Satara-Karad (Maharashtra), Rewa-Satna (MP), Eluru-Kakinada (AP), and Palghat-Trichur (Kerala) are a few examples where this has happened. You also may have observed this phenomenon at many other places.

4. Socio Economic Segmentation

Socioeconomic factors like disposable income, role of society in developing the lifestyles of individuals, industrialization, and so on, help us divide locations in clusters as the needs of customers become similar. Shahdol—a small town in MP where mines are predominant—has a different lifestyle of patients. The physicians available at Shahdol have also formed specific prescribing and dispensing habits.

Education is also an important factor. The prescription behavior of young doctors differ, depending on the university at which they have studied medical science, irrespective of their location of practice.

5. Psychographics

Based on market research, we can construct a doctor typology on the basis of psychographics. *Nine* types of doctors can be distinguished on the basis of such criteria.

(i) *Experimentalists:* Eager to try new drugs, they look at the pharmaceutical industry as a source of information and experiment confidently. Of course, they do this only when there is a low risk involved in prescribing or trying new drugs.

(ii) ***Progressive:*** Broad-minded doctors, who are keen to develop themselves, they tend to be positively disposed to clinical trials.

(iii) ***Hospital doctors/teaching staff:*** They are keen on formal methods of education (symposia, medical journals, postgraduate courses). They have a pronounced orientation towards generics and branded generics. They are not spontaneously driven to new drugs unless the hospital committee accepts new drugs.

(iv) ***Overstretched:*** Doctors are more demotivated than disillusioned when they feel overworked. They have little time for immersing themselves in scientific information about drugs. They tend to appreciate concise, sharp presentations of new drugs. They are generally above average prescribers of established drugs.

(v) ***The self-satisfied type:*** They have been successful and don't see why they should be involved for further formal education. They feel really good about themselves. They also can't work up the enthusiasm to do anything new!

(vi) ***The philanthropic type:*** They are always ready to help the society, through camps or other ways. Often, they are attached to trusts.

(vii) ***The commercial type:*** Everything in their practice is governed by commercial considerations. They will do almost anything to make money!

(viii) ***The undecided:*** They never decide on any prescription of any product by themselves. They always look for reinforcement from others.

(ix) ***The disillusioned:*** These are doctors who chose the profession for idealistic reasons but have become disillusioned by the environment. They look for new drugs as a means of contributing to the patients' health. They tend to be disappointed by existing drugs. This behavior has been observed among doctors who have come from abroad because of their liking for India as well as among these who come here to be with their families but cannot adjust to the social or professional environment.

6. Prescriber and Retailer Behavior

Several behavioral or attitudinal criteria of prescribers and retailers are responsible for the following segment possibilities.

(i) *Heavy-occasional prescribers:* We can segregate heavy prescribers from occasional ones, and scanty prescribers from those requiring extended treatment of two to three months. Several categories exist. Identifying doctors on this basis gives a direction to the sales force in their asking for prescriptions. Similarly, one can also focus on the scanty and light prescribers and try to convert them into the heavy prescriber group. It is easier to identify such doctors through Retail Chemist Prescription Audit (RCPA). There are doctors who even prescribe one tablet of Crocin at a time.

(ii) *Variety of users:* In a similar way, the market is segmented in terms of loyal and non-loyal prescribers. By focusing on doctors of both types, we can identify ex-users, potential users, existing users, first-time users, and repeat users. We can do the deal with them separately.

(iii) *Benefit-oriented:* Another approach involves segmenting the market in terms of the special benefits sought by the doctor population. This can be done by considering product-specific attributes, packaging, after use packs, different technologies like transdermal patches, and so on. Most benefits can be categorized in terms of fewer side-effects or more potency, or a combination of both. Other benefits have been developed and have become very successful. For example, oil-base topical ointment was converted into a cosmetic-base ointment with gentle fragrance. A telephone dial pack was developed for daily oral contraceptives to ensure its consumption without fail. Dispersible aspirin—Disprin—has created a history in Aspirin market. This approach, known as the benefit segmentation approach, is also the most appropriate basis of segmentation for brand positioning strategies (Wilkie and

Cohen, 1987). The approach, however, becomes difficult to implement for 'me-too' products.

(iv) *Readiness of prescribers:* A fourth approach consists in focusing on the stages of readiness of a prescriber. These stages might include awareness, liking, and intention. For example, you can segment the market into doctors who are aware of a particular drug and those who are not. The target segment could be those prescribers who are not aware of the product offering. Alternatively, you can choose, as a target segment, those doctors who have a relatively positive attitude towards the product but do not prescribe it, in the hope of converting them into prescribers.

(v) *Retailers:* Retailers can also be similarly divided into several categories:

- Those who buy regularly from one source such as appointed stockists
- Those who buy from multiple sources, i.e. from different stockists
- Those who buy from wholesales, stockists of the company, and other stockists
- Those who buy from other states as they can earn on price and tax differentials
- Those who are attached to doctors who prescribe
- Those who are attached to nursing homes/hospitals
- Those who operate both in the day and night and chain of retailers
- Those who have a chain of outlets

You can separate all these categories, and then handle them individually to maximize their support.

7. Brand Relationships—'The Inner Circle'

Many times it becomes easier to launch a line extension when we observe that a class of doctors has already established a relationship with one form. The product takes off quickly.

Similarly, it has also been observed that the known obliging doctors of an MR, can be classified in a group of 'inner circle' doctors for another MR. They can also help products to succeed.

TARGET-MARKET SELECTION

Once the market has been segmented, the choice of a viable segment is dependent on the following three key issues:

1. The marketing attractiveness of the target segment, size, growth, price sensitivity, and entry and existing costs.

2. The competitive dynamics in the proposed segment. How tough is the competition? How strongly do the competitors react to a new entrant? Is it feasible to carve out a niche in the market without strong retaliation from existing competitors

3. The strength of the strategic advantage for the target segment. In the drug industry, one often starts out with a product with given strengths and weaknesses. The task of target-market selection consists of searching for groups of customers for whom the product strengths can form the basis for a strategic competitive edge.

CASE

Nitravet[1]

Anglo-French (A.F.D.), a subsidiary of Hoffman-la-Roche, was known for its Beplex Forte group of products. The impact of market dynamics was weakening the organization year after year. The management, therefore, decided to introduce Mogadon—a sleep-inducing agent of Roche through A.F.D., since Roche was already promoting Valium and Librium (other benzodiazapines). Indian doctors were now in a dilemma as regards segregating tranquillizers, hypnotics and muscle relaxants. Now, it was risky to launch a new product like Mogadon and cannibalize on Valium. So A.F.D. decided to launch Mogadon (Nitrazepam) under the brand name of Nitravet in India. It was placed in Category Four (no price control) which gave it additional advantage.

Nitravet (5 mg) was launched in 1980, and even today, Nitravet is a leader in the 'hypnotic' market. Nitravet now is a major profit contributor of A.F.D., which has now been sold by Roche to the Kanoria group.

---

[1]*This case has been contributed by Interlink Marketing Consultancy Pvt. Ltd., Mumbai.*

The success of Nitravet during the launch period was due to its process of target-market selection and segmentation scheme.

When A.F.D. launched Nitravet for the first time in India, a majority of its field force was around 45 years. As A.F.D. was known for its Beplex Forte group, it was a familiar name to GPs. Otherwise, the field force did not enjoy any specific edge for its new product launch. However, A.F.D. drew its innate strength from the loyal GPs of the 45 + years age group.

Thus, GPs above 45 years were chosen along with orthopedics that used hypnotics for insomniac patients in general practice, and for inducing sleep after orthopedic surgery.

The basic sensitivity of GPs was carefully studied. By educating them on 'sleep patterns' and 'onset of action' of Nitravet, they were fully satisfied of the efficacy of the brand. A 'Nitravet pillow' was given as a gift to all those GPs who took up Nitravet, to act as an added incentive.

On the other side, sensitivity of orthopedics towards including sleep to the patients after surgery irrespective of disturbances of environmental impulses was studied in detail. And a separate information bulletin on trials was offered to them to make them feel confident about prescribing Nitravet to their patients after surgery.

Thus, although GPs and orthopedics were heterogeneous in nature, the benefits of Nitravet offerings were homogeneous. And the same segmentation scheme of sensitivity was applied to both.

The product was a terrific success. Nitravet continues to march ahead.

LEARNINGS

Apprehensions

Today, there are some reasons for the existing apprehensions regarding the segmentation approach:

Vision of those who wish to experiment

Faith in the segmentation approach

Practicability of the concept of segmentation

Disparity among customers

Commitment of the field force for this approach

You can overcome these apprehensions provided you decide to change the way of approaching segmentation. To begin with, you can start thinking from the customer's point of view.

Dilemma

There is a perceived dilemma between segmentation and positioning in pharmaceutical marketing. Many of us firmly believe that positioning is a luxury. In fact, segmentation can lead to correct positioning of your product. The purpose of segmentation is to develop a homogeneous group of responsive customers. Here, the focus is on customers and not on the product alone.

Methods of Segmentation

Seven different methods of segmenting the markets have been explained. All these are based on three major aspects:

Relationship of the customer/end-user and product usage

Related to characteristics of customers

Related to prescription/stocking behavior of customers

CHAPTER **8**

Positioning Towards Identity

Most of you would have heard the story of the shepherd boy who cried 'Wolf.' It goes like this. There was once a very naughty shepherd boy who used to take his herd of sheep to graze a little away from the village. One day wanting to play a trick on the villagers, he went a little further in the jungle alone and screamed. 'Help! . . . Help! . . . Wolf! . . . Wolf!'

On hearing his desperate cries, the villagers came to rescue him from the wolves. When they reached the boy, he laughed at them, and gloated over the fact that he had fooled them.

Three times the boy played the same mischief; and each time the villagers ran to his rescue. On the fourth day, a pack of wolves really entered the jungle and started approaching the boy and his sheep. The boy panicked and once again started screaming for help, this time in real fear. However, no one came forward from the village as all of them felt he was trying to make a fool of them again.

The villagers perceived the child to be a cheat, and hence, even when he was telling the truth, nobody believed him.

Positioning is usually a cumulative effect of small consistent activities which create positive or negative perceptions about a person or a product.

Only simple, appealing propositions which are consistently made can establish a strong 'positioning'. After all it's the 'perception' of the audience we are trying to appeal to. When Amitabh Bachhan took up the role in *Zanjeer*, it was not that he had decided he would be positioning himself in the minds of the public as an 'angry young man'. But he continued in the same gutsy vein in subsequent films for years together, and it was a matter of time before his fans accepted him only with that image. Things, however, became a little complicated much later, in *KhudaGawah*—people had difficulty in accepting the angry old man.

Surbex T of Abbott highlighted the need for a daily dose of 500 mg of Vitamin C. Even in those days, the daily requirement of Vitamin C was not more than 25 to 30 mg. However, the communication was so powerful that practically every doctor at that time prescribed Surbex T for patients suffering from Vitamin C deficiency.

Even today if you were to ask any one of those doctors about Surbex T, he would justify the need for 500 mg of Vitamin C. How does this kind of thing happen?

Some of you may have observed even healthy people taking Liv 52 tablets after a few pegs of whisky in the evening. Have you wondered why?

You will also find mothers giving Crocin to their children if they complain of body ache or feel feverish. Who told them to do so?

POSITIONING

Positioning is the process of establishing an object in the minds of the members of the target market in such a way that it is perceived to answer the needs of the market. Invariably, positioning refers to the identification and communication of differentiation or differential advantage.

If you start communicating a simple message consistently to the target audience, it has been observed that the product gets positioned. A good marketer does not rely on luck, hoping he would be perceived in the market as he would like it to. Instead, he carefully plans the position he wants his products to have in the minds of his customer.

Positioning can be achieved essentially by either communicating a 'differential' advantage of your product in relation to your competitor's, or by establishing a 'relative uniqueness' for your product. We will discuss both these concepts briefly below.

DIFFERENTIATION

While differentiating a product, we should see that it provides one or more key observable and measurable benefits which satisfy *four* fundamental criteria:

- The benefit differentiates the product from all others, creating a perception of uniqueness
- It is important, or can be made to seem important, to the target segment
- It is sustainable, over time, against competition
- Its qualities are easily measurable and observable by the prescriber or user

Each of these factors is vital to establish a viable positioning for any product.

Government regulations can sometimes prove to be obstacles to making claims in support of a pharmaceutical product. They can then affect a specific positioning strategy. To cite an example, an antibiotic like Tetracycline was not supposed to be given to children less than 10 years of age because it caused discoloration of teeth. Communications issued by the government constantly highlighted this message, and as a result, the positioning of Tetracycline was affected. In general, pharmaceutical trade guidelines laid down by the government are rather strict. However, there is still sufficient room for a variety of effective positioning strategies.

RELATIVE UNIQUENESS

Relative uniqueness is the perceived uniqueness of a brand in relation to its immediate competitors which may come from the brand's intrinsic qualities or processes, or just from communication to the customers. In case of Doxy-I (USV), this relative uniqueness was brought in deliberately. There were very few competitors when it was launched in 1977-78. As a new molecule, however, the product had no uniqueness. It was promoted by many as a one-a-day (OD) antibiotic. It did not work when USV started promoting it as an 'Improved Tetracycline' which provided relative uniqueness in dosage, over tetracycline and other intrinsic factor like a drug of choice for Bronchitis, Sinusitis brought success to Doxycycline.

Relative uniqueness, or rather 'perceived' relative uniqueness, is a product's only protection against generic or commodity status. In the pharmaceutical industry, relative uniqueness in most cases is related to the intrinsic as well as extrinsic qualities of the product itself. For example, the developed technology of sustained release theophylline could be an intrinsic quality. And the price of such a product could be its extrinsic quality, helping it get an edge over other theophyllines—either branded or generic.

The search for relative uniqueness for a product is often a primary task of both the marketing as well as R&D departments. Considering their interdependence, it is important that marketing and R&D or Design and Development (D&D) go hand in hand, with product differentiation becoming increasingly difficult. The need for interaction of these two disciplines has become imperative for providing a strategic edge to an organization in terms of positioning.

Relative uniqueness, value for money, relevance, and importance distinguish one product from another. A listing of all the features a product offers without this classification does not constitute product positioning. A feature becomes relatively unique only if it is perceived to be special by the customer or user. The creation of this value is the final objective of positioning.

ROLE OF ORGANIZATIONAL STRATEGY AND RESOURCES

Analyze Competition along with your Strengths

While positioning any product, the knowledge of the company's resources, commitments, and organizational strategy as well as the strategies of its competitors and their strengths is vital. It is also important to have an idea of the ease with which the company can nullify the competitor's strategy. Patent-protected drugs are the safest in competition. However, generics can pose a threat in such a situation. At the other extreme, price advantages are short-lived in mature product categories where prescription patterns are stable and product specifications are already standardized.

Sustainable Positioning

The basis for defensible positioning results from a company possessing unique skills, resources and distinctive capabilities that set it apart from its competitors. These skills may include special R&D capabilities, specialized knowledge of doctors' needs, or a privileged relationship with the trade or customers. Any of these can form the basis of a sustainable positioning strategy.

Superior resources could be in terms of financial structure, production capacity, ownership of raw material sources, long-term supply contracts, or corporate image. Thus, the art of formulating a sustainable positioning strategy lies in taking advantage of the opportunities provided by the relative strengths, skills and resources of the company.

Few years ago, Epro, a sister concern of Marico, developed a unique anti-hypertensive from natural oil—Primrose oil, which was then clinically tested by the National Institute of Nutrition, Hyderabad. Rigorous testing proved it to be an excellent remedy to lower hypertension. However, it was soon found that the entire cultivation could offer relief to a meager one lakh patients in India per annum, which meant that there was practically no sustainable advantage. Unless the company can develop a synthetic oil through R&D, it will not be able to turn the situation to its advantage.

Use Limited Features for Positioning

Claims, well supported by clinical trials, are often not taken seriously or perceived as important by the prescriber. Competing companies may make the same claims on the basis of suitable research studies or references. A laundry list of claims, on the basis of evidence provided from a plethora of clinical trials, is used to position a product in many cases. The implicit assumption is that the more the claims, the better are the chances of success for the product.

This is not necessarily true. Prescribers, although well-educated and intelligent, are also human beings and suffer, as do all of us, from limitations in their capacity to process information. A clear positioning, i.e. association of relative advantage with the product, is often more easily achieved with a limited number, say two or three, well-considered product benefits, and not an exhaustive list of product features. In the end, a product tends to get defined by its features, while, as you know, its acceptance is determined by its benefits.

Again, if a product has a strong relative advantage which is not protected by a patent, competitors will try to copy the same advantage or make it appear less important. Hence, the task of marketing is to defend, reinforce or renew the existing relative advantages of established products, and try and preempt counter-attacks by competition. This is where competition dynamics come into play. Erythromycin and Cifran are examples of one or two specific benefits being well perceived by prescribers. There is no need to enumerate several features to reinforce the utility of these brands.

Corporate Positioning

Although the main emphasis in the pharmaceutical industry is on product positioning, corporate positioning also plays an important role (Kotler, 1986). Creating and reinforcing a favorable overall positioning for a pharmaceutical company is important to *six* different target groups:

1. **Prescribers and Patients**

   To the extent that the prescription and usage of medicines involves some risk on the part of both the prescriber and the patient, a favorable company image can develop credibility and trust and serve as an important risk-reduction mechanism. Developing a company's relationship with doctors, in contrast to a reputation for hard-selling and promotion, is recognized by many companies as a worthwhile long-term investment. In Italy, unlike India where a variety of practices prevail for wooing doctors, the perceived trend has been towards unethical 'buying' of doctors.

2. **Retailers, Wholesalers, and Stockists**

   They play an important role in converting prescriptions into actual sales. Since they put in considerable investments and resources in companies, they need to be cultivated and their interests protected.

3. **Stock Market**

   The global company image is an important factor according to which players in the stock market assess the value of a company's stock. This is important to the company's shareholders, and can be crucial in the case of potential mergers, capital expansions, and takeovers. Financial muscle further helps companies provide better drugs to patients.

4. **FDA, DCI Government and Regulatory Agencies**

   Obtaining a favorable overall image in the minds of the relevant government bodies is of crucial importance to pharmaceutical companies in getting speedy regulatory approvals.

5. **Special Interest Groups**

   Unions and consumer organizations are two examples of special interest groups that should be addressed by corporate positioning to avoid or prevent actions on their part that might hinder the company's operations. This can be done by communicating the values of an organization to partners and patients. A platform to exchange ideas can be evolved. Mediware from Lupin, Sandoz Times from Sandoz, Wockhardt Times from Wockhardt, and Mediscene from Kopranare examples where a dialogue had been established with the customers.

6. **Employees**

    Corporate positioning is an important vehicle for improving the loyalty of current employees, and for attracting the best new employees from a competitive executive market.

The substance of corporate positioning depends on the target market, and includes information on the company's experience, safety record, its image as an innovator, its specialization and leadership position in specific therapeutic areas, and its commitment to basic research and development or other aspects of business. The corporate image of a company is the net result of all the experience, impressions, feelings, and knowledge that people have about a company. Corporate position building is often most visible in journal advertising, but to be effective it is important to promote to coherent image through all media inclusive of press coverage, and the behavior of the management must match with those exposures.

TYPES OF PRODUCT POSITIONING

Traditionally, positioning strategies in the pharmaceutical industry have been exclusively built around the 'technical aspects' of the product. Nowadays, at least in India, it would not be incorrect to say that a large number of new pharmaceutical products do not have a real relative advantage based on the product itself. It is becoming vitally important to broaden the concept of the product in order to create greater scope for alternative relative advantages. A 'breakthrough' new product (e.g. a cure for breast cancer) will surely have a strong and clear-cut differential advantage. But introducing a 'me-too' product is what poses a much greater challenge to the marketing specialist. In the case of Piroxicam as well as Tinidazole, Pfizer was successful in positioning its products although it was perhaps the last to enter the Indian market. In Indian market we can position pharmaceutical products using *ten* different approaches. These approaches can be classified into *four* major areas.

1. Product attributes, galenical forms, life-cycles and function-related
2. Customer and end-user related

3. Competition related
4. Marketing-mix related

1. Natural Positioning

Natural positioning is when a brand is positioned using a specific product property to match a deeply felt, unmet need of doctor or patient. So what 'natural position' could the aforementioned antihypertensive have aimed for? Among the product's dominating secondary benefits was greater renal safety. And that, as physicians realize but rarely articulate, is an unmet need. There are many doctors who worry about compromising the renal function of their hypertensive patients while treating them. Overall, the number of hypertensive patients who are at renal risk is perhaps only one-tenth of the patients in the broad category. So why lower one's sight? How can one justify relinquishing the chance of capturing a big share of the elephantine mild-to-moderate market?

Well, initially, ensuring trials of such new drugs is essential to elicit customer response. And that is what sharp positioning does.

The range of indications for the drug can always be widened later on, when the brand has established its credibility and the doctor is seen willing to explore new uses.

Most pharmaceutical products go through the above path till stage 5 (Figure 8.1). The idea of unmet needs hasn't yet entered. Unmet needs range from specific product benefits to lack of side effects, drug interactions, drug's profile will include parameters like effectiveness, side effects, toxicity, tolerance, drug interactions, compatibility, and so on. Devising a strategy based on these is important. Yet most organizations skip stage 6 and go straight to stages 8 and 9, and then on to stage 11. They miss the benefits of natural positioning. Let's look at what natural positioning does.

(i) *Lowers barriers, increases acceptance:* Physicians are usually traditional and do not switch well-managed patients to new therapies. They evaluate a drug positioned to compete with long-time favorites far more strictly. However, a naturally positioned drug speaks of unmet therapeutic needs, and gets more attention.

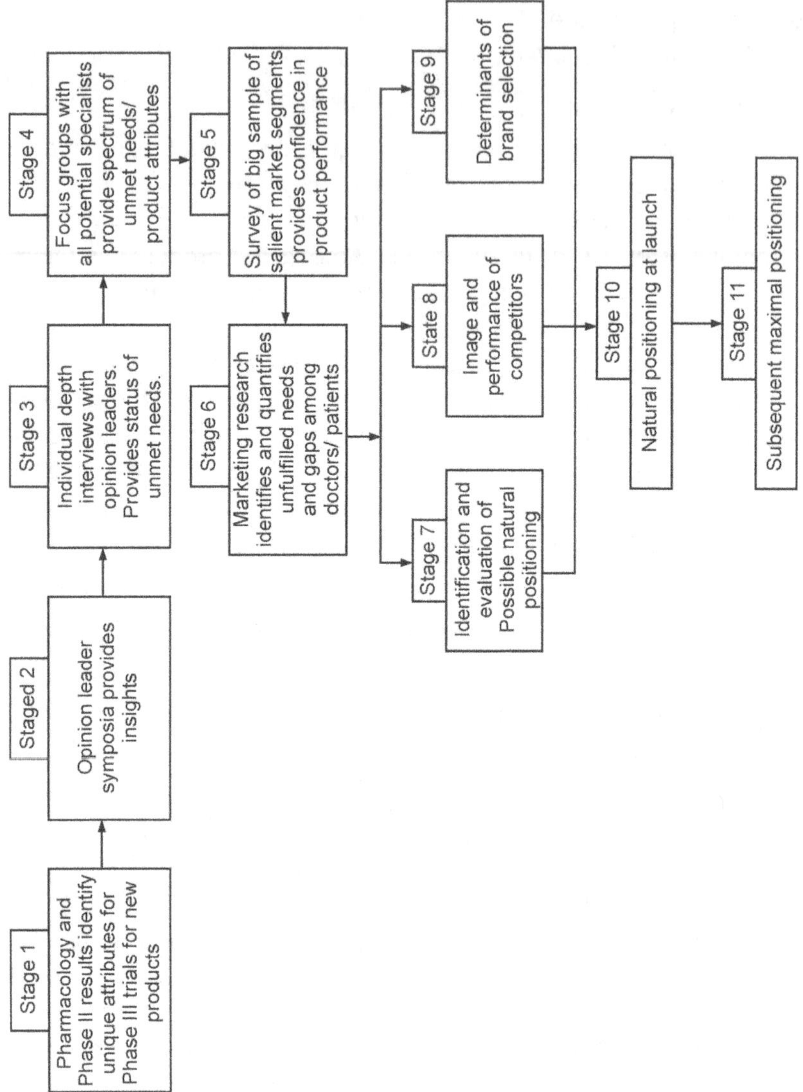

Figure 8.1 The path of natural positioning

This is even more so in a category constrained by unavoidable side effects. For instance, Asprin is a standard anti-rheumatic but it results in blood loss if taken regularly. Though relatively tolerable, all other anti-rheumatics (Brufen, Voveran and so on) also produce side effects. Given this market scenario, any new product which talks about reducing the agony of patients, and does so, will be warmly welcomed.

(ii) ***Reduces the cost of launch:*** In most cases, natural positioning strategies cost less to execute. The communication reaches a focused target.

(iii) ***Raises product credibility***: If a drug promises what it can deliver, it wins the faith of doctors. Chloromycetin and Cifran proved themselves as typhoid treatments. Both are useful for many other indications.

(iv) ***Resolves apprehensions of doctors and patients***: Those who suffer from ulcers and rheumatism present doctors with a problem. A category of drugs effective for rheumatism has the potential of aggravating ulcers. A product to solve this problem, and positioned as such, will find a huge market immediately.

(v) ***Reduces price sensitivity***: It is evident that a specialized agent in demand is a premium over a me-too. A breast cancer drug can fetcha higher market price than a general one that acts on a variety of tumors.

(vi) ***Builds base for better penetration***: A strategy that gives the product a natural position in the specialist's mind can be followed up with an effort to encourage general physicians to try it. In pharmaceutical products, specialists can influence general practitioners.

(vii) ***Gains cooperation from regulators and the government:*** Reporting on well-targeted and well-documented trials for specific needs is likely to get prompt FDA approval. On the other hand, seeking labeling for a host of indications could prolong the procedure.

(viii) ***Boosts profits***: Since the marketing program is more efficient, you can expect a higher profit margin for the first few months than would be possible with a strategy that seeks a big market slice straightaway.

2. Positioning with Respect to Use or Application

'Once-a-day' is a favorite positioning approach. Feldene (Pfizer) in the international market and Pirox (Cipla) in India were positioned as the first once-a-day, non-steroidal, anti-inflammatory drugs for arthritis. Aten (Kopran), Tenormin (Torrent), Presolar (Cipla), and

Betacard (Torrent) entered the Atenelol market by offering cardioselectivity among available betablockers. They were the second to offer the once-a-day regimen. However, their differential advantage lay in cardioselectivity and once-a-day convenience. Drugs may also be positioned as first-line, second-line or third-line therapies.

A broad range of galenical forms can also be grouped under this type of positioning strategy. A good example is that of Wockadine which was first introduced as an antiseptic in the form of 100-ml solution. An ointment form was released later for cuts and wounds; the jar followed for acute burns and then came the gargles for night-time relief. Finally, it was given to surgeons to scrub their hands before surgery.

3. **Positioning with Respect to the End-User (Type of Patient)**

Drugs have great flexibility. They can be positioned as most appropriate for minor or major degrees of a disease, acute or chronic sufferers, adults or children, old or young, for a particular ethnic group, or even as an adjuvant to treatment. Although it may be tempting to target all possible markets, a more disciplined focusing often helps establish a particular drug in the mind of a prescriber for a specific alternative, even if it is eventually going to be used in a wider range of cases. At the same time, another viable approach would be to aim for a broad spectrum of applications.

In the international market, when GSK launched Zinetac as the second H_2antagonist, rather than taking Smith Kline's Tagamet head-on, it defined a broader patient target. To carry out this strategy, a larger sales force was required, which was provided through an agreement with Roche for the US market. In effect, GSK managed in flank rather than attack Tagamet, and succeeded in significantly expanding its market.

In contrast, in Indian Zinetac did not face any opposition from Cemetidine. However, they had to really work hard to overcome the competition from Omeprazole in a systematic way.

The ACE-inhibitors Capoten (Bristol-Myers Squibb) and Aceten (Wockhardt) developed the market segment catering to patients with severe hypertension.

4. **Positioning with Respect to a Competitor**

   The differential advantage can sometimes best be established, be explicitly or implicitly taking the competition as a reference point. This is a useful way to piggy-back on the good image of a competitive product while adding a plus. Combiflam of Roussel is a good example of riding the image of a competitor. Roussel positioned Combiflam after Brufen of Boots (an analgesic) but enhanced its image by adding paracetamol.

5. **Positioning with Respect to a Product Class**

   Inderal (betablocker), Cifran (antibiotic), Daonil (antidiabetic), Zinetac (H_2 antagonist), and Aceten (ACE inhibitor), were positioned as the first drugs in their respective new product classes.

6. **Positioning with Respect to Marketing-Mix Variables**

   Price is one of the key variables in positioning generic products as well as branded products. As mentioned before, different parts of the marketing mix can be used to give the product a distinct slot in the mind of its target audience.

   Packaging could be another variable. Packaging in India is outdated. Much work needs to be done to take advantage of this factor. Many new options have opened up today. Probably, limited margins have not allowed companies to have fancy packaging for their products. (In fact, cartons were discontinued for most products in the 1980s). But cost-effective products can revolutionize markets. For example, the use of specially designed dial-shaped oral contraceptive packs enhances utility—the customer does not forget to take her tablets, being able to see each of them from outside on the dial. Perhaps the next ten years will see this variable being fully exploited.

   The *size and quality* of the field force could be the third variable capable of giving an important and sustainable edge to a product. Ranbaxy demonstrated this with Cifran by creating a distinct image, while Searle tried to achieve similar results by effective co-marketing with GSK for Equal. Elders capitalized on a talented sales force, by licensing-in good products from other international companies.

   Hospital-related and health-care pharmaceutical products pursue positioning strategies based on instant delivery, frequent-buying patterns, and custom-made service, as Royal Chemists in Mumbai have been doing.

7. **Positioning Based on Appeal to the Senses**

An attractive design making a favorable visual impact, a pleasant smell and taste, smoothness of powder, and an attractive brand name appeal to our five senses. We can position our products by using any one of these 'sense-appealing' alternatives.

A novel method was used to promote an old product, Citralka (an alkaliser). It was shown that red litmus paper dipped in it turned blue. This illustrated the fact that although it acted as an alkaliser, Citralka was acidic in nature. It was important for it not to be alkaline, since the stomach is acidic. (When the medium is acidic you must give a compatible product.) On the strength of such demonstrations, Citralka established itself as a compatible product for the stomach, and was readily accepted as a cure for burning micturition and other acidic disorders common in summer. This activity was carried out in clinics by MRs to position Citralka— although it was acidic in nature it could relieve burning micturition.

Hematinics like Dexorange and RB Tone, were promoted by reinforcing flavour, odour, and taste.

The 'micro fineness' of particles of an active ingredient (like sodium chromoglycate) was demonstrated by opening the capsule in the presence of doctors, who were requested to feel the smoothness of the powder, by touching it. It was important to provide extreme fineness to the product as it was to be inhaled by asthma patients.

GSK successfully used another technique in-clinic by incorporating a telephone number in the visual aid. The number indicated the dosage schedule of one of their products, for example, the number 65432 would indicate six tablets for day 1, five for day 2, and so on.

All these are in-clinic activities. Hence, the MRs need to be trained meticulously to ensure desired impact and differentiation.

8. **Positioning based on Outside-the Clinic Activities**

Public demonstrations helped establish products such as Ferradol and Protinex (Pfizer). The MRs were asked to prepare milk shakes at street corner for physicians and patients. In many physicians' conferences, these demonstrations were carried out successfully to remind them of Ferradol, and also its likeable taste.

9. **Positioning based on Products Life-Cycle States**

   A classic example would be the way Brufen shielded its market share by continuously shifting its positioning from anti-rheumatic to anti-inflammatory to analgesic, and even focusing on its low antipyretic action, as it progressed in its life-cycle.

10. **Positioning by Galenical Form**

    In India, patients and even a certain class of doctors are of the view that a drug in the injectable form provides speedier relief as compared to oral administration. Even among oral forms, capsules are perceived to have greater strength than tablets, while liquids are supposed to be only meant for geriatric and pediatric cases. And usually pessaries are not commonly used in India owing to cultural taboos.

INNOVATIVE POSITIONING APPROACHES

There can be *seven* possible approaches, as described below.

1. **Bringing about a Paradigm Shift in the Minds of Doctors**

   Cadila brought about a change in the mindset of doctors by using hemoglobin powder for the first time in its product Haem-up. Earlier, all hemoglobin preparations had the image of being a blood-product.

   Zedex, a cough suppressant from Tridoss, introduced the idea of a non-antihistamine cough syrup changing the paradigm that a cough preparation had to have an antihistamine in it.

   A shift to the use of beta-blockers from the traditional antihypertensive treatment involving Serpentina was brought about by ICI through Inderal.

   Basically, these shifts in paradigms were brought about by replacing existing beliefs or attitudes with new ones.

2. **Continuity of Therapeutic Group for Different Target Patients**

   A company can have a series of products in one therapeutic group in an attempt to hold on to several segments with one product category and different brands. This approach involves a risk, but the possible benefits can be very tempting. In such a situation, it is important to adopt an appropriate multiple-segment strategy involving different segments simultaneously.

A good example is that of Parke-Davis who introduced products in the B-complex and multivitamin therapy category by launching Abdec for infants, Paladac for children and adolescents, Myadec for adults, Natabec for pregnant women, and finally, Myadec C for old patients. Torrent too launched a number of cardio-vascular products for diverse patients by hypertension with varying complications.

3. Confronting the Competition

At one point, Ampicillin with its unique cost-effectiveness had almost driven out other competitors. Even, Amoxycillin took a lot of time to come anywhere near it. Of course, openly denigrating competition is generally ill-advised in view of the risk of adverse reaction. But within limits, weaknesses which opposition may have can be brought to the target's notice and used in easy way competition.

You can also compare competitive products to your own to establish the distinct cases in which your various products may be considered ideal.

Oil- or alcohol-based ointments were improved by using a cream base instead to enhance their relative quality. Manufacturers of skin ointments also use this method to differentiate their products.

Relative price difference is observed in paracetamol brands. For instance, generic paracetamolis available at ₹ 0.7 per tablet where in Crocin costs ₹ 1.06 per tablet.

4. 'Me-too' Positioning

Developing relative quality and relative price is the key issue for any generic or 'me-too' brand. Many such products have captured regional markets and put a check on nation-wide brands.

5. Carry on Business (COB)

Brands without patent protection confronted with generic competition always face a dilemma: Should they reduce their price (i.e. re-position towards the competition on the price dimension), and if so, by how much? Or should they become defensive and lose their share?

Ciprofloxacin manufacturers and marketers were at a crossroads, as the prices are dropping almost every second month. All of them were facing a dilemma. Should they follow others, or take a lead, and drop the price further? Or, were they to carry on their business and take what comes? Marketers of Roxithromycin and Diclofenac were also facing the same dilemma.

The best way to deal with such a situation is to hold on to the target market or segment, and slowly provide relative uniqueness to them at the same price keeping the same quality. This takes time, but works.

6. **Commercial Edge Positioning**

   In India, the three-way price war involving Band-aid (Johnson & Johnson), Hansaplast (Beiersdorf), and Dettol Plaster (Reckitt Benckiser) led to an interesting situation. The maximum beneficiaries were the wholesalers and dealers as they obtained products at about ₹ 0.30 per plaster and sold at a price of ₹ 0.75 per plaster, which made for a huge margin of profit. This shows how organizations lose out when they focus all their attention on wholesalers alone.

7. **Positioning through Mnemonics**

   This is a very different positioning slant. All the activities are related to project a 'mnemonic' as a reminder of a brand. All the benefits are projected through the mnemonic. Over a period of time, the mnemonic directly provides for brand recall. Anacin is an excellent example for providing brand recall with four spread-out fingers. Trika is another brand from Unichem which used this positioning method to establish itself.

MEASURING PRODUCT POSITIONING

For developing a sound positioning strategy it is important to measure the current position of the products already in the market. The process of measuring product positioning involves three steps:

1. Identifying the perceived relative value in terms of product offerings
2. Determining how competitive product offerings are perceived vis-a-vis your product (perceived uniqueness)
3. Determining how the target market evaluates these value-based product offerings (importance)

1. **Identifying the Perceived Relative Value in Terms of Products Offerings**

   Listing the product offerings that compete with each other is often more difficult than it appears to be (Day, Shocker and Srivastava,

1979). For example, aspirin is prescribed for headaches, migraine, premenstrual pain, as a preventive for heart attacks, and for several other common conditions. Does not include aspirin (and other aspirin-like drugs) in the definition of the market for each of these conditions?

In most cases, there will be a primary group of competitors and one or more secondary groups.

One approach to this definition of market boundary is to get hold of a list of appropriate drugs for each condition. A good market research organization can do this for you. Managers do not always find this a satisfactory solution since certain drugs are prescribed for several conditions and the data may not list all the drugs for all conditions for which they are prescribed. However it can provide you the list of relevant drugs.

A second approach is the development of product-condition associations. A sample of prescribers might be asked to recall the condition for which a certain brand was last prescribed. This can be done through a qualitative or quantitative study, or a combination of both. For each condition, prescribers are then asked to identify all the brands they consider appropriate.

These two approaches suggest a conceptual basis for identifying the competitive environment of products. One of the Indian organizations did try to explore this second approach to redefine positioning of its hematinic in the existing competitive market.

2. **Determining Product Offering Perceptions—Perceived Uniqueness**

Objective characteristics of the competing brands can be determined from objective product information. The perception of these brands by the target market is, however, far more difficult to measure.

Doctors are constantly besieged by various stimuli from competing products in the form of literature, samples, gifts, special offers, advertising, calls by representatives, and so on. And given their own background and experience, individual doctors perceive the various product offerings in their own way. Limited exposure, selective and distorted perceptions, limited memory, and limited information-processing capacity mean that vital gaps develop between the objective facts and the subjective perceptions of the product offerings. Predetermined images such as the 'halo' of a particular company can severely bias product perceptions.

The perceptual nature of positioning complicates the measurement process, because subjective, cognitive constructs are more difficult to measure and compare than the objective physical characteristics of a product. This is for two reasons: one, because objective features are specific, and two, because they can be measured unambiguously. However, perceptions are, by definition, subjective and differ from one prescriber or patient to the next, owing to personal idiosyncrasies and experience, and change over time as the result of many influences, including the activities of the competitors, such as the launch of a competing product.

A number of methods have been developed to help capture the perceptions of products. Broadly defined: they fall into two categories: compositional and decompositional methods.

Compositional methods are based on the belief that prescribers can decompose their perceptions of brands into separate attributes and can evaluate each of the brands on the basis of these attributes. This can lead to a method like semantic scales (Wilkie and Pessemier, 1973).

Although used frequently in the pharmaceutical industry, this method has significant weaknesses. First, is the risk of omitting important attributes from the analysis. For instance, in the case of cancer therapy, 'nausea and vomiting' and 'restlessness' might be important attributes in the context of the therapy as a whole but may not be considered in the analysis of a product. Although one can never solve this problem entirely, methods do exist to reduce this type of error. One approach for creating an exhaustive list of attributes is to ask prescribers to identify the two most similar brands from a set of three competing brands, and to explain why those two brands are similar and different from the third. This exercise is repeated with all combinations of brands so that it becomes likely that all significant differentiating attributes are then likely to be revealed. An alternative approach consists of asking prescribers which of the two brands they prefer and why. As this is done repeatedly for all combinations of brands, it becomes unlikely that important criteria are missing.

The second problem is in a sense a result of the first: the methods cited for generating an exhaustive list of attributes usually produce lists of such length as to make them impractical, and which include many overlapping attributes that really refer to the same underlying concept. Logic and judgment or statistical methods (e.g. factor analysis) can subsequently be used to reduce these redundancies. In general, doctors use few characteristics (between two and five) to discriminate between competing brands. It is often difficult to identify these crucial dimensions directly from the doctor.

Third, the semantic differential method assumes that the doctor can decompose the brands into a set of attributes, and that while evaluating a brand, he (or she) integrates all that information. Psychological research, however, tends to show that such a model is often unrealistic and that the semantic differential approach might not be an appropriate method for capturing doctor's perceptions of competing brands.

Decomposition methods are generally better adapted to dealing with the perceptual measurement problem. These methods are based on the idea that people have global perceptions of objects, which they are not necessarily able to decompose.

The first step in such an analysis is to identify the positions of the products relative to each other, and then, as the second step, to infer the underlying dimensions which span the global perceptions. Perceptual maps, as a typical decomposition method, use as their input, the doctor's global comparisons between competing brands. Subsequently, they try to represent these global perceptions graphically, via a perceptual map (Green et al., 1988).

	A	**B**	**C**
Similarity	Benadryl	Solvin	Zedex
Soothing	+++	+	+++
Cough suppressing activity	+++	++	+++
Taste	Palatable	Palatable	Palatable
Similarity	AB	BC	AC
Soothing	4	4	5
Cough Suppressing acitivity	6	6	8
Taste	4	5	6

Figure 8.2 Perceptual map for three brands of cough syrups

An example will help illustrate this concept. Suppose you want to understand the relative positionings of three brands of cough syrups, such as Benadryl, Solvin, and Zedex:

The starting point of the analysis would be to ask the prescribers how they perceive the similarities among these three brands. The question can be posed in terms of overall similarities and not in terms of similarities with regard to specific attributes (Figure 8.2). Three comparisons have to be made: AB, AC, and BC. Suppose a scale of 1 to 9 is used, where 1 implies very similar and 9 implies very dissimilar perceptions. Also, suppose the similarity judgements are given as in Figure 8.3.

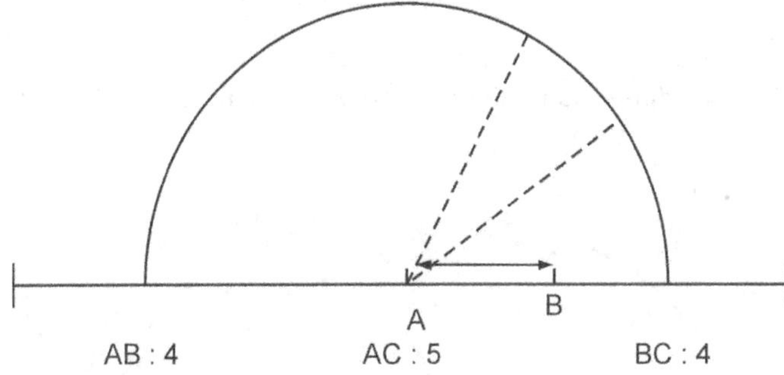

Figure 8.3 Similarity judgements

The simplest graphical representation of these similarities would be in a one-dimensional space, i.e. on a line. If A is arbitrarily located in the middle of the line, B should be at a distance of 4 (either to the right or the left of A). Now, C has to be located at a distance of 5 from A and also 4 units from B. It is clear that these two constraints cannot be satisfied if C is placed on the line. This implies that the given similarities cannot be represented in one dimension. Therefore, at least two attributes (dimensions) must be important to the prescribers to differentiate between A, B, and C. If BC were 1, then one dimension (attitude) would have been sufficient.

A solution is, however, possible in two-dimensional space. B must lie on a circle around A with a radius of 4. Similarly, C must lie on a circle of radius 5, around A (Figure 8.4).

If you choose a point B on B's circle, C must lie on a circle of radius 4 centered at this point. You can then find satisfactory locations for C by choosing the two points of intersection of appropriate circles (Figure 8.5). Of course, these points are not unique. You could rotate the positions of B and C in an infinite number of ways (e.g. by turning the sheet of paper).

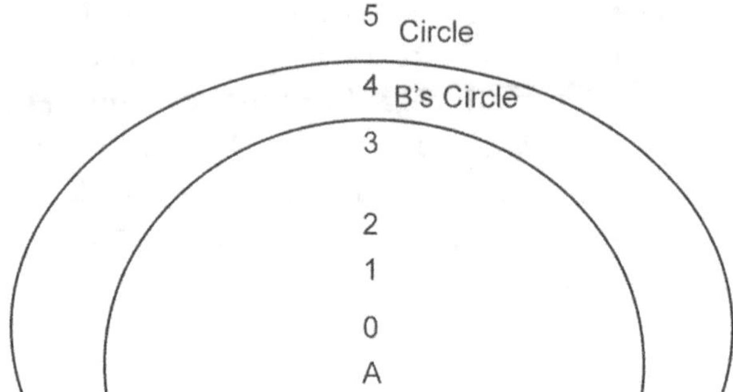

Figure 8.4 Two-dimensional solutions to overall similarities of three brands

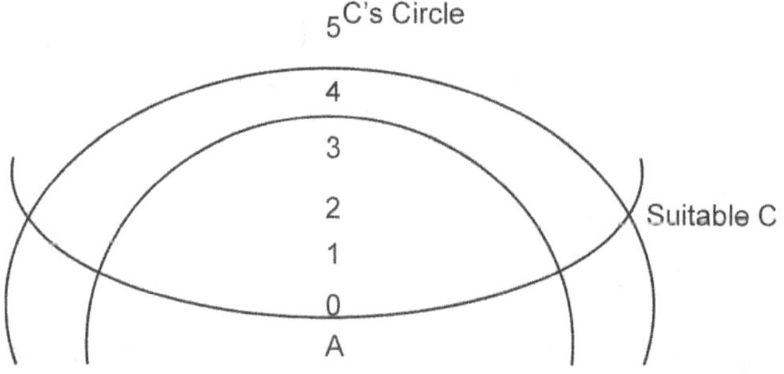

Figure 8.5 Suitable locations for C

If more than three brands have to be positioned, the task becomes progressively more complicated and special computer programs are necessary to deal with the complexity. The principle, however, is exactly the same as with three brands.

A variety of mapping techniques have been developed, such as the multi-dimensional scaling techniques, to deal with the complications which arise with higher dimensionality, and the interested reader will find a detailed discussion of the methods in marketing research literature (Green and Tull et al., 1988).

Such a competitive map is extremely useful for understanding market dynamics. These maps can also help in deriving the underlying dimensions (attributes) that differentiate the prescribers' product perceptions. This identification is subjective and is done as follows. On the horizontal the order of the brands as one goes from left to right is C, A, B, E, G, D, and F. In the vertical dimension, from top to bottom, the order is A, E, B, C, D, F and G. What are the attributes that might classify the brands in such an order? Perhaps, we can call the horizontal dimension 'potency' and the vertical, 'side-effects'.

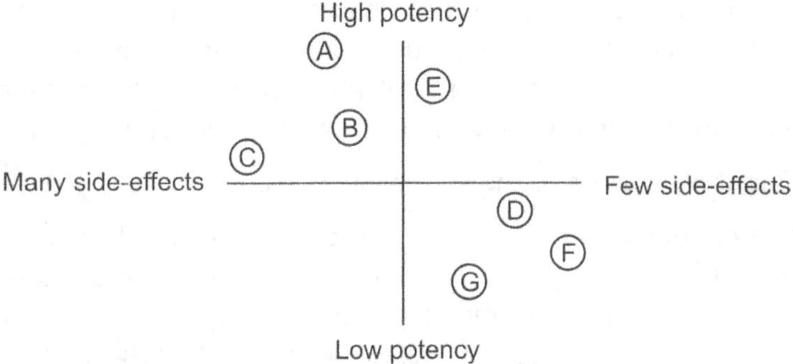

Figure 8.6 A competitive perceptual map

This interpretation is necessarily subjective, and therefore, introduces some bias. This is inherent in the method because we started with the idea that doctors have global views of the product offerings. Therefore, these global views have to be then reconstructed and decomposed to derive the implicit salient attributes. Once the important discriminating attributes are identified, perceptual maps can be a useful vehicle for the positioning and repositioning of product offerings.

If you want to develop a product that can compete with the successful product E, you can see from the perceptual map that the new product has to be positioned as a drug product having high potency, with average-to-low side-effects. You can plot the perceptions of physicians of varying positioning statements concerning a proposed new product on such a map, to guide your future communication strategy.

Furthermore, you can use perceptual maps to identify gaps in the market that can be potentially useful for the positioning of a new product or for the repositioning of existing products.

Perhaps prescribers are not interested in a particular area of the perceptual map, but interested in such gap like lesser side-effects, speed of action, etc. where an opportunity exists. In this manner, perceptual maps can be useful for uncovering strategic windows in the market.

Finally, perceptual maps can be a useful instrument for monitoring the evolution of the positioning of competing brands over time. By deriving perceptual maps at different points in time, you can trace how the prescribers' perceptions change over time. You can also check the success of repositioning exercises for existing brands by analyzing perceptual maps before and after the repositioning.

3. Target-Market Evaluation of Product Positions

The target-market evaluation of the positions of different product offerings is a crucial step in studying positioning. How important are the perceptual dimensions and what is the ideal product for the target market? Your answers to these questions will depend on how you measure the prescribers' perceptions.

Perceptual maps can provide some insight into the question of the ideal product. The concept of an 'ideal product' can be introduced into the data collection for perceptual maps in the same way as any other existing brand. Based on the similarity rating of each existing brand with the prescribers' ideal product, the ideal product can be located on the perceptual map in the same way as an existing brand. The ideal brand derived via perceptual maps refers to a 'realistic ideal'. The prescriber is not asked to describe his ideal product, but to compare all existing brands to his ideal brand. Some of the existing brands will be located closer to the ideal than others. This is a realistic approach, and has considerable intuitive appeal.

Perceptual maps can also be used to derive the relative importance of the salient perceptual attributes; for instance, in the case used for illustration (Figure 8.7), potency and side-effects. Special techniques (e.g. PREFMAP, Green et al., 1988) exist to superimpose iso-preference curves on perceptual maps. These iso-preference curves encircle the ideal point (or points) and indicate that all brands located on the curve have the same level of appeal to the prescriber.

All these three basic techniques—perceptual mapping, preferences, and target-market evaluation for understanding communication of brands—provide us clarity of positioning by helping us evaluate our basic statements of positioning.

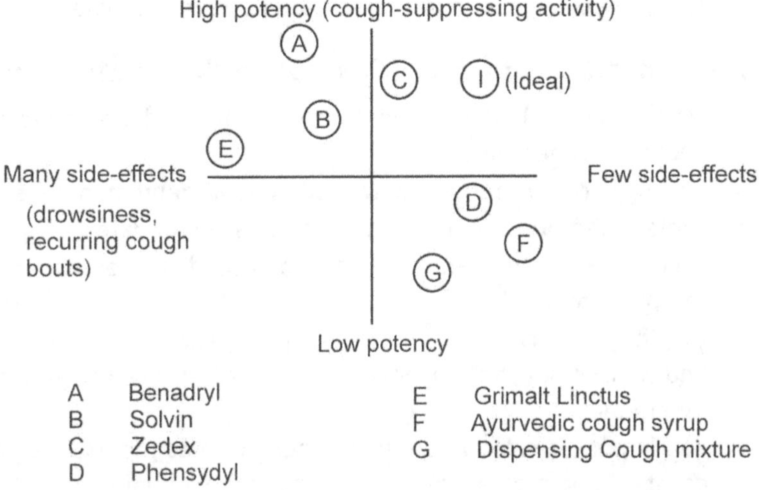

Figure 8.7 Perceptual maps for identifying relative importance of salient attributes

---

CASE

Using a Mnemonic for Positioning—The Story of Trika*[1]

The brand name Trika is an acronym for 'Triozolo benzodiazepine for calming anxiety'.

The following were the salient product features of the product Trika:

- Anxiolytic agent: calming effect
- Triozolo Benzodiazepine: pharmacologically unique over Diazepam/Lorazepam
- Usage: In case of anxiety, and for agitated and restive patients; in anxiety associate with depression; and in panic disorders

---

[1]*This case has been contributed by Mr. A.K. Jain, Former Executive Director, Unichem Laboratories ltd. and Dr. L. Ramaswamy, Managing Director, Sotax India Pvt. Ltd.*

The Mnemonic: Monarch Butterfly Resting on Fingertip

- Large aggressive butterfly depicted resting on a finger tip
- Symbolizes sunny carefree days full of tranquility, elegance, and poise
- Thus, the product and mnemonic are perfectly matched

Activities Undertaken to Establish the Butterfly as a Mnemonic

- Mailers dispatched with the 'butterfly' logo and a detailed story about the mnemonic
- Visiting cards with the butterfly logo for MRs and managers
- Large mnemonic provided on all reprints and updates
- Unique, attractive and specially designed sachet covers for samples provided
- All gifts, such as pens, key chains, playing cards, memo pouches, and pencils pouches, strongly reminding the receiver about the mnemonic
- Yearly pocket calendars/school labels used as inputs to provide constant and regular 'reminders' about the mnemonic

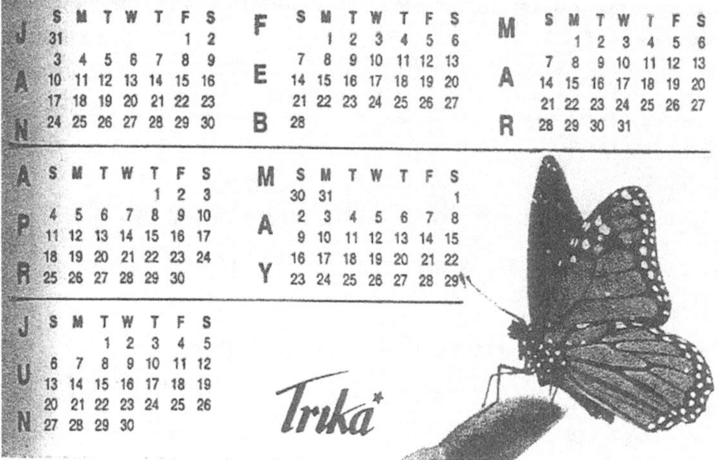

- Large, attractive and glossy posters of the butterfly and its association with Trika
- The butterfly was a constant feature in all communications to the customers—on all pages of LBLs (leave-behind leaflets), 'Thank you' cards and letters, New Year cards, Trika update books, etc.

- Butterfly painting competitions were organized to drive home the mnemonic to the family, and thereby ensure their involvement

All these activities and inputs helped establish the mnemonic for Trika in a short period of five years. Doctors associated the butterfly with Trika, and hence, its brand recall was strong.

In addition to the excellent mileage derived from the perfectly matched mnemonic, the enthusiasm, involvement, and commitment of the field force that detailed and sold the mnemonic and the brand Trika contributed to the success of the launch.

LEARNINGS

Positioning is usually achieved through *identification and communication* of a differentiation or unique relative advantage over competitors.

It is important for a pharmaceutical product to receive the backing of corporate positioning. This synergy helps speed up the positioning of a product. The synergy is one of brand and corporate equity.

Corporate positioning is dependent on corporate strategy and resources. At the outset, it is essential to study the competition in order to determine the amount of resources required to gain sustainable advantage. Strategy can then augment the risk of committing these resources.

Good corporate strategy usually *creates a desired favorable response among internal and external customers.* These categories include employees, vendors, suppliers, customers, trade, etc.

Product positioning has *four* distinct categories related to:

1. Product attributes
2. Customer/end-user
3. Competition
4. Marketing mix

There are certain innovative positioning slants on the basis of shifts from conventions. These may be classified as follows:

- Shifting attitudes of doctors
- Shifting target patients

- Shifting response to competitors
- Shifting forms of business
- Shifting focus from product to intangibles of product

It is equally important to measure positioning. This measurement gives us a clear picture of your own response to positioning. A few techniques like perceptual mapping and target-market evaluation are useful in this respect.

CHAPTER 9

Communication and Promotion Impact

ONCE UPON A time a Brahmin received a goat as a gift. Delighted, he placed it across his shoulders to carry it home. On the way, he was spotted by three thieves, who eyed the goat with greed and envy.

'It would be nice to eat that goat,' said the leader.

'Yes,' agreed the others. But how were they to get the goat away?

It was the third thief who finally devised a plan. As the Brahmin walked along with the goat on his shoulders, he was met by the first thief.

'Oh, good morning, Sir!' said the thief politely. 'Why do you carry a dog on your shoulders? A Brahmin should not even touch an unclean dog. I really am surprised.'

'But I too am surprised!' echoed the Brahmin. 'This is no dog. This is a goat which I have received as a gift.'

'Don't be upset, Sir!' said the thief. 'I am sorry for what I said. But I only told you what I saw.' And he went his way.

The Brahmin walked on, wondering a bit. He was soon met by the second thief.

'My good Sir!' said the second thief. 'Why do you carry a dead calf on your shoulders? It is a terrible thing for a Brahmin to carry a dead animal.'

The Brahmin was most surprised. 'A dead calf!' he cried. 'What nonsense! This is a goat, can't you see?'

The thief shrugged his shoulders, 'Who am I to question you, Sir. If you want to carry a dead calf, it is your business.' Saying this, he walked away.

The Brahmin was all the more upset now. What sort of a goat was this, he wondered. He kept staring at the animal on his shoulders to make sure it was indeed a goat.

Soon, along came the third thief.

'I beg your pardon, Sir'! he said. 'But why do you carry a donkey on your shoulders? It is not right for a holy man to carry an unclean animal.'

The Brahmin was completely confused now. This animal was some sort of a devil, he thought. To appear once as a dog, next as a dead calf, and finally as a donkey.

He decided to get rid of the goat once for all. And casting it aside, he went home alone.

The three thieves, of course, gleefully claimed the goat, and had a sumptuous meal.

Our minds are indeed very susceptible to any kind of communication. Even without a credible source of communication and with only exposure to different media can influence the mind. You can, therefore, imagine the impact communication can have if you use a credible source and also an appropriate media mix. Pharmaceutical communication requires both these to be effective.

COMMUNICATION IN THE PHARMACEUTICAL INDUSTRY

The totality of the communication process influences the way in which different audiences perceive an organization. In the pharmaceutical industry there are two types of communication: (i) interpersonal, and (ii) impersonal. Selective attention of doctors, noise created by competitors and the environment, selective perception of brands, and so on, are a few barriers to any pharma communication process. The source and credibility of communication is very important for every pharma brand.

Interpersonal communication sources are either formal or informal. Among formal sources, other fellow physicians, influencers, guides, co-workers, pharmacists, and professors provide additional credibility. In the case of informal sources, the family, neighbours, and non-professional friends influence the choice.

In impersonal communications, reference of college and university for physicians, corporate image of brand, brand image of a product, and government influence the communication impact.

THE TASK OF COMMUNICATION

The way to communicate with the target market and the communication message itself depends largely on the kind of product and the prescriber's involvement with it. A distinction can be made among the types of products, depending on whether the prescriber perceives a high or low risk for prescribing the product category, and on the degree of rational decision making he or she may exercise.

The risk dimension represents the level of prescribing risk, degree of uncertainty about the innovation, and the prescriber's clinical interest in the product. The 'rationality' dimension represents the level of rational arguments available to convince the physicians of the product's effectiveness. For some product categories, the prescription decision is based on rational arguments, whereas for some others less rational approaches, such as company and product loyalty, impact of the product on the patient's self-image, habit, etc. prevail.

The following *four* types of product categories (Figure 9.1) have implications for the kind of communication message and choice of media.

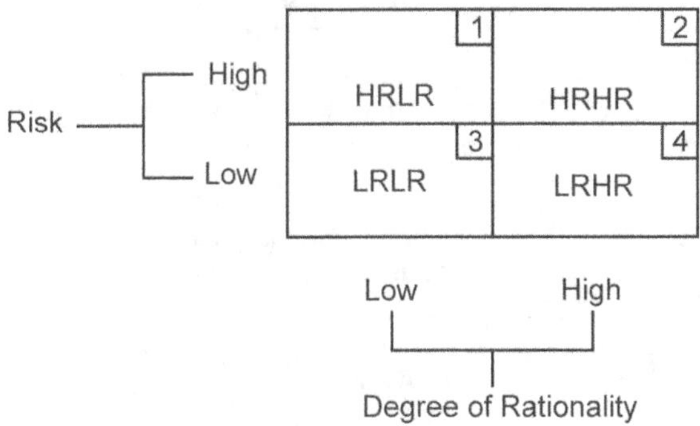

Figure 9.1 Four types of products categorized by doctor's perception about risk and decision making

1. **High Risk Low Rationale (HRLR)—Reassure**

   Symposia and group presentations are crucial to provide peer group support and personal assurance for the prescriber. Journal advertising and other print media should provide more emotional support for the prescriber.

2. **High Risk High Rational—Inform**

   Specialized detailing, hospital presentation, and clinical symposia are important vehicles for convincing prescribers of the added value of a product. Advertising with long copy format and argumentation giving additional information should be used for this purpose.

3. **Low Risk Low Rationale—Generate Feeling**

   The prescriber is not very interested in detailed information about this type of product. Simple messages via third-order detailing, journal advertising, and promotional activities seem most appropriate here.

4. **Low Risk High Rationale—Habit Formation**

   Reminding the prescriber with simple messages is important for these types of products. Direct mail, journal ads and other less expensive media can be frequently used for this product category.

Most pharmaceutical prescription products fall in the second ('inform') category, and the task of the manager here is to guide the prescriber through a set of stages described in the 'hierarchy of sales-effort approach', shown in Figure 9.2.

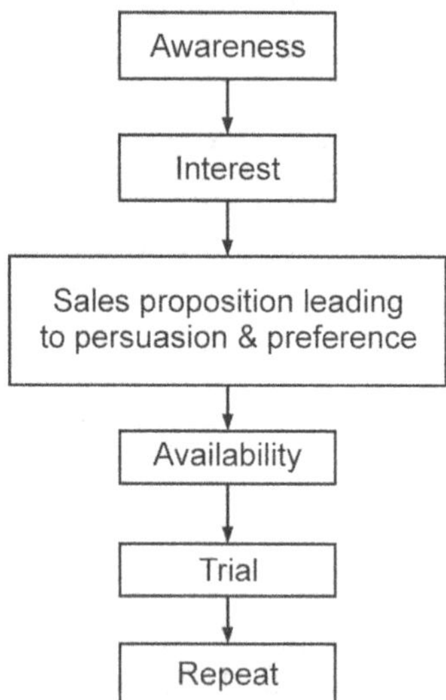

Figure 9.2 Stages in the sales-effort approach

(i) ***The awareness stage***: Most prescribers become aware of most new pharmaceutical products, or at least those put into the market by larger companies. The key task at this stage is to achieve not only passive awareness, but 'top-of-the-mind' awareness. Prescribers have a limited capacity to process information, and limited memory space. Coupled with the proliferation of new (mostly 'me-too') products and new product extensions, gaining 'top-of-the-mind' awareness often requires the use of heavy marketing artillery. Conferences, symposia, journal advertising and detailing efforts have to be used. The current trend is to use promotional activities aimed at the final consumer. Cipla is one company, for example, which has been able to capture 'top-of-the-mind' awareness through the use of symposia and seminars. The Mickey Mantle (ex-baseball star) promotional campaign by Novartis for Volteren in the USA generated substantial 'top-of-the-mind' awareness not only for prescribers but also for patients. Clinical trial activities also contribute to generate 'top-of-the-mind' awareness with opinion leaders.

(ii) ***The interest stage***: When confronted with a specific health problem of a patient, the prescriber usually considers very few therapeutic alternatives. To enter this evoked set of alternative products is an important step in building a market position for a drug. Information about the benefits of the product are very important at this stage.

The sales force, combined with supportive journal advertising and samples, are crucial communication media at this stage.

A MODEL FOR EFFECTIVE COMMUNICATION

Our company, Interlink Marketing Consultancy Pvt. Ltd., has tried applications derived from Dr. Osgood's model and promoted many products to doctors. This model helps the marketer to build up his communication strategy.

The model works beautifully. Let us take an example of a product like Zedex which is different from other traditional cough suppressants, being anti-histaminic in nature. At the message level, if Zedex had tried to provide a combination of measurable attributes and signs of cough in the communication message, chances were that even after the entire communication was over, the doctors were likely to be reminded of Benadryl; and thus the interpretation of this communication would have only yielded a prescription for Benadryl.

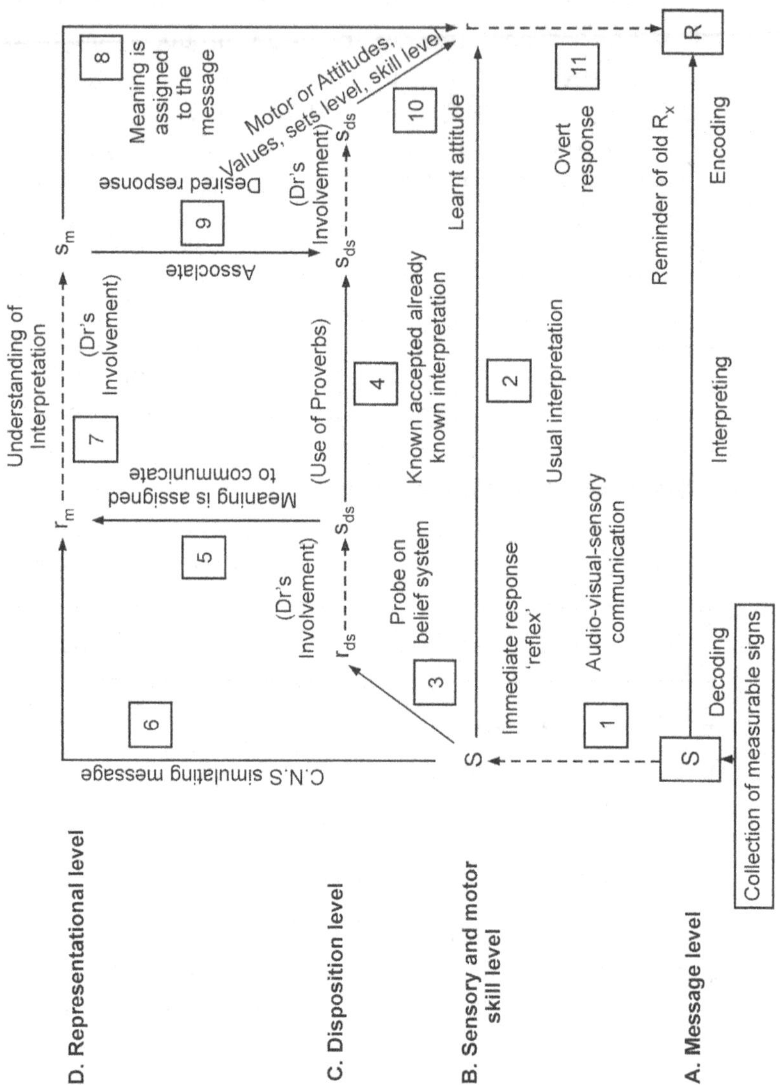

Figure 9.3 Modified design on the basis of Dr. Osgood's model

The second possible stage of getting the message registered was at the sensory and motor skill level. So the communication had to lead to this stage. This could be done by drawing attention to the appearance and taste of the product. Yet the immediate response or reflex of the doctor was to prescribe Benadryl as he was not yet attuned to the new product.

The third possible stage was at the disposition level. To make an impact, the communication had to reach this level. So a 'question' was posed to the doctor and a doubt about Benadryl was cast in his mind, on the basis of established technical confirmation. Although Benadryl was prescribed for coughs, its ingredients showed it to be only a 'cold therapy' during allergic manifestations. There was no ingredient in Benadryl except ammonium chloride which helped expectoration. Thus, its basic value was questioned. The message reached successfully. New attitudes and values were formed and the doctors were now well-disposed to consider Zedex in place of Benadryl.

Yet, for prescriptions, one needs to still go to the fourth level of representation. Hence it is important to provide a central nervous system (CNS) stimulus. This can be done by appealing to one of the senses. And the meaning assigned to the message thereby communicated. So the feeling of coolness throughout the respiratory tract one got after taking Zedex due to its high viscosity and texture was highlighted. This was also demonstrated. The doctor was requested to try Zedex in the presence of the MR. The cooling effect the doctors experienced took them to the representational level. They appreciated the novelty of the experience.

Zedex took the market by storm. You can also perhaps use this model to develop a communication strategy for launching your new product.

EVALUATION OF PRESENT –DAY COMMUNICATION

The goal of communication, even when travelling a circuitous path under the guise of 'education', is to achieve the uncritical acceptance of a preconceived message, and captivate the mind of physician. Basically, every pharmaceutical company is trying its best to obtain a 'share of the mind' of the physician for its brands. The success of communication depends on many factors—the choice of the molecule, the timing, the strategy, the competition, the preconceived message, the promotional material, the physical promotional plan, the technology, and the process of communication of the message to the physician in a captive mood. It is therefore important to evaluate the existing system and technology of communication and see where improvements can be made.

It is usually seen that when patients provide their case histories on the insistence of the doctor, he usually concentrates on verbal, nonverbal and observable clues in relation to the basis of condition of the patient.

Suppose a patient shows all the symptoms of hypertension. The doctor tries to gauge the seriousness of the condition with his professional tools. If he is apprehensive, he sends the patient for pathological investigations. On the other hand, he also treats him with, say Diazepam, to eliminate the causes of stress and strain. Through his investigations and clinical facts, he arrives at a specific diagnosis. If he cannot, he refers the patient to specialists. However, once he makes the diagnosis, memories in the recent as well as remote past play a vital role in prescription. Prescription is by and large a reflex action.

The deficiencies in medical literature, the limited time available for a physician to keep himself abreast of developments, and shortcomings in his education have provided a splendid opportunity to communicators in the pharmaceutical industry. Many have communicated products on the basis of ethical medical value. However, many have also quoted medical references out of context and tried to justify their marketing claims by even inventing some references on their own. Many have used neurolinguistic models to influence the doctors. But what ultimately works is a scientifically surveyed communication pattern.

PERSUASION

The process of persuasion is the keystone upon which all civilization rests. It accounts for our orderly system of living. If it were not for persuasion, we would not be very different from the cave man. We would still be wielding the club to get by physical force, the necessities of life.

We have progressed far from the days of the cave man. To some extent, the principle, 'survival of the fittest,' affects our civilization even in modern times. Only the definition of 'fittest' has changed. The survivors of today—who have the greatest share of the rewards of life—are not necessarily people of physical prowess. They are individuals who have learned the art of persuading others to think and act as they desire, who are able to convincingly sell their ideas to others.

Today, effective communication is a challenge to any communicator. In pharmaceutical communication there has been no major and tested alternative to the medium of medical detailmen. As it involves human beings, this medium is prone to distortion of the persuasive message. So, the development of a proper media mix is a necessary task for every pharma marketer.

Effective communication and a judicious media mix are thus integral to pharmaceutical communication and promotion. In today's competitive market, without these aids, it may not be possible to persuade a physician to change over to prescribing a new product.

While a lot of published literature is available abroad through studies conducted by Ben Gaffin and Associates, Ferber and Wales Associates, Caplon and Raymond and Noyas, there has been very little published literature in India about the physician and his sources of information about medicines. Some individual organizations may have made their own studies, albeit discreetly, considering the competitive nature of the Indian market, but without any common matrix to judge the perception of doctors in India, the very notion of effective communication may be elusive.

Designing such a matrix would involve examining issues such as the attitude and values of doctors, the health consciousness of patients, cost of medical care, social cost of illness, cost of social benefits like government health schemes, and cost of promotion. The most you can do immediately is to analyze the situation as carefully as possible to make sure that the various functions of this communication system are not overlooked, check out the reactions of the people who use it, and arrive at your own judgment.

Among the available media, detailmen stand out distinctly as the most effective medium for creating awareness of new or existing medicines. Conversation with doctors, especially with opinion makers and general practitioners, has been mainly responsible for influencing the flow of prescriptions (Figure 8.4). The frequency of visits at properly designed intervals of an expressive detailmen can create an impact on the physician's mind. Journals, direct mail, other colleagues, conventions, hospital usage, shelf space allotted to the company products, 'high tea' seminars conducted by pharmaceutical companies, conferences among selected physicians to discuss the issues of medical practice, audio-visual aids, public sector advertisements, newspaper columns about drugs, consumer or patient movements (as have taken place in parts of Kerala and Gujarat), and so on, have been important in influencing physicians. We will take them up, one by one, for a detailed study later in the chapter.

When we take a serious look at the practicing physician's job situation together with the loads of information about drugs that are available to him, it is easy to see that communication channels leading to the physician are overloaded. In the Indian context, where more than 16,000 organizations simultaneously operate, all that is left is a loud NOISE. What then are the options left for the physician? He can completely ignore all communications reaching him, he can randomly select those which he can attend to, or he can allocate some of his time and effort so as to gain only that information which is useful to him.

Personal communication by the sales force is absolutely necessary to convince the prescriber to use a particular brand. The effective use of the sales person gives the real differential advantage to the brand.

Does this not provide a new dimension to the thought processes of a practicing marketing person? Can he cut through the NOISE and expect positive effects of this communication? Can a marketing person use a proper media mix to communicate his message to physicians for better results? These are questions you need to ask yourself.

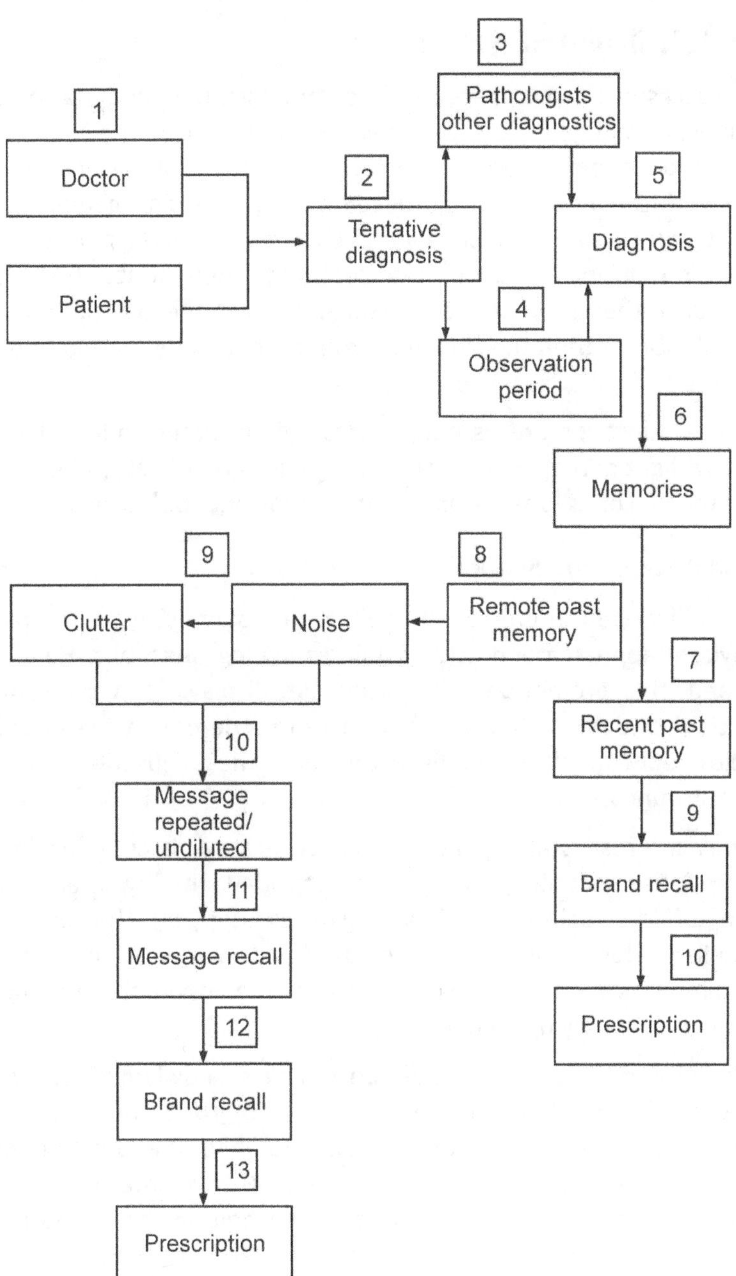

Figure 9.4 Flow-chart of prescription

INFLUENCING THE PHYSICIAN

The success of pharmaceutical communication and promotional activities, to a large extent, depends upon how much they influence the habits and beliefs of prescribing and dispensing physicians. In other words, ethical promotion has become an influencing game, directed towards attitudinal and behavioral changes. But which is the most crucial influencing factor in the communication strategy? Is it the technical authenticity of the message, or is it the psycho-behavioral manipulation attempted in the promotional copy, visual aid, and literature?

These questions are essentially strategic in nature and not ethical. They highlight perhaps the most exciting issues on the ethical promotion scene today. Let us look at some of the important approaches.

Medical Education School

The 'medical education' school looks rather skeptically at the psycho-behavioral approach and asks certain searching questions. How is and MR and the promotional literature he displays perceived by the physician? Should an MR be different from a detergent salesman? The 'medical education' school believers raise these questions on many ethical grounds.

Their interest is also purely strategic. Strategy is coloured by their assumptions concerning the physician of today. The physician thus is a victim of the colossal technical gap created by the burgeoning technology. Hence the followers of the 'medical education' school feel that communication must be dominated by medical information to keep physicians regularly up-to-date.

The physician today is rapidly becoming a knowledge user. As the quantum of medical knowledge increases and grows in complexity, the media that carry this knowledge also multiply. The problem of the physician today is not access to knowledge but the interpretation of it for his own use. The copy and visuals must help in this function. They must interpret and inform and not excite and manipulate. In other words, when the physician has to be made to choose between concepts and ideologies and not merely between Brand A and Brand B, the tools of the MR have to be different from that of a detergent salesman.

The 'medical education' school essentially sticks to scientific communication. It processes hard-core technical facts and authentic evidence, and presents them in an acceptable and meaningful form. It skips the irrelevant gimmicks and emotional appeals.

Psycho-Behavioral School

Advocates of the 'psycho-behavioral' school, on the other hand, assert the ascendancy of a marketing man over the medical expert in the medical communication function. In their scheme of thinking, the medical experts report to the marketing man, bending medical facts so as to serve the marketing man's copy theme. This school has thrown open a 'Pandora's box' of the 'hidden persuaders'. Its practitioners seek to probe the secret recesses of a physician's psyche, playing upon his nascent ambitions and hidden fears. They conjure up esoteric visuals in their 'glossy' layouts and coin 'clever' slogans to fit 'cute' copy.

To the best of our knowledge there is no convincing research evidence to suggest which of these two schools is the most effective. Nor is there adequate data available to indicate the number of companies which practice the 'manipulation' philosophy, or the measure of success of reputed companies that have followed the 'medical education' approach. It remains to be seen which approach will ultimately dominate the ethical marketing scene in India. Perhaps a good balance would work.

As a marketing person involved in ethical promotion, you must reflect on the following points: Must marketing communication yield prescriptions? If getting prescriptions is the objective, should communication be dominated only by medical information or only by the creative inputs of marketing and detailmen, or should it be a balance of both? Can persuasive ethical marketing communication ignore medical facts?

Along with the proliferation of products and technology and the segmentation of types of prospects, there has been a tremendous proliferation of media. There are new kinds of media, new developments in the traditional media, and new uses of media. Increasingly, the new media are being used for targeting pharma markets. You can't use them all, but you need to know the wide range of choices that exist in order to make the most intelligent and cost-effective selections. And because there are so many choices, there is a need for greater accountability and a means to measure comparative cost-effectiveness.

The traditional MR still remains the most effective medium of promotion to doctors and hospitals, but with the advent of many media you should explore other choices also.

Edsel Ford II, the general marketing manager of Ford's Lincoln-Mercury Division, complained in a talk to an auto-writers group that he didn't know of an advertising medium that was effective enough for reaching out to women. He pointed out that 40 per cent of new cars sold were registered in the names of women, and an additional 50 per cent of sales were strongly influenced by them. Ford expressed his reservations about women's magazines being the only answer. 'I believe there is another way.' He said, 'but I don't know what it is?' The case with the pharma industry is similar.

The Enticing Web

Communication has power to lift a product to soaring heights. But if you look at some of the practices prevailing today to promote pharmaceutical brands, you will find that pharmaceutical companies are designing grand schemes no less intricate than a spider's web. The enticing web they weave appears to first confuse and then capture the prey—the unwitting physician.

The methods are resorted to when companies are unable to face competition. The efficacy of these methods is questionable. They may yield short-term benefits, but could in the long run spell disaster for a professional company. When the rot sets in, there is no stopping it. If company A gives one kind of inducement, a competing company B will try and better it; this kind of one-upmanship can go on. There is no end.

COMMUNICATION MEDIA AND THE PRODUCT LIFE-CYCLE

One of the most crucial aspects of the marketing strategy of a pharmaceutical company is effective communication with the target market. Usually, a variety of means of communication comes into play—the sales force, journal advertising, direct mail, conferences, samples, gifts, newspaper advertising, free-standing supplements, cable TV, teleconferences, videocassettes, videomagazines, and telemarketing. Given the nature of pharmaceutical products, personal communication with prescribers is a key factor for success. The sales force of drug companies is, and will be, together with the quality of their products, the most important factor in obtaining successful product penetration and sales.

If you keenly observe, the importance of the various media varies over the stages of product lifecycle; yet the success or failure of a pharmaceutical product is determined in the early stages of its life cycle. Here, for pharmaceutical products, the pre-launch phase needs to be emphasized. Indeed, even before the product is actually launched, the target market has to be prepared for the product's introduction, the sales force has to be trained, and word has to be spread about what is to come.

Judicious use of all other media, inclusive of journal advertising, direct mail, and other promotion avenues, is useful to prepare for successful launches for giving advance information to the target audience. Conferences, clinical-cum-promotional trials, and symposia are also similarly most important at the prelaunch phase.

Conceptually, if you examine the impact of each medium at different stages of the product life-cycle, you will perhaps get the following matrix.

The importance of the different means of communication at every stage in the product lifecycle is illustrated in Table 9.1. After the pre-launch stage the sales force dominates the other media in the introductory and growth stages of the product. Later in the product's life, the more impersonal mass media become important; more so because they are less expensive. You will observe that during the pre-launch and launch phases, the sales force is extremely important. However, as the product life-cycle progresses, the use of other media in combination is essential. You can perhaps get some ideas from this basic concept and develop a communication mix on the basis of the needs of your product.

Table 9.1 Importance of each medium at every state of the product life-cycle

		Stage of Product Life Cycle				
No.	**Media**	**Pre-launch**	**Introductory**	**Growth**	**Maturity**	**Decline**
1	Sales force	2	1	1	2	-
2	Journal advertising	4	1	2	3	-
3	Mailings	3	4	3	1	-
4	Conferences and symposium	1	2	3	4	1
5	Clinical trials	1	2	3	4	-
6	Promotion trials	1	1	2	-	-
7	Samples	2	1	2	-	-
8	Gifts	1	1	2	3	-
9	Newspaper ads	1	1	-	2	1
10	Free-standing supplements	1	1	-	2	-
11	Telemarketing	1	1	-	-	1
12	Video conferencing	1	1	2	3	-
13	Digital marketing	1	1	1	2	-

Let us take each one of these elements and find out how companies have used them for their products, either selectively or collectively.

1. Sales Force

The ability and commitment of MRs to promote their organization's brands and communicate the desired message to the doctors is a very crucial factor for their effective performance. The MRs have to totally involve themselves in their work and become both the message and the medium. If they don't, and function only as the medium, the message gets lost and they end up logging empty hours in the field. A more detailed discussion on the tasks and motivation of the sales force is provided in the next chapter.

2. Magazines and Journals

Can magazines survive the video revolution? Earlier revolutions in communication suggest that they can and will. In fact, the public is buying more magazines than ever before, and their prices are soaring.

Movies didn't kill stage plays. Free music on radio didn't kill recordings. Free films on television didn't kill rural theatre. And television viewing did not kill listening to the radio or reading magazines, newspapers, and books.

More specialized magazines create credibility among readers. If you use them as an advertising medium, you may pay higher cost per page, per thousand readers, compared to a large general magazine, but you will greatly reduce wastage as the medium is audience-selective.

A dental association magazine, an ophthalmic surgery magazine, or a general practitioners' magazine may give you a change to address readers who are more emotionally involved in reading their publications. They may keep the publication for a longer time than they keep the local newspapers.

(i) *New technology*: In 1985, France's leading news weekly, Le Point, published what was called the first electronic print advertisement. It was a four-page IBM ad that lit up and played music. A year earlier, a software company had bound an actual demonstration disc in the pages of a computer magazine. Many magazines did carry a gramophone cellular disc which could be played and heard for specific messages. Innovation in technology does provide an edge to magazine ads. The experiment to impregnate paper with the product's flavor and fragrance was tried in India for a good-flavored Ampicillin, but the fragrance could not be retained.

In Britain, magazine publishers were attaching free samples to their front covers. For example, 'surgical gloves' were attached to the back cover page of a magazine which reached surgeons.

(ii) *Customized journals and magazines*: The *General Practitioner (G.P.)* and *Pulse* have been outstanding successes in the UK in the field of ethical journals in promotion. In India there are few journals like *JAMA (Journal of American Medical Association)*, *Indian Practitioner*, *BMJ (British Medical Journal)*, *IJCR (Indian Journal of Clinical Practice*, which play an important role in the promotion of pharma products.

3. The New Direct Mail—'Direct Response'

Traditionally, direct mail has been used by marketers seeking direct-response inquiries or orders from customers. An astonishingly underutilized form, direct-response mailing has a great future in India. It is important to select target prospects and establish direct communication with them in such a way that they prescribe your product for patients. This method augments the visits of MRs to the select group of prospects.

A direct-mail piece is not just an impression, it is a whole campaign. Viewed in this light, it may be your best media bargain, whether you are promoting curative or palliative therapy. The success of Cipla has shown us that direct-response mailing can give equally sustaining results. The mailing was then coupled with samples and gifts. The unusual success of the Cipla campaign prompted courier companies to explore the pharma market in India. It was a powerful campaign and resulted in a tremendous direct response. Even the envelopes caught the physicians' attention and compelled them to open them. Inside were personal letters to the physicians.

When Sandoz decided to experiment direct-response mailing for one of their old anti-hypertensive products, Visken, they selected the target market of old GPs. Visken of Sandoz received a phenomenal response of 15% after the first mailing of its series. Instead of asking for a direct prescription, the mailing provided an impetus to ask for more information about Visken. As a reward, a reply-paid offer of a premium medical book at a concessional rate created special interest among physicians. The response of the second mailing was overwhelming, and many physicians sent drafts and cheques for the offered book.

4. Conferences and Symposia

All of us need recognition in one form or another. Doctors are no exception. Even they would like to be heard, and their views discussed.

Conferences and symposia are appropriate occasions where doctors can be given an opportunity to speak. Companies organize such conferences to have some pretext to make the acquaintance of doctors—their most valuable customers.

Conferences also are vehicles for pharma companies to make doctors aware of new applications and products. It is needed an excellent medium to obtain a captive audience.

5. Clinical Trials

This is also a very useful medium for new chemical entities before they are launched. A handful of 'influencing' doctors from selected hospitals recognized by the Drug Controller General of India (DGCI) can be given the molecules before launch to study its effects and side-effects in detail *in vitro* and *in vivo*. These trials are basically conducted before the launch. After the launch, such trials are conducted to reinforce the indications or for new indications.

6. Promotional Trials

When the scientific data for communication is less and the information on diseases, like those in tropical areas, is rare internationally, a company resorts to promotional trials. Clinical trials prove the utility of particular drugs. They also have promotional value. Syn of AFD, SpasmoProxyvon and Wotinex of Wockhardt, Intestopan of Sandoz, all had resorted to promotional trials. Special customer groups were selected. A protocol was prepared by medical department and the chosen group of physicians were given samples for promotional trials. They carried out trials on 10 to 12 patients and submitted their reports to the companies. After tabulation and calculation, reports were prepared and used for promotion.

7. Samples and Gifts

Otto Kenyon, one of the founders of Kenyon & Eckhardt, once said, 'Sampling will establish a good product faster or kill a poor one quicker than any other form of advertising.' Sampling is undoubtedly one of the oldest and most powerful techniques for overcoming the reluctance of skeptical physicians to change their prescribing habits. But, is it essential to sample when the product is established? How often is a sample required by a physician who has started prescribing the product? When would one say the physician is prescribing enough? As a medical marketing person, such innumerable questions must have crossed your mind several times. You may have also temporarily resolved your conflict. But just think, isn't it unfortunate that we are still tradition-bound in terms of sampling?

If you sincerely look at the activities of those who give and take samples, you may perhaps even start questioning the utility of sampling. It has been observed that sampling which ranges from 5% to 25% or more of a company's promotional budget is rarely distributed judiciously. The amount of samples to be distributed is normally worked out only from the point of view of coverage of doctors or only on the basis of activities of the field staff, or sometimes, only to keep up with the competition.

An informal conversation with doctors about sampling will reveal varied reactions ranging from 'Sajaa do . . .' (a Hindi expression implying decorate or fill up my shelf with samples) to 'What can I do with so many samples?' to 'I don't require them . . . please take them back?' to 'Only so few units, I need more for my personal use!' How can you ever plan your sampling strategies when there is no standard to go by.

How does one prevent the waste, abuse and misuse of sampling? This is a nagging question every marketing chief would like an answer to.

The problem gets further complicated when one wants to introduce new products. In that case, either sampling gets undue importance and takes away a chunk of the budget, leaving very little for other promotional inputs, or is carried out mechanically. Traditionally, costs are incurred without any planning or subsequent cost-benefit analyses.

Waste is always present to some extent in any human activity. As such, reducing waste should be one of the fundamental goals of any effective organization. The questions you should be asking yourself are: Is sampling producing waste or winning over prescriptions? Are we in a position to evaluate the effectiveness of sampling? How do we decide a sample plan which produces prescriptions?

(i) *Using innovation*: Way back in 1967, several programs were launched in the USA to help the proper management of samples. They were launched under brand names like Clinic Script, Scrip Letter, and Mediscript. One of the programs for a product named Arlidin through Mediscript became so popular and successful that physicians, pharmacists, retailers, and patients were tremendously benefitted. As a result, approximately eight out of ten physicians using Mediscript advised their patients to renew the original sample prescriptions. Programs like Mediscript give an important role to dispensing pharmacists or retailers in sampling. We can think of other innovative programs that could involve all the players in the game of creating demand, like the physicians, pharmacists, retailers and patients, without misusing, abusing, and wasting the most important and costliest aid. In-house agencies could study the utility of samples and validate the same from time to time. Often, the role and perception of samples for one organization or for one therapeutic group is different from those for another organization or therapeutic group, for example, insulins versus a cough product. The cost of this in-house 'cell' would certainly pay for itself by reducing wastage and misuse.

Organizations in India like Cipla, Pfizer, Unichem and Cadila, to name a few, innovatively utilized sampling funds in other activities which involve physicians more than samples.

The problem of sampling in India is no longer exclusively economic, its emotional overtones need to be smoothened out before you can attempt any unusual changes.

8. Newspaper Advertising

Not everyone in India has used this avenue fully. IDPL, Wockhardt, Torrent, and Zieta are a few who took advantage of this medium.

The biggest advantage of newspaper advertising is the potential it offers to reach your message to the target market quickly and without distortion. Both total market coverage (TMC) and selective market coverage (SMC) are by choosing the right newspapers. In the early-1970s, Wockhardt used newspaper advertising for Flabolin, an anti-obesity drug, without mentioning the product/brand name. It helped Wockhardt to seek the opinion of patients about the product. IDPL floated a contest for doctors to match bulk raw materials with the names of companies to provide 'recall' of IDPL products. Torrent started using the newspapers to announce their new product introductions. Zieta used this medium for its launches. Through this ad, it gave an opportunity to greet doctors and family physicians by their patients. All approaches were innovative using only the newspaper medium.

Advertising in dailies is also helpful for adding weight to a national campaign that has a foundation on network television, especially for OTC products. Possibly, this could be done innovatively for ethical pharma products too. Newspaper advertising enables you to focus on the prospects in major markets where sales are developing. The retailers too gain confidence in stocking your products in large quantities if they are advertised in newspapers. Not far back, Kopran reduced the price of Lokit (omeprezol) and advertised through the dailies. The response to the sale was almost overwhelming.

9. **Free-Standing Supplements**

Free-standing supplements (FSS) now slip out of the weekend newspaper in every major city or town in India. They offer an opportunity to use quality color printing and to display an entire catalogue of sale merchandise. It is a matter of time before the subtle use of this medium reaps benefits. Journalists use this forum for providing case studies and discussing the success and failure of brands. Readers find these discussions appealing, and awareness about ailments like AIDS and cancer can be increased through write-ups. Many articles can appear on the nutritional role of vitamins, tuberculosis, gastroenteritis, and so on, to help the general reader take precautions to improve his and his family's immunity. These write-ups are also useful for those who promote drugs for such diseases. Ayurvedic drug companies have already started this type of promotion activity.

10. **Telephone Marketing**

While you will still search for an ideal means of communication, the telephone became India's largest communication medium. Using this medium, you can call on prominent doctor all over the country within a span of one hour as all of them are usually available at the same time in their clinic. The message can reach 25 top physicians in India within an hour. You really have no need to travel all over and meet them personally.

If you have not been maximizing the use of the telephone in marketing the product, service, or business you are promoting, you are in danger of being left behind. And if you are accustomed to thinking of telemarketing simply as calling up somebody to sell something, you are missing out on a good deal. Inbound telemarketing is as important as outbound telemarketing, perhaps more so for many businesses. And now it is easily within the capability of almost any business. This is possible when you know the physician personally.

Wipro baby soft soap and powder were promoted to GPs and gynaecologists over the phone in Mumbai. The script was properly formulated. It was rehearsed well. The detailing was given by women through phone calls to all doctors whom Wipro wanted to call on. This phone call was followed by promotional gifts. It worked. In another case, a well-known organization used the medical advisors of the company to make these calls. This was also successful.

(i) ***Outbound telemarketing:*** If you are thinking of using telemarketing to contact prospects or customers, here are several important considerations.

- Each call will cost you much less than any other media, and if successful, will produce about ten times greater results. However, this kind of success in calling lists of doctors is usually possible only when the caller has already established a cordial relationship with the respondent.

- Outbound telemarketing has been used successfully in magazine subscription renewal campaigns and to remind doctors to continue the prescriptions of medicine brands they are already prescribing.

- Outbound telemarketing has been used successfully in magazine subscription renewal campaigns and to remind doctors to continue the prescriptions of medicine brands they are already prescribing.

- Outbound telemarketing is a job for a professional agency. They will be able to write a skillful and professional phone script for their trained operator and, through feedback from respondents, will refine it to a high level of effectiveness. And there should be significant cost advantages compared to paying your own line charges and full-time operators whose work load might vary widely. You can also employ a few physicians to contact the customers. Using specialists in the medical teams is already in practice. So you should certainly not have a problem in employing them in your telephone marketing team.

- Other things being equal (which of course they never are), the higher the price, the greater the sales resistance. So there is no magic solution, but a professional telemarketing agency and a well-designed text can provide a realistic answer.

In telemarketing, as in any other business, nothing succeeds like success. There is no limit to the future of outbound telemarketing because the customer wants it and likes it.

11. Television

Malayala Manorama in Kerala developed a hard-hitting campaign against television to prove the sustainability of the print medium along with the use of television in corporate image promotion. The advantages of focused interpreted information from print media was bought to the forefront to counter-attack the clutter and interruptions due to ads on television. The concentration on serious aspects can be broken on television but the print media provides a captive concentrated time.

Although the print media is likely to dominate the scene for some time, television has also been innovatively used in corporate image promotion in India. The equity market also requires this kind of initiation. Medical quizzes and other special programs featuring specific therapies on television can also boost the corporate image.

12. Group Detailing

The era of the individual medical practitioner is ending. The responsibility of medical care is shifting from the GP to teams of doctors. So campaigns, using multimedia presentation tools perhaps, can be aimed at groups of medics and shown in wards, nursing homes, and so on. This can be very cost effective.

If we target dermatologists and GPs for a brand and aim for prescriptions from the two groups in a 4:1 ratio, and end up getting in a 1:4 ratio instead, we see no reason to worry so long as the overall volumes are achieved. What this really means is that we are interested purely in sales, not brand building.

13. **Digital Marketing**

Technology has prompted drastic changes in the marketing world over the past decade, and pharmaceutical marketing has not been excluded from this evolution. In the past, doctors were limited to offline materials like journals and references for accessing medical information and news. But those days are long gone, and with just a click of a mouse or touch of a screen, physicians have access to all of the resources they need to stay abreast of the latest knowledge in the field. Internet-savvy physicians are no longer an emerging group – this market is at a saturation point, as nearly all physicians are online for professional purposes weekly or more. In fact, the average physician now spends a full work day (eight hours) per week using the Internet for professional reasons, a substantial jump from only 2.5 hours.

Mobile technology has played a significant role in increasing physicians' dependency on online resources – 64% of doctors own smartphones and are using them to supplement their desk or laptop computer usage to be "always on." Also, mobile devices help physicians to access clinical resources at multiple points throughout their day, even to at the point of care. Currently, physicians prefer to conduct easy tasks such as information checking on mobile devices, while leaving more complex activities like CME for completion on their PCs. But as mobile browsing capabilities improve, physicians will start to use smartphones for more advanced activities than just reference purposes.

As a group, physicians have acclimated themselves to advanced online activities, such as watching streaming video and listening to podcasts, at a much faster rate than consumers. Doctors are also catching the social media fever. Many are collaborating in online communities designed specifically for healthcare professionals.

Pharmaceutical companies are offering physicians online customer services such as customer service portals, live video reps, interactive detailing, and e-sampling. Sales reps are also "digitalizing" their in-person visits with tools such as tablet PCs.

ADVERTISING AND BRANDING

Creative product management teams often complain that they do not know 'how to win' advertising impact. I do not have any actual evidence but logic suggests that any creative team knowing that its work is going to be pre-tested will work even harder to excel.

What does it take to excel? Are there any guidelines or principles which, if followed, can enhance target audience response?

Indeed there are. And any one may be prompted to say, 'I already knew that.' Of the many who 'know,' some apply them consistently while others seem determined to learn the hard way.

It is interesting to observe that all those who have taken the guidelines into consideration have most certainly received applause from the audience. How does this work in the field of pharmaceutical advertising? There is no magic involved, just basic medical communications theory.

(i) ***Objective of communication through advertising:*** Many advertisements miss the objective. They start with them all right, but over time, in the process of being created, the ads get skewed. Many lose their focus midway and the brands end up looking alike. Today, all those selling cetirizine have a problem defining the objectives of the communication. The ads are made in a hurry to inform the doctors they are meant to target. All of them communicate the 'once-a-day' theory, common to all brands selling the formulation.

(ii) ***Copy focus:*** The most persuasive arguments conveyed by a winning ad need to be a direct reflection of one's primary copy strategy, instead of some subordinate copy. I have stressed the need for copy focus, especially on important issues. Once achieved, the arguments should play on the target's mind as reasons to prescribe the brand. If they don't, either the ad has not done its job properly or the copy strategy is off the mark. It might be placing primary emphasis on ideas that don't warrant attention. In sum, it all comes back to the appropriateness and strength of one's strategy. If one makes use of the right arguments, they should make a strong contribution, provided they have been properly showcased in the advertising. Radiopaque, an imaging product from Dabur, is a good example.

Getting the lead idea across to 50 per cent of the audience is excellent. Only fantastically well-focused ads get their point across to more than three-quarters of ad readers. But unfortunately, these are only exceptions.

Too many ads have suffered from the 'too-many-cooks' syndrome, with an advertising-by-committee approach designed to incorporate everyone's ideas. With a whole lot of ideas being squeezed into each ad, one often winds up saying nothing.

Concept research done upfront should help an advertiser narrow down the available claims into a hierarchy, a ranking of approved arguments from the highest to the lowest potential. Efforts need to be made to concentrate copy content on one or two strong arguments, with a decidedly subordinate role given to the remaining copy points. Only through such an effort is true copy focus likely to result.

When one's product is new, physicians will prove to be remarkably patient in their willingness to wade through and absorb a broad range of information. But once prescribing levels cross the 20 per cent mark, one needs to focus prominently on just a few key claims if one expects physicians to register them well.

On the other hand, pharmaceutical ads cannot be made the way you formulate an adline for, say, a mint with a hole. This is a complex job. Whenever possible, try to avoid simply telling readers what a particular product is for. Laying stress on indications without sufficient emphasis on patient-oriented benefits, such as reduced side-effects, safety, dosages and so on, leaves you pretty vulnerable. Unless, of course, your product happens to be the only one capable of treating the indications.

This does not mean that equal emphasis be placed on a laundry list of copy claims. Far from it. From concept research done earlier, one should know which arguments have the greatest merit (or appeal to a particular group of doctors), and it is those that deserve to be in the forefront.

(iii) ***Skills in developing headlines:*** Our analysis always focuses on the merits of large, bold headlines. The best ones are those people relate to faster, and directly convey an important idea. An example of a straightforward headline is one for Minirin from Ferring Pharmaceuticals, 'Bedwetting is an universal problem',' it says.

Caution is urged, however, when a play on words or a clever visual is employed. The physicians tend to be literal-minded, and headlines which are tricky, smart or too subtle may zip right past her or him without being appreciated. This guideline is more relevant in circumstances related to a serious or life-threatening disease. One can be granted more latitude in less critical categories.

Relating copy length to sub-heads, lead-ins and bullets need to be examined as well. How many times has an ad loaded with meaningful information simply looked like 'too much work' and repelled its audience? All too often. But that does not have to be the case. Long-copy ads (even those with hundreds of words) are not automatic losers. They can, and often do, outperform shorter ads. Physicians, given well-organized text, will devour lengthy copy, especially when the ad makes good use of sub-heads, lead-ins and bullets.

Use of many short paragraphs rather than a few lengthy ones ease the reader's path. Sub-heads in bold typeface help tell a reader what is coming next and, if well-written, can arouse curiosity or suggest the importance of the message that follows. Boldface lead-ins in paragraph text, originally a trademark of photo-journalism caption in *Life*, remain a quick and successful means of drawing a reader's attention and keeping things moving.

Above all, one should avoid the temptation of squeezing lengthy texts into a type size so small that middle-aged and old physicians may have difficulty reading it. Finally, one should not be afraid to ask why an ad's text has become lengthy. Is it long because it must be or is it because it has been put together by a committee and everyone's interests are being served? If the latter is the case, the copy may have no focus.

(iv) ***Illustrations that work:*** If one has a choice between a large, individual illustration and several smaller ones, our analysis of pre-test results suggests that one will be much better off with a single illustration, which are quickly understood and related to the text of the headlines. The ads should preferably be in color, but the modest added costs of only a second color rarely produce a measurable return, with results typically at about the same level as that of black-and-white visuals.

(v) ***Full disclosure:*** Some physicians want to read good ads. For those who do (do not yet feel they already know all there is to know about a product), why not make it easier by using more space between sections, with readable sub-heads, larger type and so on?

(vi) ***Type of ad:*** Message ads versus reminder ads: do not expect a reminder ad (promoting an established product and using fewer than 25 words) to do the job of ads that actually say something specific. That may happen now and then, but overall, message ads (with 25 or more words) elicit the best physician response. They do better in generating an audience, gaining an advantage on the measure of high prescribing interest, and tend to convey more by way of newsworthy information.

(vii) ***Flawless execution factors (initial and long term response):*** On all occasions except one, the element of physical presentation of one's ads should generate considerable immediate response. That exception maybe for an introductory ad for a new product, when the news itself (especially in an important category) will so dominate physician reaction that there will be a little mention of the ad's creative execution elements. That does not imply a criticism of the presentation but simply illustrates the temporary dominance of the news. Once the newsworthiness ebbs, the element of physical presentation (colour, illustrative content, and so on) become quite critical in generating an audience. The more the presentation response, the better it is, provided the margin between favorable and unfavorable reactions is substantially positive. No other factor can be expected to be more in capturing an audience.

Surprisingly, a successful presentation will even contribute to later expressions of prescribing interest. When that happens, it is a bonus, but a truly outstanding ad campaign that supports prescribing interest will be described as 'informative', 'educational', 'easy-to-read' and 'professional', while winning praise for colour, illustrations, or even graph or chart.

But while one is at it, one should make sure that such text is not immediately heavy. Showing it all in close proximity will give the impression of massive copy tonnage and turn away many potential readers. The age-old expression-'a place for everything, and everything in its place'-applies here.

So much for the design of ads for print media. Equally important is the selection of publication where you wish your ad to appear. Depending on the kind of drug-bulk generic, speciality, branded product- and the type of physician you wish to target, your need to select an appropriate publication. This brings up the contentious issue of advertising in medical publications.

ADVERTISING IN MEDICAL PUBLICATIONS

The claimed readership or circulation of various medical publications is an issue of debate amongst pharmaceutical marketers. Such debates challenge the basic need of advertising or airing pharmaceutical brand messages through such publications. As there is no foolproof method to arrive at the exact relationship between the claimed readership and the direct expenditure on advertising in the publications, pharmaceuticals marketers feel uneasy in investing in such activities. As such, budgets for such promotion are very low and are not given priority in the total brand plan.

But before we go into the usefulness of advertising in medical publications, it is necessary to examine how pharmaceutical marketers target their audience. We know that marketers look to target their audience. We know that marketers look to target speciality doctors and GPs with their brands through a team of MRs who visit them. GPs account for almost 70 per cent of all doctors in India, so they form an audience for even the highly specialized products (unless the product is meant for very specific cases such as cancer-oncology).

Conceptually, there is no arguing that you need to expose your specialty brands to only the specialist. You would need to promote an infertility product specifically to those gynecologists who treat infertility product specifically to those gynecologists who treat infertility cases (and leave out GPs altogether). But look at it another way. There may not be more than 15 such gynecologists in any one MR's territory. For example, a company may have 700 MRs or 700 'territories' in India and 1,40,000 doctors to reach out. If you were to follow the policy of exclusivity, you would be promoting your specialty brand to just 10,500 doctors who qualify as gynecologists (7.5 per cent of the total). However, a good GP who exclusively treats female patients (very likely in class II and class III towns) may get left out. Also, few organizations have an error-free, updated, list of specialists and GPs since yearly updation is a costly affair, in each territory, the 'target segment' is really defined by the MRs and not by the brand manager.

Perhaps GPs have no role in treating infertility expect to refer the patient to a specialist. However, in almost all specialist fields, the follow up of patients is usually done by GPs. So, while precision targeting might work for other brands, the infertility product is better off covering both GPs and specialists. Yet, pharmaceutical marketers end up putting all their eggs in the one basket of MRs.

This is not to imply that pharmaceutical product management teams do not wish to rationalize the exposure they give to each of their brands. They do. The crucial difference between them and the brand managers of consumer products is that the latter tend to look at the media mix in its entirety, thereby putting themselves in a position from where they can analyze the resultant brand exposure at the end of the day. They believe that over time exposure turns into awareness, preference and trial, which helps to establish the brand (if, of course, the product meets its promise). Fine-tuning is done all the time.

In contrast, pharmaceutical marketers tend to be absorbed more by the means than the ends because a large part of the promotional budget usually goes towards giving away product samples and paying MRs- both of which are fixed costs. Given this situation, it is inevitable that the other promotional avenues are given a short shift. Even when market changes place a premium on adaptiveness , the 'MR-centricism' makes it harder for them to reorient the marketing mix in line with the changing market dynamics.

The pharmaceutical market in India is thus in a state of transition. A lot of churning is taking place and new ideas are being thrown up. The case of promoting a brand that is useful for specialists but not for GPs, for example, has raised the issue of placing ads in periodicals. Marketers typically eliminate (or choose) publications on the nature of periodicals. But the practice may take a different turn if pharmaceutical marketers see the wisdom in making a distinction between their primary and secondary target segments, and tailor their programs accordingly.

Major Issues

How effective are ads in these publications? The question encourages one to examine the following issues:

- Usefulness of medical publications
- Methodology to review and appraise readership/circulation

(i) *Usefulness:* Unlike customer brands, pharmaceutical brands need what in medical parlance is termed 'ethical handling', which means that the message must reach doctors and only doctors. Spillage is not permissible, since superficial knowledge reaching a non-target group could cause confusion and conflict.

In the Indian context, it is essential to continually educate doctors on medical issues. For one, medical information keeps growing (and changing), and Indian doctors are not bound by any stipulation (as they are in developed countries) to continue their medical education through their professional careers. An MBBS degree holder of the 1960s or 1970s in India can continue to practice without any further formal authorization. In developed countries, non-compliance to CME (Continuing Medical Education) and failure to secure credits at appropriate intervals can lead to cancellation of the authority to continue the practice. Hence, the utility of high-quality medical publications is beyond question.

In medical publications, relevance is everything. Invariably, magazines which are not sufficiently useful to the target audience are forced to shut down. It is extremely difficult to provide high-quality value to doctors for years on end.

However, marketers should not worry so much about determining the magazine's precise usefulness to doctors, so long as the frequency of publication is maintained and it has subscribers. A reasonably large subscription base - depending on the specialization – is evidence of genuine usefulness.

Are these publications financially viable? The useful ones are. In general, for a niche publication, the ratio of production cost, marketing costs and profits should be 3:2:2. Any publication with this ratio must be useful to both the readers and the publisher.

(ii) ***Review and appraise:*** As of now, there is no foolproof method to review and appraise the readership of a publication in India. However, there are many ways to approach the problem. The most widely used among these in the West was the ad-page-exposure (APX) study method.

The scenario in the West was quite like India's for many years before APX methods were evolved to study the utility of such magazines. Although these studies became an accepted form of readership confirmation, individual studies were to take charge of syndicated studies later on.

Medical TV Programs

Marketers recognize audio-visual communications as forceful and more personal. Such communications involve little work on the viewer's part and provide good clinical summaries. Also, they are inexpensive for the physician and available in a convenient setting.

Globally, televised medical programs are quite popular. In the US, pharmaceutical marketers use TV in the following ways:

Special Programs

These aim to deliver medical education to physicians. Often, their contents are based on medical meeting or symposia, the publication of research papers, or new knowledge in the management of diseases. Most of these are produced under third-party editorial supervision. Many are produced in collaboration with academic or scholarly groups that select the participants and approve the content. With independent editorial control, Category I CME (Continuing Medical Education) accreditation is available for physicians.

For the marketer, producing a program entails communicating a message in a tailored environment to a national audience of physicians. Doctor Television Channel, MediBizTV, and Medical Channel are some of the widely watched medical networks.

Programs have been produced in every conceivable format and length. The longest was a two-and-a-half hour, live phone-in program requested by the Food & Drug Administration (FDA) at the time of licensure of the first HIV ELISA test. Usually, special programs last 30 minutes, since viewership of half-hour program are better than for longer ones. Companies that have a commitment to medical TV and study its impact regularly produce special programs.

Unlike TV ads, the cost of such special programs can be amortized by producing and distributing their DVDs or by developing spin-off sales.

Ongoing Serials

To maximize viewership, medical TV networks provide a variety of programs directed at key physician groups. In developing these, they create general medical serials. For instance, *Physician's Journal Update, Cardiology Update, Family Practice Update* and *Infectious Disease Update,* enjoyed a broad based primary viewership when they were launched decades ago.

Networks optimize their programming mix by balancing serial programming (with known target viewers) and special programming (which get sponsors).

In India, however, things are moving in the opposite direction. There are no special serials in India which target physicians unlike the print media where there are special publications for physicians. But such films are produced for private screening. In fact, marketers have since long recognized the impact of audio-visual production capabilities are improving, many firms are using DVDs as gift for physicians. However, while filmmakers are comfortable with medico-social DVDs, which often have the feel of any other documentary; they are not trained to work on films involving intensely scientific details. Also, unlike in other countries, marketers in India are not promoting patented products. So, no one wants to spend megabucks on high-quality programs.

Government Issues

Special TV programs for doctors are subject to the Food Drug Administration and the Drug Controller General of India (FDA and DCGI) regulations concerning promotion, labeling, and scrutiny as are all other communication media. Producers of medical media content, even when sponsored by marketers, want their output to be viewed as scientific communication rather than as a promotion activity. Physicians have to trust the fact that the information is not biased. For this, an authority has to certify that the issues dealt with are independent, objective, balanced and have scientific rigor. Balanced communication involves giving coverage to the sponsor's rival products, and ensuring that there are enough viewpoints on every issue. The target audience, remember, is highly discerning.

The USFDA guidelines divide medical programs into two categories: (i) those that are developed independently and meet USFDA guidelines, and (ii) those that do not follow USFDA rules. These are said to be under the control of the sponsor and must meet advertising standards. Even sponsor-controlled programs must be fair, mention the major side effects and say where the prescribing information is available. These cannot deal with products yet to be approved or with unapproved indications for an approved product.

The FDA and DCGI guidelines are a starting point for the Indian pharmaceutical industry to debate issues related to medical education. After all, the authorities and pharmaceutical companies have the same goal: informing the medical profession about new products, procedures, equipment, and so on. If a workable system is created, sponsors will receive value for their investment without compromising the integrity of medical education.

Editorial Issues

The logic behind free exchange of information is the continual and quick communication of medical advances is essential. TV is an ideal medium for providing this. Restraining medical communication works against patient care, particularly in India, where medical facilities are inadequate and updated information is scarce. However, sponsorship for commercial interest raises tricky questions. Promotion and scientific exchange issues need to be handled separately. Even in programs with respected experts and independent editorial supervision, content that is favorable to a sponsor tends to appear quite often. Is it valid scientific news or covert advertising? The separating line should be clear, else the credibility of the program will suffer, which would impair the very idea of medical TV.

Production Issues

After the decision is taken to use medical TV, there are points to consider when deciding of the format. 'Should I produce a special program?' If you have a simple message to get across, it is better to air a commercial on a program that is likely to deliver the appropriate message to the target audience 'Should I produce a program with individual editorial control or a controlled-editorial program that can be tailored to my product?'

Another consideration is that TV is different from our media. Strategies that work in print, lectures or in symposia can fail on TV. It is crucial that the experts and the host have good communication skills. There is nothing worse than a program where the experts cannot encapsulate their conclusions, and where the host is unable to conduct interviews or read a teleprompter properly. Shoddy productions ruin everything.

So, make sure that the budget is adequate. Does it include adequate money for, say, field location shooting? Does it cover studio, set and art direction costs? Find out how many computer graphics will be produced, what special effects will be used, and make sure that professional writers, medical editors, and on-camera talent will be included. All such elements add to the cost, but if the program doesn't have any interesting and valid creative envelope, you'll be disappointed.

India needs continuing medical education, not least because many doctors do not find time to read traditionally produced documents and pamphlets. The vibrancy of TV can overcome this problem. It is time the medical fraternity approached the government with a proposal for medical TV.

Desk-Top and In-Clinic Media

Let's face it. Marketers are crippled by a lack of flexibility, the lack of direct influence on sales compounds their woes. Marketers of consumer products can rely on their promotional; efforts to a considerable extent because they influence the consumer directly. Pharmaceutical marketers, on the other hand, can only empower their MRs with the right promotional tools to influence the doctor's prescription behavior. Even when successful, the response time is painfully long.

What tends to happen is the following. The pharmaceutical marketer commits funds for brand promotion at the start of the product cycle, which is at least two or three months in advance, and just waits for favorable results from the field. With so much competition at the promotional level, the money required keeps rising. And over time, the marketer finds that the expenditure becomes fixed in nature (not varying in accordance with sales).

Need for Flexibility

Pharmaceutical marketers, therefore, need promotional media which allow them to be flexible. Desktop reminders, for example, are seen as an important and long-lasting promotional medium. These innovative desktop knick-knacks serve as brand reminders, but are they flexible? Perhaps or perhaps not. The question to ask is: Does the doctor need constant reminding? And if he does need extra reminding, will the knick-knack be in a position to recover the money that has been spent since there isn't anything that the marketer can do to tie its functioning to the brand's ongoing needs.

Take diaries for instance, which are a much used promotional option. Many organizations had started giving annual diaries, but this didn't prove to be a flexible option. They became an expectation each year and routinely ate up a part of the budget. Likewise, after launching calendars, both Cadila and Alembic tried to keep these promotions flexible but must have paid the price for it.

Promotional items differ vastly in their utility. Experience, however, does suggest a few basic criteria a marketer can follow while selecting these:

- It should be exclusive to the brand.
- The less 'promotional' it appears, the better.
- It should be credible in nature.
- It should bind together the trio- the brand, physician and patient- in a relationship that maximizes everyone's benefits.

The best ideas, however, are those that don't take a permanent place on the budget documents month after month, year after year. Parke Davis, for example, came up with a simple but brilliant and inexpensive gift for pediatricians. It was just a small plastic arm-circumference measuring tape. The pediatrician could measure the arm circumference of a child, and if the tape crossed the green mark into the red zone, it indicated the child's need for better nutrition. This tape was distributed as a reminder. Not only that, every pharmaceutical company needs to adopt an image of being an innovative company on the whole. Product-and-need specific thinking has been growing. And copying rivals is on the decline. The emphasis is clearly on achieving more with less money. As in any other field of human endeavor, such a tall order can be met through some truly innovative thinking.

Many look for variety in their media selections. You can't limit yourself to just one medium. Physicians are all different, and all respond to different media. Besides, one should try influencing the rest of the medical staff too, not just the doctors.

Measuring Results

Finally, what marketers should pick is what is actually showing results. Desk-top and in-clinic media are more 'targetable' and more measurable than other promotional tools. In the West, prescription pad fans claim to have done numerous studies that have shown their effect on brand awareness, product recall, message memorability, and so on. Some studies have also shown positive effects on sales and market share. However, in India, formal independent research has never been done. So, individual companies rely on their own experience and learning. The objective, typically, is to raise the frequency of brand exposure. Repetition seems to be the goal. When choosing a vehicle, don't rely exclusively on the suppliers of the materials. Carry out your own market research. Don't spend even one promotional rupee on media that aren't giving adequate returns on your investments.

Marketers in India are still not doing this as rigorously as they should. Most often, a set of managers do the creative thinking and get pleased with its efforts once something interesting has been created, while the field staff is then just required to go and exploit the benefits. Innovation is important, but there's no excuse for not keeping a sharp and scientific eye on how productive the ideas are.

PUBLIC RELATIONS AS A MARKETING TOOL

Pharmaceutical marketers in India use public relations (PR) as a marketing tool. Many of them mistakenly think PR entails sending out a few press releases, holding some press conferences and conducting some events when the company launches a new molecule or product. In reality, PR usually ends up making a point at very personal level. Its impact in the industry is seen at several levels, affecting doctors and brands.

However, it is important to understand that the promotional mix for any brand or organization is dependent on various things- advertising, personal selling and PR. Overuse of personal selling in pharmaceuticals through MRs and limitations on advertising pharmaceutical products due to FDA restrictions, present an opportunity to explore the role of and exploit PR in the pharmaceutical industry and exploit it fully.

PR covers a broad spectrum of activities- from internal communication to external publicity, and also financial reporting, PR's major task is to build a one-to-one, positive, effective, motivating, and self-reassuring relationship with the consumer through mass or individual media. It encompasses brochures, industry booklets, mailing, catalogues, corporate communication devices and websites. All of these have their importance as marketing tools.

At a company I know, the chairman is interested only in the use of PR for financial affairs. He is not really interested in furthering the interests of the company's products. He just wants to increase the perceived value of the company which, in turn, can help it in the financial markets. This results in a very limited use of such a powerful tool as PR.

Some years ago, Cipla was forced to make use of PR tools when its major communication medium, the field force, turned uncooperative. The company conducted meetings for not more than 10 customers at a time and ensured that thousands of such meetings took place at different locations in India. This helped Cipla in building one-to-one relationships with its organization in creating a positive platform for direct response communication.

PROMOTING STRATEGICALLY

In the pharmaceutical business, most companies work on monthly, bimonthly or quarterly promotional cycles, and promotional resources are carefully allocated to ensure that the efforts of the company's MRs bring in maximum sales. Most organizations bring out 'strategy guides' who provide details on inputs, information on competition, approaches to detailing, and sometimes, a chart on incentives. But they rarely mention anything on using 'cycle strategies', for getting sales.

Strategies are much more than plans to achieve goals. They differ from operating procedures because they are drawn from changing market situations and are thus alive and dynamic. Since it is more like playing a game than following the yellow line, operating strategically demands the creativity and financial muscle. It calls for an integrated and combined effort of the sales and product management teams. Unfortunately, few companies are aligning their forces.

Innovative detailing can bring the horse to the water, but it requires in-clinic sales promotion to make it drink. Physicians may be predisposed to prescribe, retailers to retail, and MRs to detail a whole range of products. But if the clinic promotions do not focus their attention on a particular product, at a particular time, in a particular place, and do not provide the incentive to prescribe, retail or detail at the right moment, the entire exercise could become futile. It would be like losing a patient to opportunistic germs in the recovery ward after having performed a successful heart operation.

If pharmaceutical sales promotion has to achieve a multiplicity of objectives, it is because it follows a multi-pronged approach. Each and every scheme should start by specifying one or more of the following objectives to be achieved. Time spent thinking through the objectives, and relating them to the overall marketing strategy is time well spent. Because this is the level at which managers could be working at cross-purposes without even knowing it. Some examples of objectives are given below:

(i)   Related to physicians
- Instituting prescriptions
- Creating a new set of prescriptions from physicians
- Retaining prescriptions of existing physicians
- Widening the loyalty base of physicians to repeatedly prescribe the same brands
- Widening usage of the products in terms of indication and patients
- Deflecting attention prices of competitors

(ii)   Related to chemists
- Increasing repeat purchase and retailing
- Gaining display at the shelves

(iii)   Related to MRs and field managers
- Increasing volume of sales to achieve and surpass the targets

- Increasing involvement and pride in a product to promote through personalized incentives.

Targets need to be qualified to make them measureable, and then the marketing team can take steps to achieve them by developing comprehensive sales promotion plans.

Changing Behavior and Attitude

Those who advocate direct person-to-person sales promotion argue that this form of promotion is effective because people's behavior changes first and attitude's follow. However, in a study sponsored by the America Marketing Association, more than six out of ten (63%) marketing managers believed that marketing works by changing people's attitudes or their beliefs (or both) first, and that behavioral changes follow. Fewer than two out of ten (17%) believed that people's behavior changes first and then, changes in their attitudes and beliefs follow.

It is best not to go by generalizations. Consumers vary, and so do products and strategies. In pharmaceuticals, if a product is tangibly different and clearly superior to its competitors, a promotional strategy will almost always work. If a company introduces a low- calorie diet formula that smells better and looks better, then patients or healthy people will unquestionably relish more than the competitor's product. Therefore, if the marketer can motivate people to buy it just once (or may be twice), it can change a person's buying behavior straightway. The brand would enjoy annuity.

But take the coffee category, where few consumers can distinguish one brand from another. In fact, in most food categories, a manufacturer must do something dramatic to have a product that stands out in terms of taste. Few customer's taste buds or senses of smell are sensitive enough to detect product differences. Therefore, with most food products, including soft drinks and beer, a marketer needs to build a psychological identity. Loyalty in these categories is often built on a foundation of attitude and outlook towards life, unless manager opts to make the product a me-too and sell on the strength of distribution. This insight is equally applicable to the pharmaceutical industry as well, where differentiation levels range from one extreme to another.

Providing Promotions a Direction

In the case of pharmaceutical brands, pioneers in therapeutic group areas (or need categories) tend to maintain a firm lead even when duplicates arrive. There is also an opportunity for new players to enter and thrive. For instance, a relatively unknown company then, Panacea, launched a new molecule, Nimesulide an anti-arthritis product. Through the strength of its sheer promotion, it made a mark for itself within just two years. When a product is outstanding, the marketer should use sales promotion to help prescribers 'break the force of inertia', and to motivate them to try and prescribe the better brand. The following conceptual model can give some direction to sales promotional inputs at different levels of brand distinction.

Table 9.2 Relative product superiority

Product/Service superiority (compared to competitors)	Percentage of all products/services marketed	Strategic implication for marketers
'Very high' an outstanding product	5	More total promotion to build trial
'High', a good product	15	A mix promotion/detailing
'Normal', and average product	16	More detailing/positioning
'Low', a bad product	12	Product reformulation/redesign
'Very Low', an awful product	3	Product discontinuance

Of the hundreds of pharmaceutical brands stocked on any retail shelf, not even 20 percent are likely to be doing well in terms of 'volume' and 'acceptability'. Volume measures mass acceptance (by doctors) and acceptance measures the level of actual prescriptions. Most of the pharmaceutical products on the retailers' shelves have nothing going for them in terms of product superiority. This does not mean that sales promotion will not work for these products. In fact, marketers of these products ought to be placing greater emphasis on detailing to doctors and using in-clinic promotions. What differs is the strategy. If a brand is average (or inferior), the promotion team must figure out some appeal (such as low price) and shape the sales promotion message around this proposition.

The real issue is that while pharmaceutical sales promotion may be effective, it is not necessarily efficient. The company may be giving away more promotional inputs than needed to generate consumer trial. Many firms, if and when they analyze their samples-to-sales ratio for a brand, get astonished and alarmed that they have actually delivered more free samples than the actual sales.

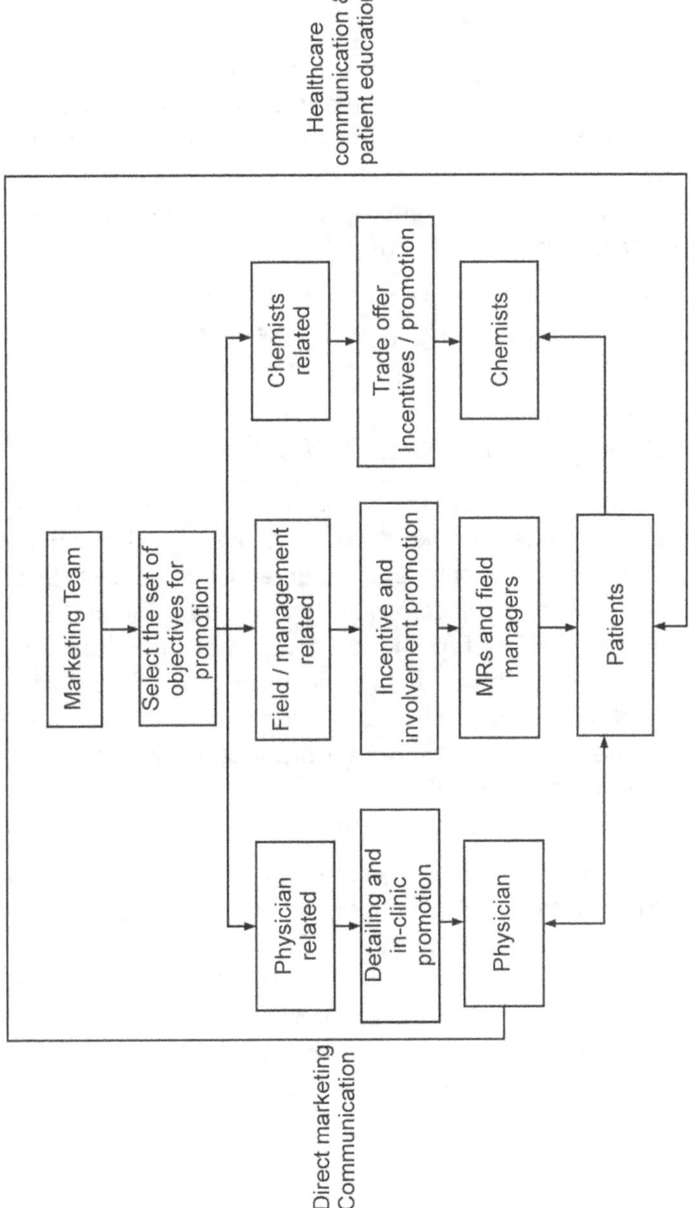

Figure 9.5 Promotional flowchart

Let us examine how to make promotions cost effective. Take a look at the promotional flowchart shown in Figure 9.5. Once you have set your objectives, you can develop a scheme on the basis of the flowchart.

Some pharmaceutical marketers prefer approaching patients directly. This is done through such activities as patient education programs, and is common for such chronic and distinguished diseases such as asthma, diabetes, hypertension and tuberculosis. In the case of AIDS and cancer, it is very important to educate the patients as also their families. There are a wide variety of educational methods being used which we looked at earlier. In general, patients appreciate selfless advice (keeping business interests out of the picture).

There is yet another development that has taken place with the advent of polyclinics and nursing homes. Besides the doctor and patient, the technician is also assuming an important role.

CLINICO– PROMOTIONAL STUDY

A clinico-promotional study is usually done by pharmaceutical companies which need to take decisions concerning their own products and how they are to be sold. Every marketer needs the help of results from an economic clinico-promotional study when he has to substantiate the claims of his brands, and demonstrate how the product is differentiated in a crowded pharmaceutical market. For example, Syu (AFD), a protein (nutritional) product, conducted a clinico-promotional study among adolescents at different orphanages, and over a period of time, established the weight and height benefits to a highly convincing degree. This then became a platform for its promotion.

The only way to properly execute an economic clinico-promotional study is through the thorough understanding of a drug's properties, the disease for which has been approved, and the marketing issues involved (such as positioning, pricing and the bill payer's willingness to pay). It is important to understand that economic clinico-promotional studies, while helping decisions on money matters, are not exclusively designed to deliver knowledge to be used mainly for economic reasons.

Health economics, on the other hand, is almost purely about placing values on clinical outcomes, and it is the valuation that provides us with the economic data. This might sound quite simple, but there are significant issues, that must be addressed in designing these studies.

Data variables, patient surveillance and follow- ups differ significantly from the traditional clinical trial.

Ground Rules for a Successful Clinico-Promotional Study

(i) ***Pay-offs:*** It is important to look at the expected pay-offs of such a study right at the beginning. The objectives of such an economic clinico-promotional study are usually manifolds and they justify any one or more of the following marketing decisions:

- Pricing decisions
- Repricing decisions
- Promotional stances
- Specific quantification of product promises
- Credible nature of date on file for the future
- Regulatory approval

As this kind of study is usually done *in vivo* (by taking patients from nursing homes or hospitals), it has a real-life basis. Many studies were conducted before the launch of an anti-amoebic, Metrogyl (JB Chemicals). Promotional efforts for this brand using these studies as the base were quite successful even though it faced competition from big multinational brands. Similar was the issue with Entazezol (of Boots- Knoll) which was promoted on the basis of the results of numerous such studies to justify its efficacy and safety. Clinico-promotional studies have assumed greater significance in India today with market-driven products becoming predominant in India and medically driven products taking a back seat.

Marketers of norfloxacin-tinidazole combinations recently conducted studies all over India and generated sufficient data to show that the stools of patients suffering from diarrhea carried both microbes and protozoa. Because the combination works on both, the data was used to make the right- efficacy safety pitch.

The objectives of an economic clinico-promotional study must be very clearly stated. When the objectives are broad, the results can lead to changes in resources devoted to different modes of patient treatment and care. The time spent by various health professionals and the time spent in various hospital or clinical units, medications and supplies can all change. The monetary value of these resource-use changes must be weighed against any difference between the costs of alternatives in use. After learning the most effective and efficient way to use a product, a savings in resource use plus any increase in patient satisfaction can greatly out weight a product's cost.

(ii) ***Target group***: In most cases, no single economic clinical trial methodology can satisfy all groups in a realistic time frame. One can address any one of the following target groups depending on the need of the brand and that of the organization:
- Society
- Healthcare provider's, such as doctors
- Hospital administrators
- Patients
- Government

(iii) ***Protocol:*** The most important things to remember throughout the protocol development process is that traditional clinical trials are often done in an artificial environment. Clinical tests to evaluate efficacy and safety performed during traditional trials are not necessarily performed in the real world. Such tests can lead to artificially inflated costs for the comparator drugs. Also, many of the traditional clinical are performed on homogenous groups, which gain is not truly reflective of a real practice.

The message here is that a traditional study is not done in the real world, while an economic clinico-promotional study is an observational one. If the protocol meets the objective of tracking a real world situation and not confounding data with artificial costs, while maintaining safety and efficacy, it will meet the criteria for an economic clinico-promotional study.

(iv) ***Selection of site:*** Choosing sites for an economic clinico-promotional study is not really very easy. Potential sites must be filtered carefully. Investigators must be quite experienced with comparator drugs in order to preserve a real world environment. The administrators of the site must not only be able to capture all economic data associated with the delivery of care but also be willing to share cost data on overheads too.

The location of a study should not be determined merely by the willingness of clinicians to participate nor should it be conducted because of the availability of patients alone. Rather, it should be done after weighing all the factors. Some important criteria for site selection are given below.

- Availability of adequate facilities to carry out the study
- Maintenance of SOP related to the study at the site
- Availability of staff to document, implement and follow up the study
- Existence of the dispensing monitoring process and control system
- Availability of staff experienced with such a study (full-time or part-time) to provide insight
- Well- entrenched cost accounting system

Economic analysis requires some additional criteria, such as size of the facility and general data on the probability of outcomes. Typically, academicians and clinicians are a good start. Depending on the therapy that is being evaluated, data generated from these settings can be extrapolated to a broader group within a category.

(v) ***Critical success factors checklist:*** To understand whether these criteria are met, the following checklist of critical success factors should be considered to evaluate the study:

- Clear, quantifiable protocol
- Clarity in addressing the perspective in protocol
- Parameters to observe clearly defined results while working on the protocol
- Practicability of the study to be carried out in the environment in which it needs to be conducted
- Statically correct sample size for carrying out the study
- Cost-effective time frame to conduct the study through researchers
- Resolution of alternate treatment issues
- Controls or prescribed behaviors in the protocol reasonable in relation to the real-world behavior
- Inclusion or exclusion criteria to represent real-world practice
- Proposed economic analysis for efficacy and safety

Such clinico-promotional studies require an alliance among product marketing, medical research and regulatory affairs of the organization. Such groups need to be formed in every organization as 'task forces' to clarify the positioning of the product and substantiate the claims and promises which product marketing makes to the doctors so that they can prescribe their products to patients.

PR AS PART OF PHARMACEUTICAL PROMOTIONAL MIX

While exploring the use of PR tools in pharmaceutical marketing it is necessary to ensure that PR complements and is coordinated with the rest of the company's efforts. Operating in a vacuum without overall back-up can send conflicting signals, which can harm corporate credibility.

For years, PR has been trying to establish its role in integrated marketing. But because the effectiveness of PR cannot really be measured or quantified, marketers often fail to see its value as a promotional tool.

There are two major utilities of PR as a marketing tool. One, it is a prerequisite to direct response marketing, and two, it allows quantification of subtle, yet firm, consumer related objectives of marketing at a one-to-one level and measures the same. PR became a prerequisite to direct response marketing after the suc-Touch's 1-2-3 service in Mumbai.

Yet, this is just the tip of the iceberg, considering that there is no limit to what people want to know and the tribe of people who value super-quick delivery of information is expanding. However, there is no reason that a regular phone service can't run this kind of 'tip-off' business. The reason that cell phone operators are taking the initiative is that they gain directly from increased airtime usage.

Through value addition, operators may even carve themselves a special identity based on their area of specialization. The question then is: What do people want to know and how much will they pay for it? Operators claim to be watching usage patterns, attitudes and needs that could help them fine-tune and create new add-on services.

After considering the success of Cipla in using PR techniques, many organizations tried to follow the same path, but without using PR as a platform. They started exploring 'obligation', 'direct marketing' and other tools. For instance, US Vitamins, with its financial power, tried to make customers (read doctors) happy by obliging them in many ways. Torrent and many other pharmaceutical companies also felt the need to do something similar. So over time, customers became greedy and the pharmaceutical industry contributed to making them greedier. As a result, the bargaining power of doctors today knows no bounds.

Objectivizing and Measuring PR Effectiveness

There is a reason to believe that PR can actually be measured for effectiveness, just as advertising can. The basis is to undertake an analysis that is far more rigorous and sophisticated than what is usually done. Any pharmaceutical marketing company that wishes to exploit PR for its advantage must define its objectives. One may want to build an image of quality and competitiveness through R&D and other competencies. Another may want to target the government and the bureaucracy, since eight ministries regulate the pharmaceutical industry. Yet another may want to target the insurance companies, or build a service image for the organization to influence bulk customers, or build relationships with decision-makers and in-between to get to hospitals, or win over the trust of doctors, or heighten credibility and reliability among patients.

So, a pharmaceutical company must prioritize its objectives and then work out the PR budget. At the end of the year, it must also measure the impact of the PR efforts against these objectives through available research techniques. Once the objectives are clear, evaluating the effect on the target group later is that much easier.

Difference between PR and Advertising

Clearly, PR is not the same as advertising. It is a far more interactive process. If prepared with adequate feedback mechanisms, the marketer can immediately see if the particular form of communication seems to be responding to specific messages of positioning a brand. The marketer can document that information and keep a finger on the pulse all the time. It may also show that the marketer has other important messages that simply are not suited to the audience.

At present, one can choose between 47,000 different media vehicles in the US alone, each one of which can carry a story of the safety and efficacy of your new product or molecule. A company such as 'Public Relations Data Systems' in Norwalk, Connecticut, analyzes these stories in terms of what messages they have managed to communicate about the company. Was the message positive or negative? What would be the message's equivalent advertising value? I am not sure whether one can analyze pharmaceutical stories through Public Regulations Data Systems, but for consumer products it has been happening regularly.

When aimed at media coverage, it is possible to show, for example, that the target media mentions of a particular company increased by a specific percentage from one quarter to the next. Moreover, following the launch of a reasonably priced PR program, researchers may tell you that the bulk of the second quarter's stories concerned the company's new product and that a few of them were highly positive.

One of the interesting result of this type of work is that it helps in establishing the PR's message equivalent advertising value - the dollar value of the space in magazines, or airtime on radio shows, and so on – that the company received for 'free' from media vehicles. Also note that editorial coverage, since it is perceived to be unbiased, tends to carry a great deal more of creditability as opposed to paid-for advertising.

In India, PR efforts are still at a nascent stage since they are dwelling in the area of 'activities'. India pharmaceutical marketers haven't given much thought to objectivizing and measuring these efforts.

Many have tried the impact of PR efforts only with corporate communications and financial markets. Results were quick, whether positive or negative! These efforts were *de rigueur* before a share issue.

Efforts on PR are subtle and specific. They deal with mass communications in a cost-effective way. Among the interesting decisions to take is which vehicle to get the message into. Smart PR can use various innovative means to send its message, particularly if the regular mass media vehicles begin to lose their appeal. Subtlety and sophistication can be employed to enter new avenues. There is much potential in PR for pharmaceutical marketers to explore.

We have till now looked at promotion and communication through alternative media, that can be used besides traditional detailing. Let us now turn to sales promotion through detailing which still remains the backbone of any promotional effort, and other new avenues.

Medical Practice of Tomorrow

The era of the individual medical practitioner is waning. Medical practice in India is undergoing revolutionary changes. Since the last few years there has been a profusion of 'nursing homes'. The responsibility of medical care is rapidly shifting from the general practitioner to teams of doctors grouped around a specific locality or speciality.

Besides, physicians are becoming more acutely aware of the amount of time they spend in functions that do not require their medical skills. Clearly, the doctor's time has become too valuable to spend in other than medical-related areas. It's quite natural to assume that he is now in the process of becoming as efficient in the use of his time as the most efficient businessman.

The complexity of competition is putting more pressure on the doctor's mind and hence he has to keep himself up-to-date. The physician of tomorrow will need to share and information on an even larger scale if he is to be successful.

The availability of diagnostic centers and polyclinics along with nursing homes and hospital chains is definitely inducing physicians to form teams and work together.

Patients too are looking at facilities more critically. A polyclinic or nursing home would certainly be better equipped than a GP's small clinic. There is also the question of credibility—a patient would much rather rely on a specialized group, than on an individual.

Yet another group of individuals is ushering in a change of profound significance in medical practice—the technicians. They will play an increasingly important role and will form groups and teams along with ancillary medical personnel.

Clearly, new spheres of influence in medical practice are emerging. In such a changing professional society which is likely to depart completely from the traditional one-to-one relationship, can techniques for communicating information to doctors and influencing them remain one-to-one?

Just as the manufacturers selling to the industrial market have to reach a number of specialists in addition to purchasing to agents, so will it be necessary for pharmaceutical companies to communicate with several groups and teams inclusive of technicians. Can the creaking, antiquated detail system cope with a situation of such magnitude?

Communication between the ethical pharmaceutical companies and the physician or team of physicians must turn to 'new' communication technologies to meet the challenge.

CASE

Multimedia Communication from Cipla[1]

In May 1991 when Cipla started operating through direct mail, it became the talk of the industry. Everybody was looking at the experiment. However, Cipla took the conscious decision of augmenting promotion and communication by personal and impersonal media. This gave birth to a multimedia approach.

Direct Mailings An operative database was prepared to undertake massive mailings. Courier services were pressed to give added boost to entire campaign by spreading the message through the special 'timely' service.

Prescription Watchers In May 1992, Cipla got some of their management trainees to stand in front of leading chemists of a given area and record prescriptions for a week. They would return to their office, sit with their regional managers and analyze the data, pick out important doctors, competitors and products, and organize mailings through courier. Specific mailers on products based on the information obtained from the survey were sent. It was also important to meet these doctors. A private viewing of video shows promoting their products was arranged, and thus a personal rapport with the doctors was established.

Video Magazines/Cassettes Around 85 video cassettes on various topics were prepared. Gatherings of a few doctors varying from 8—15 at a time were arranged in a five-star hotel with cocktails and dinner. After these video shows, prescription watching was organized to analyze and ascertain the impact of the video shows. The dispatches and mailing were continued as earlier.

Doctors' Meeting, Conferences and Symposia When it was decided in June 1991, to arrange gatherings of doctors, it was difficult to chase the doctors and get them to attend the meetings. Managers from Cipla booked venues and dates of the Indian Medical Association (IMA)

---

[1]*This case has been contributed by Interlink Marketing Consultancy Pvt. Ltd., Mumbai.*

meetings and followed up with the doctors month after month. They then started taking specialists from metro towns to address the IMA gatherings. Cipla also sponsored various symposia, such as on allergy by the Indian Academy of Allergy, and nephropathy by speciality chapters of nephrology, gastroenterology and urology. It was essentially Cipla who formed the Urology Association and sponsored their monthly clinical meets. The attendance at these meetings and symposia swelled over time. From December 1991 to January 1993, Cipla sponsored the meetings of the Society of Obstetrics and Gynaecology, once every two months. Each meeting was attended by about 150 doctors. Cipla also participated in the Indo-Singapore Gynaecology Workshop held in Bangalore by way of giving away delegate bags and prescription pads.

LEARNINGS

Communication

Communication is essentially a process which influences the audience. The basic task of communication in the pharmaceutical industry is largely dependent on the degree of risk and rationality. Effective communication is dependent on the way your message is received at the disposition level. A well-disposed mind will receive the message in the right frame. You can definitely evaluate the impact of the communication on the basis of prescription.

Persuasion

Personal communication by the sales force is absolutely essential to convince the physician to prescribe a particular brand. There are two schools of thought as regards influencing physicians for prescriptions: (i) medical education school, and (ii) psycho-behavioral school. It is difficult to choose one, as other unconventional promotional tools are used by companies.

Media Mix and Product Life-Cycle

The importance of the media is dependent on the stage at which the product is. There are *twelve* different media which can be used to influence physicians. These are:

1. Sales force
2. Magazines and Journals

3. The New Direct Mail
4. Conferences and Symposia
5. Clinical Trials
6. Promotional Trials
7. Sampling
8. Newspaper Advertising
9. Free-Standing Supplements
10. Telephone Marketing
11. Television
12. Group Detailing
13. Digital Marketing

Other promotion methods include advertising and branding, advertising in medical publications, medical TV programs, desk-top and in-clinic media, PR and clinico-promotional study.

CHAPTER **10**

Execution Prerequisites

Shivaji was the first to challenge the might of Bijapur and Delhi. This was a signal to his associates, countrymen, and subjects that it was possible for them to be independent leaders. Then he founded a state and showed his people that they were capable of administering a kingdom with all its complexities.

He thus, proved that they could build nations, find state, defeat enemies, conduct their own defense and maintain navy fleets. Also, that they were equally capable to protect and promote literature, arts, commerce and industry.

He operationalized and institutionalized many policies, which according to him, would help keep the morale of his people high as well as instill discipline among them. Different policies for different types of behavior were operationalized.

Once, while bringing home the riches and spoils after their victory over Kalyan, Vasai, and Surat, Shivaji's officers also brought along the daughter-in-law of the Subedar (officer-in charge) of Kalyanalong with them. She was so beautiful that they all had unanimously agreed to present her as a gift to Shivaji.

She was brought to the court and presented to Shivaji. Seeing her, Shivaji exclaimed, 'Oh, what a beauty, I wish my mother had been so beautiful . . . I too would then have born beautiful.' 'He at once freed her, and accepted her as his sister. After giving her the due respect that should be given to a lady, he sent her back to Kalyan with guards.

Through his own example and behavior he was thus able to guard one of his most dearest policies, namely to ensure that nobody would show disrespect to or enslave other people's wives, mothers, or sisters. They all would be treated as one of their own.

Many of the policies laid out by Shivaji are cited even today. A few examples are given here.

- This state is a gift of God; it will prosper as He wishes it. Let us commit; as He is with us.
- The Treasury is the life of the state. Protect it. Increase it.
- Never waste funds, never allow relations to waste it, never remain without a sword.
- Those who are talented and honest, scientists, and people without any addiction, should be always picked out and rewarded adequately. They should be kept happy and requested to work for the state and the king.
- Traders and merchants are symbols of prosperity of the state, and so the kind should choose his trade policies carefully.

Shivaji's strength lay in being able to thus operationalize his strategies. When strategies are formulated and understood, it becomes essential to operationalize them through internal organizational processes. Every forward-looking management needs to pay adequate attention to this process of operationalization of strategies so that any possible hindrances can be overcome.

When you start operationalizing any strategy, you need to examine the objectives and policies. One part of the objectives is usually spelt out while formulating the strategies. The remaining part needs to be taken care of by involving those who are given the responsibility of implementation. Processes like Management by Objectives (MBO) which even today retains its relevance, or annual planning, or annual budgeting can prove useful aids for achieving these objectives. Policies are also equally crucial for orienting the behavior of implementers toward a particular direction.

ADVANTAGES OF POLICIES

Policies provide objective guidelines for establishing and controlling ongoing practices and operations in a manner consistent with a firm's strategic objectives. Well-formulated policies perform several definite functions, and many companies have found that adherence to the policies provided for:

1. A uniform code of practice and behavior
2. Automatic decision making

3. Continuity of decisions
4. Effective communication
5. Protection from pressures of expediency
6. Indirect control over independent actions
7. Counteracting resistance to chosen strategies
8. Successful implementation

1. Uniform Code of Practice and Behaviour

Different codes of practice and lack of uniform behaviour, particularly in large organizations, lead to feelings of envy, resentment, frustration, and disappointment among the sales force and customers alike. Take a situation where one regional sales manager asks for regular reports and the other managers don't. The field staff of the manager insisting on reports would not like such discrimination; they would think unkindly of their manager and may even refuse to send in their reports. Most people, be the customers or representatives or managers, wish to be treated equally without any show of favour or discrimination. Managements must therefore frame policies that can ensure uniform behavior and bring about professionalism in the organization.

2. Automatic Decision Making

One of the more important functions of policy is to serve as an aid in decision making. A good policy is like, a previously made, well thought out decision, and finally now applied to problems in a similar context. There should not be any procrastination and the decision should be more or less automatic.

The bulk of routine field sales problems in any organization can be handled by the application of a well-enunciated field sales policy. Thereby, the field manager has time to deal with more crucial customer problems and need not to be bogged down with ordinary matters which produce internal tension and irritation.

However, policies should not be blindly applied without the use of judgement. There can always be exceptions, and field managers and in fact the entire field staff must be trained to recognize when it is not appropriate to apply a stated policy. A policy can be a guideline, and not an inflexible rule.

3. Continuity of Decisions

At the same time, there is always need for uniformity of decisions over a period of time. Discontent can result from unexpected changes of policy. Policies help bridge the gap between changes of management and prevent needless interruptions in successful operating procedures. It is sometimes seen that in few organizations there is a total reversal of earlier management decisions. Such organizations are seldom successful and lose credibility. On the other hand, in more successful organizations the basic operating policies remain essentially the same, despite changes in the top management.

Take some of the multinationals operating in India, such as Pfizer, Novartis and Sanofi, as examples. Each succeeding manager in these companies is well schooled in the company's policies, and hence leadership can be assumed with little noticeable change.

Continuity of decisions does not imply that policies do not change over time. They most certainly must be altered to adapt to the changing realities. However, uniform policy does provide for stability in the organization's outlook.

4. Effective Communication

Written or stated policies are one single means by which the management communicates its decisions to all levels of the organization.

Policy statements let everyone know what is expected. They are particularly useful for helping new employees quickly grasp what is expected of them and what they can expect from the management.

5. Protection from the Pressures of Expediency

To most people, the most pressing problems are those that immediately confront them. The seriousness with which a problem is considered is often a direct function of its proximity in time. People tend to discount possible problems in the future. Many managers fall prey to competitive pressures and ask their distributors and stockists to deal with such problems in a manner not in keeping with company policy. This sometimes leads to future problems.

For instance, suppose competition gives a 20% trade offer for a particular product. The manager then compels or convinces the distributor to convert his 10% share of the scheme into different slabs, and tries to make it more attractive by offering the same scheme in kind.

6. **Indirect Control over Independent Actions**

To achieve their targets, many field persons unilaterally resort to last-minute sales. A cooperative stockiest may not mind retiring the documents once in a while. However, if this becomes a habit, the stockiest may begin to resent it, and may send the consignments back.

Many organizations learn from these mistakes. They then try to monitor such independent actions through a policy whereby only those orders which are duly signed and stamped by the stockists are executed. No other orders are accepted. In this way you can directly control independent actions which are not in congruence with the company's strategic decisions.

7. **Counteracting Resistance to Chosen Strategy**

Had there been no policy of 'transfers' of the field staff, it would have been difficult for GSK to transfer their MRs. Although every appointment letter does carry a clause for the transfer of every field person, very few companies can adhere to it in practice since they have never acted on the policy from the beginning. GSK, on the other hand, has been consciously following a policy of transferring their MRs on a regular basis. As a result it is not perceived as a malpractice, or punishment, or a deviation from a practice. As a strategic decision, it is perhaps important to promote a person from within when the person is exposed to more than two territories. The experience certainly widens the field person's perspective.

8. **Successful Implementation**

The success of implementing strategies in most organizations is due to a set of proven policies. This is not to say that any policy is superior to 'no policy'. The key term here is *proven policy*. There can be bad policies which if followed could ruin companies. And policies that have been sound in the past can be ill-advised if there have been changes in the environment of the firm. Sound management is continually alert to the need for policy revision, but does not make changes without conclusive proof of their advisability. Responsible management is reluctant to abandon a policy that has been sound over a period of time in favor of untried, unproven alternatives.

A classic example would be of Reckitt Benckiser (Consumer Division) that redefined their 'stock-on-shelves' policy. As a result, many distributors started getting more return on investments, which they were looking for eagerly. With one change in policy they were able to elevate the morale of their distributors, who in turn helped them recapture the share of a few products in the state of Andhra Pradesh, which had become difficult to protect otherwise.

Policies can help build discipline and a sense of responsibility among the field force. Activity norms and appraisal parameters can be provided to the field staff for this purpose. When each representative is aware of the norms, and the management as a policy appraisal allows each of them to take stock of their behavior vis-à-vis the norms, they all learn. This brings about responsibility in their behavior and also helps managers maintain discipline in their teams.

Very often, companies who develop excellent marketing strategies spend very little time in operationalizing them through proven policies. Many organizations, even today, struggle at the policy level and the management always takes ad-hoc decisions or backs the productive decisions and practices. Sometimes this type of behavior ruins the future of the organization as these decisions turn out to be useful for a very short term.

For example, in one organization for the purpose of bridging the gap between the 'target' and 'actual' sales, a new strategy of 'institutional sales' was evolved. A few MRs were promoted from the sales and they were now operating as field managers for institutions. Although there is a gestation period for institutions to yield results, the entire process was rushed through.

When the orders were procured by the managers, the issue of payments, mode of channel, etc. began posing problems. The stockists were also not ready to supply to these institutions as they were finding it difficult to recover the dues. So they began turning down the orders. The orders were then directly supplied to the institutions from the depots. Since the existing MRs had not been covering these special institutions and hospitals, the field managers now found the field force inadequate to cover all of them. Their problem was compounded by the fact that since their force had been newly created without much field force support, they were unable to get the cooperation of the existing MRs or exercise control over them. Over a period of time, the outstandings began to mount to more than 180 days. You can imagine the loss the company may have suffered in terms of time, money, energy of the entire field force, along with the frustration of these newly promoted managers. Eventually, the promoted managers were absorbed in the existing organization. Through this incident, you can perhaps realize the dangers of trying to implement strategies without laying down clear policies.

Not only is it important to formulate good, well-though out policies, it is equally important to communicate them to the entire team, and ensure that all concerned have understood them. Once laid, down it is also equally necessary to adhere to these policies.

TYPES OF POLICIES

Field force policies can be characterized along several dimensions. They may be:

  (i)   Strategic or operational,
  (ii) Stated or unstated,
  (iii) Covert or overt, and
  (iv) Implicit or explicit.

Strategic versus Operational

The top management makes strategic policies that guide the entire enterprise along selected routes. Baidyanath, for example, in addition to its strategic policy of making only Ayurvedic products, also pursued a policy of expanding its sales volume and profits by investing in its own wholesale-cum-retail outlets in different cities in India. They appointed one vaidya at a retail outlet and over time they got the required per day sales with the help of his free diagnosis and prescription. Later, they sold the outlet lock, stock and barrel to any entrepreneur who then ran the shop from there on. While buying the shop, the new owner inherited exclusivity of Baidyanath stocks. Over a period of time, although he bought products of other companies, the ratio of Baidyanath sales to that of other companies remained 80:20. Thus, with this process Baidyanath was able to maintain a near monopoly situation.

Operational policies are guideposts that are established to carry out strategic policies. Many times they take on the appearance of work rules. In this typical example, the location, space, appointment of the vaidya, and stock management, till the stock is sold, form part of the operational policies.

Stated versus Unstated

Choice of either stated or unstated polices mostly depends on the circumstances. To improve the morale and provide incentive to your sales force, you may adopt a selection policy of promoting from within. Only a stated policy can achieve the desired result in such a case. There are other times, however, when it may be wise not to state a policy that nevertheless is operative, as in a firm that follows a policy of going outside to hire top executives. While some may be able to discern the policy from the firm's actions, many cannot be sure of it. All unstated policies are confirmed by employees when they observe the actions of the management.

Covert versus Overt

While a policy may not be stated, it may still be obvious because of the management's overt actions and behavior. Indeed, polices of most concerns can be detected from their actions. For example, it seemed to be the policy of GSK to depend on inexperienced fresh college graduates for sales recruits; its overt hiring behavior made this quite obvious.

At times, the management does not want certain parties to know the actual policy on a given matter. Perhaps the law is involved, or it could be a matter related to competition. Or the management may want to conceal its policy to protect its interests. Near about the late 1970s and early 1980s, Abbott helped their field staff get jobs in other organizations discreetly.

Implicit versus Explicit

When the management and union sign the charger of demands, both of them explicitly establish many operational policies after deliberate thought and premeditation. Other practices without an explicit decision being made are implicit in nature. That the MR should call on twelve doctors and five chemists per day may be the explicit policy for many companies; but it is also implicit that each of these doctors should be on an 'agreed', select list. To be on the list, they should, for example, have potential to prescribe, and may be over a period of two to three visits should actually start prescribing.

Basic Policies for Operationalizing Strategic Decisions

We can identify *four* major policies that can provide strength to each implementer while discharging his duties in the marketplace.

1. Field sales policy
2. Distribution and trade policy
3. Pricing policy
4. Promotional policy

Each of these four policies is equally important for fostering implementation, and are described in detail below.

1. Field Sales Policy

Some of the major contributions to resourceful implementation come from the field staff. Organizations which formulate relevant policies can ensure discipline among its workforce. Even exceptionally motivated field staff without self-discipline, over a period of time, can become demoralized. In order to ensure adequate productivity and discipline, there are *ten* important policies that need to be formulated relating to:

(i)   Selection, induction and training
(ii) Travel and conveyance
(iii) Development on the job
(iv) Appraisals
(v)   Promotions and career planning
(vi) Financial responsibility
(vii) Manpower requirements
(viii) Norms
(ix) Feedback and communication
(x)   Termination

(i) ***Selection, induction, and training:*** It is essential to develop the profile of the field staff hierarchy inclusive of MRs. Usually, I have observed that it is only the managers who fill up the vacancies and the MRs are left out, if there is no laid down policy and procedure. As an organization, you need to decide on the following issues before selection:

- Age range
- Education
- Fresh or experienced; if experienced, for how many years and in which kind of organization
- Family background and family size
- Communication ability
- Track record
- Values and attitudes
- Achievements
- Competence and potential

If you can resolve these issues and develop a policy for the process of selection, it is likely that you will be able to acquire an asset for your organization. While implement the policy, you may also add time frame and quality of work for those who are likely to be selected.

Induction is the next step, which is very crucial, as at this stage, you induct an outsider and make him imbibe your organizational goals and values. A properly laid down induction policy reduces irritation and future possible non-compliance to regulations.

As pharma selling requires depth of product knowledge, and other related knowledge in medicine, pharmacology, biology, and zoology, training assumes a major role. While this kind of functional training is vital, behavioral training is also essential as each member of the team needs to develop expertise in handling people, inclusive of customers.

In my opinion, while planning the marketing mix, you must invest adequately in training of your sales force. Strong promotion and communication have failed due to lack of skilled MRs and managers. Policies for such training need to be well-formulated and implemented.

(ii) *Travel and conveyance:* Although pivotal in maintaining high motivation levels among the MRs, some organizations do not take travel and conveyance polices seriously. These policies need to be reviewed every three to five years with changes in the environment and organization size. While these policies should be reasonably easy to implement, they should at the same time be flexible enough to accommodate human issues. Once you operationalize your strategies through good policies of travel and conveyance, day-to-day irritations can be eliminated. In organizations where there are no set policies, adhocism prevails, leading to tension and loss of morale among the field staff. On the other hand, with sound policies you can hope to inculcate a sense of responsibility in each member of your team, and ensure their compliance.

(iii) ***Development on the job:*** For any quality job in India, supervision is the key. Supervision assumes meaning when the subordinates learn on the job. The learners also begin to respect the supervisors when they see the problems on the job being resolved in their presence. Since on-the-job development is different from simulating situations in the classroom, this process provides credibility to the techniques and guidance being provided by the supervisor. Here I am not limiting the meaning of 'supervision' and 'supervisor' to only front-line managers and MRs; it encompasses the hierarchy. So, even the managing director is to play the role of a supervisor in relation to his vice presidents. At this level also, development on the job is very crucial as each vice president while being an expert in one's own area of specialization may have a lot to learn about other areas. Thus, formulation of policies and procedures that can derive benefits from development on the job are essential.

(iv) ***Appraisals:*** Continuous appraisal helps managers to evaluate their subordinates. In pharma field management, as the superiors and subordinates meet each other often, appraisals normally do not take place regularly. Even the appraisals of those who are on probation are not perceived as tools to manage them. It is imperative that greater emphasis is given to awareness, usage and benefits of appraisals, and guidelines provided to all superiors on how to conduct them. If necessary, the training inputs can themselves incorporate a cohesive strategy of implementing appraisals for the development of human resources.

(v) ***Promotion and career planning:*** You need to decide whether a vacancy should be filled from within your organization or from outside when you plan for manpower expansion. This policy decision has implications for getting the right type of people. Many times, it is important to prepare career plans for those employees who wish to get a feeling of fulfillment by remaining in the organization by hoping to achieve their 'dream' positions. This motivates them to give their best to the organization. This also reduces the turnover of managers and MRs.

(vi) ***Financial responsibility:*** This has a direct bearing to the power an executive has in relation to the financial resources of the organization. For example, there are a few organizations which allow yearly budgets for regional managers to spend on ad-hoc souvenir ads. Once the budget is provided each manger tries to scrutinize the opportunity of maximizing that amount through adequate selection. Similarly, a policy framework can be provided for many areas of day-to-day decisions, and some responsibilities can be given to the field staff also.

(vii) ***Manpower requirements:*** All multinationals usually plan for this resource very carefully as they look upon it as an asset acquisition avenue. It is unfortunate that it sometimes becomes a liability. However, experience has shown that if human assets are developed properly, you can really create assets for the organization. It is essential to have policy guidelines to develop manpower inventory, skills inventory, and future requirements depending on the needs of the market.

(viii) ***Norms:*** These provide guidelines to all about the extent of activities to be carried out in the market. The norms could include calls on doctors and chemists, their order booking, etc. They help MRs, managers, and the management evaluate the impact of the events taking place in the marketplace. The norms must be in tune with the coverage, productivity, and strategies. They must also relate to results, which are usually reflected in the targets or budgets. Written expectations of results are thus useful for the MRs and managers to determine the extent to which they have been successful, and what more they should do.

(ix) ***Feedback and communication:*** All organizations, depending on what they wish to control and communicate, design their formats accordingly. These formats require basic guiding principles which can only emanate from the policy framework. Otherwise, a plethora of reports and systems would be evolved which would lie unused or partially used.

(x) ***Termination:*** A policy to terminate the service of employees on grounds of indiscipline, misappropriation of funds, and other integrity-related issues is essential to maintain discipline in the organization.

2. Distribution and Trade Policy

India is a trading country, and it is so vast that if adequate availability is not ensured, the marketing efforts go waste. All organizations, inclusive of OTC consumer products, give a lot of emphasis on the depth and width of distribution. The distribution coverage is dependent on the coverage of doctors and retailers.

As changes are taking place in retailing, there is a decrease in investments in retailing due to the overservicing of stockists, wholesalers, and distributors. As cash transactions take place at the retail counter, and the trade credit varies from three days to three months, retailer investments have come down drastically. The stock levels of a metro-city retailer range from 0 to 3 days. Many times the patients carry the prescriptions with them while going to work and purchase the medicines while returning home. So, a really good strategy is needed to tackle the issue of availability of stocks at retailers.

The wholesale market is also very strong in India. Many retailers replenish their stocks from wholesalers. Wholesalers are keen in earning more as they do business at lower margins, but are able to have faster rotation of money. Therefore, wholesalers prefer to buy and sell those products which move faster. If your product is wholesale sensitive, you need to decide on a specific wholesale strategy. The cases of Dettol Plaster and Hansaplast can certainly throw light on the benefits and limitations of wholesale strategy.

Distributors or stockists need to be financially sound. Above all, they must cater to the markets by giving suitable credit terms and other services. Thus, selection and appraisal of stockists and distributors become crucial issues in managing them.

It is equally important to clearly specify a distributor's role to enhance the width and depth of distribution. You need to ensure adequate return on investment for them so that they can involve themselves in your franchise.

As a strategy, you must also look at the costs of distribution; many times this cost hinders the availability of goods in deeper interiors of India. The monthly turnover and size of the order are both important factors in deciding a cost-effective system of distribution. On the basis of turnover, you must develop different categories of distributors/stockists so that other polices of stocks, order collections, catering, service level, etc. can be properly evolved and implemented.

3. Pricing Policy

In the olden days of prescription, drug industry pricing played only a secondary role for the prescriber and user. Novelty, therapeutic advantage, and effective sales promotion had a much more crucial role in determining the success of prescription drugs. The increased importance of generics, and technology breakthroughs, however, has made the drug markets, or atleast some of their segments, more price-sensitive. For the drug company, of course, the price of a drug, i.e. its gross margin, is vital for its profitability.

In India, pricing is basically done on a cost-plus basis. The percentage mark-ups are determined by the government for category I products (essential drugs), and category II products (other products of widespread use as per the needs of the country). However, the prices are adjusted for the decontrolled category as a result of competition in the market. This then depends on the technology, ambitions of competitive players, the staying power of various competitive products, and the decision taken for getting a specific profit, which may be even less than the norms.

The prices of new drugs and drug price increases are controlled by the government in most countries through direct price controls or reimbursement schemes, or both, or through the control of corporate profits of pharmaceutical companies. Elsewhere, price control systems range from controlling the return on investment on supplies to the National Health Service (e.g. UK), to controlling the mark-up pricing structure based on the production cost (e.g. France) to controlling prices with reference to prices in the home market of the company or assorted baskets of other international prices. The exceptions where governments do not control the prices are the USA, Canada, Germany, the Netherlands and South Africa. However, as a result of the ageing population and the inelastic demand for pharmaceutical products, governments in the developed world have seen health costs increase beyond their ability to meet them.

In most countries, the government pays a major part of the health bill, and since drugs represent a significant share of this bill, governments have a direct interest in keeping the drugs prices under control. In India, however, each patient pays for the total treatment. Each country thus has a unique pricing mechanism.

(i) ***Pricing strategy:*** Take a look at the following examples:

Stangen used pricing as a strategy when it wanted to improve the volume of Norfloxacin and establish itself. All other competitors were at around Rs.7 to Rs.9 per capsule. However, Stangen priced Norilet (Norfloxacin) at Rs.3.85 per capsule. This 'relative price' advantage put them ahead of Ranbaxy and Cipla and created an image of providing 'value of money' in the consumer's mind. It also resulted in lowering the 'cost of goods sold' for the others, as many were buying the basic drug from Dr. Reddy's Laboratories. This can happen through either high volume or economies of scale or through a technological breakthrough, or both. In this particular case, it started with a technological breakthrough, and now, perhaps, it has been possible to reduce the prices because of economies of scale.

As a result of the implementation and impact of GATT and TRIPS, patents tomorrow could drive out small competitors. Pricing, then, would assume a crucial role. It would require working out different price structures encompassing the consumer price index, wholesale price index, hospital price index, and the retail price index. The average sales price would also have to be determined, and then the average margin calculated. The R&D and overhead costs would also have to be taken into account. At the same time, the government too can play an important role in regulating the pricing of patented products.

Wockhardt used high technology in manufacturing baby foods for infants who had 'milk allergy' to launch its range of baby food products. It was able to dissuade other small manufacturers to enter the field as the investment in technology was enormous, and succeeded in achieving near-zero competition. Nobody except Raptakos Brett (R.B) had hi-tech food products. Earlier, Raptakos Brett had a monopoly in the Indian market. Everybody kept away till Wockhardt jumped into it with high investment.

In 1990-91, Ampicillin was not available. Hence the usual way of providing trade bonus offers to maintain the sales and demand was not possible. But Alkem kept its focus on bonus offers and took a conscious decision to reduce the price in order to gain market share in areas like Bihar. Thus, when the products of others were becoming scarce, Alkem could maintain adequate distribution. Paracetamol in generic form is today available at Re 0.50 per tablet while Metacin or Crocin (branded paracetamol) is priced at Re 0.94 per tablet. They usually use the pricing mechanism to increase volume; they are also price sensitive to dealers.

If you examine the different examples we have just discussed, you will be able to appreciate the various implications of pricing which can affect business. As Figure 10.1 illustrates, to evolve an effective pricing strategy you need to consider the various internal and external factors, evaluate your strengths and weaknesses, before finalizing your strategy. If your organization ventures into buying over technology to produce bulk drugs and formulations with R&D facilities, you have to incur high investment. This high initial cost can affect your pricing. However, if you are able to achieve economies of scale, you can reduce the cost, further, if you patent your product, there is again a cost increase. Thus, these internal factors directly relate to cost and affect your pricing. On the other hand, external factors are related to governmental controls, trade practices, paying capacity, competitive ability to reduce or increase the prices, and of course the changing business environment. An understanding of these internal and external factors can give you an insight of your *constraints* and *opportunities*. The right pricing strategy will be a balance of both.

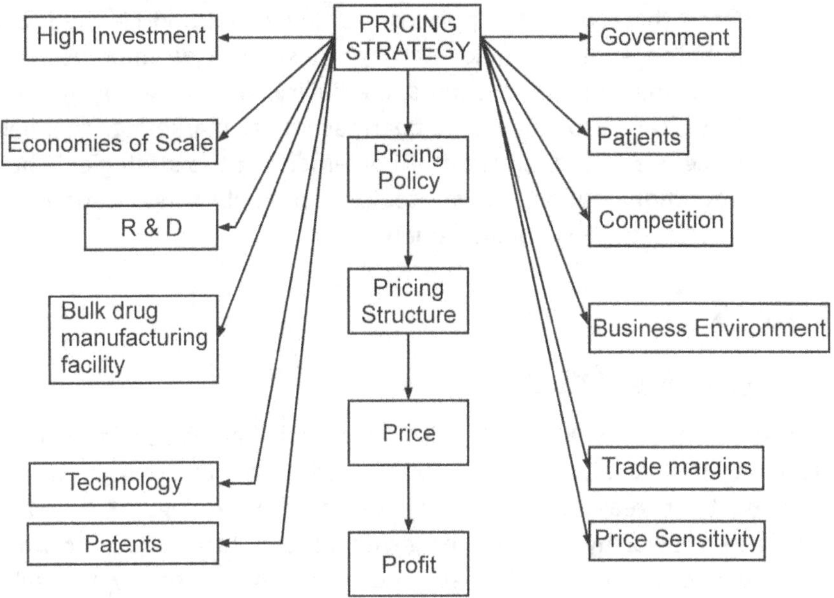

Figure 10.1 Factors for evolving an effective pricing strategy

4. Promotional Policy

Since the 1970s, GSK has made a conscious decision that all MRs will promote all products to all selected doctors. However, all those who have entered the market today expose only one product to one doctor, and thereby justify the need of prescription from the doctor. Both these policies have worked.

This implies that as an organization you must develop promotional policies which will encompass the following aspects:

- Number of products to be promoted to a doctor
- Time spent on each product
- Multimedia or single medium approach
- Trade promotion
- New product promotion
- Old and prescribing products promotion
- Sampling
- Other giveaways
- Individual v/s. group practices
- Cyclewise plan and guidelines

Once these basic *ten* policies are developed and clarified, and adherence of the field staff to these policies improves, the discipline, cost-effectiveness, credibility, and impact of the field force can also go up. In pharmaceutical marketing, the field force is a crucial element in implementing the strategies. Thus, operationalization of strategies can help organizations to improve the level of implementation.

TACTICS

The Importance of Tactics

Many fine strategies with highly desirable goals have failed for want of proper tactics. A sales manager formulated a new compensation plan designed to increase both sales as well as the earnings of the sales people—both worthy goals. But he gave no thought to tactics, and when he tried a director frontal attack, he was admonished by the sales people who were apprehensive of the new plan.

Thus, since the successful execution of a plan often depends more on the tactics employed upon than their intrinsic soundness, the developer of a sound plan should be tactically adept. Many talented young executives have been thwarted in their ambitions because they operate under the naïve assumption that right is might. Frequently, they are done in by people of lesser talent who are more proficient in the use of tactics. It is not enough to devise wise strategies; they must be implemented with proper tactics.

We do not like to discuss the use of tactics; in our society it is not quite acceptable. It gives the impression that you are manipulating people. Indeed, most tactics focus on manipulating people or structuring situations. Moreover, many tactics, when improperly applied, are considered unethical. Some administrators probably would be more willing to talk about their private lives than about the tactics they use in reaching their goals, and for good reason. It is usually best for other people to remain unaware of the tactics you are using. Therefore, it is up to you as an individual to learn about tactics through experience, on your own. Nobody is going to teach them. This is perhaps one reason that good administrators develop relatively slowly.

A noted writer on management recently said, 'Tactics bore me. I'm only interested in strategy. That's the determinant of success!' However, in field management observation, experience and logic indicate otherwise. Suppose a sales manager has been told to cut the costs of sales by 10%. There are many different plans that he could adopt; some admittedly more likely to succeed, and some more difficult to institute. But it is the tactics that the manager ultimately chooses to achieve the plan that will determine whether or not it works.

Tactics are the tools of the implementer, the tools used to carry out the firm's strategies and plans. A skillful implementer not only possesses a wide range of tactics, but knows when and how to use them.

Tools

Tactics themselves are amoral; they are neither good nor bad. And there are no perfect tactics. In any situation there is no one best set of tactics that can be used. Many tactics may work, some better than others. Many others may fail, some more surely than others. Many implementers mistakenly use the same tactics repeatedly, regardless of the circumstances. They get into a habit of using their favorite tactics because these have worked for them previously. Success reinforces the habit. But success can make you repeat tactics mindlessly. There comes a time when the tactics do not work; and usually that is the most critical time.

The classic example of the implementer's inability to vary tactics is the forceful, hard-hitting executive who uses strong, authoritarian tactics to climb up the ranks. The executive will discover that at the top such tactics are not effective in dealing with others of equal ability. New tactics are needed for the new environment. The manager who is unable to make the necessary tactical adjustments fails.

As tools of implementation, tactics can be used like a hammer to pound nails or smash thumbs. In themselves, the tools are neither good nor bad. It is up to the manager to learn how to use them properly.

Tactical Evaluation of a Situation

The crucial element is in deciding which tactics to use in a particular situation. Take the case of a manager of a field force that is unionized. In making his tactical decision, the manager must decide how to collaborate with the other party in the situation, whether through peers, subordinates, customers, or competitors.

A sales manager faces a number of considerations when deciding upon a tactical plan or course of action. Some of the more critical elements in this tactical model are discussed below.

(i) *Stakes:* How much money is involved? If the stakes are high, more forceful tactics may be needed than if the matter is inconsequential. On minor issues, many managers might choose to ignore the adversary. Suppose an association of physicians asks you to sponsor more than Rs. 5 lakh for their conference—high stakes. There is a possibility of you incurring this expenditure and not gaining much advantage from it; your competitor may display tactical skills. Recently a 'high power' organization sponsored a seminar spending more than Rs.20 lakh. The sales manager of the competing organization registered along with his medical director for the same conference and they stayed in two different suites at the venue. During the day they spent time with their 'core' doctors and in the evening they entertained the same doctors in such a way that they could build up a rapport with 30 core physicians from all over India in three nights.

(ii) *Personalities:* People react to situations in different ways. Some adversaries are belligerent and combative. Any direct action that would antagonize them might prod them into doing exactly what the manager does not want them to do. In such cases it would be better to use various indirect tactics. Other people are more passive and less apt to take offense at tactical actions. The relative belligerency of the other person's personality is only one of a multitude of character traits to be considered in making tactical decisions.

You must also recognize your own personality characteristics. It would be foolish to try to bluff your way through if your acting skills are suspect. Some managers find that their personalities are better suited for dealing with other people on a one-to-one basis rather than in groups. In their tactical maneuvering, they try to avoid group meetings. Many companies have stopped conducting meetings of large groups of doctors. They now call smaller teams to avoid conflicts between two schools of thoughts held by specialists.

(iii) ***Power bases:*** The power held or perceived to be held by both parties plays a pivotal role in tactical selection. The manager who has a strong power base, an unassailable one, can make more forceful tactical moves. On the other hand, a manager who does not possess any power over his subordinates must use other tactics.

Power is also elusive. One may have it one day and not the next. I have observed in many organizations that many front-line managers who wish to get their MRs to implement organizational norms cannot exercise their power if those MRs ignore their instructions. Many managers get shocked when their MRs refuse to act on their instructions, and question their authority. Tactically, if the manager is weak, MRs also 'manage' their managers. It is important to use all powers a manager has.

(iv) ***Future relationships:*** You cannot treat a doctor or a retailer you hope to do business with again in the same way as one who is served only once. Often, I have observed that the rule, 'Decisions should be tough, behavior need not be', works better when you deal with distributors, doctors, and MRs. Imagine a situation where the distributor is earning but does not wish to provide necessary service. You may have to be assertive enough to protect future relationship. You may observe a change in his attitude.

(v) ***Urgency:*** In the case of pending collections, it is essential to tactically stop the consignment and recover the payment first. If quick action is needed, direct, forceful tactics may have to be used.

(vi) ***Probability of success:*** Tactics have different likelihoods of success in different situations. Some managers become so enamoured with a certain type of tactics that they try to use it in situations in which they do not work. Because of their intrinsic nature, many managers ignore formal communications and use informal and verbal routes. When the going gets tough, it becomes too late and they cannot then document anything. So, the possibility of success lessens.

(vii) ***Personal skills:*** Some people can do certain things easily, others cannot. The manager who finds it difficult to detail his product to the doctors may find other ways of accomplishing the same task. A person who does not talk well resorts to written communication. Managers should use tactics at which they are adept.

(viii) ***Legal considerations:*** Some issues end up as a legal liabilities. If the firm ends up in litigation, because of, say having affixed increased price stickers on existing stocks, the selection of tactics should be made carefully. The data should be accurate and the details must be provided to the authorities.

(ix) ***Values:*** The manager's personal values play a key role in tactical selection. You should not do things you don't feel right about. There are managers who take up the task of developing subordinates as a challenge. These personal values add to providing commitment to people.

(x) ***Impact on others:*** Whether or not any manager is directly leading his team, he is still a leader. The actions and inactions of the manager affect the team. If the manager always plays a passive role, and takes time to react to competition, it will affect his team members, and the team as whole will also lose its reflexes.

Thus, a manager has many things to consider in selecting the tactics for a particular situation. The greater the issue, the more carefully should these factors be weighed.

ETHICAL DIMENSION OF TACTICS

Mr. Nani A. Palkhiwala, in the introduction to his book, *We the People*, powerfully states: 'We as a nation suffer from fatty degeneration of conscience. The tricolor fluttering all over the country is black, red and scarlet—black money, red tape and scarlet corruption.' Although we as a nation are trying to overcome all these aspects, deep-rooted systems can't be removed overnight. These systems percolate to all levels of society, and doctors are no exception. How can you expect them to be different from the changing society? MrPalkhiwala further describes two major defects of our society—a lack of a sense of fairness, and a lack of moderation.

These same defects seem to have pervaded many of our pharmaceutical companies. The practices have basically evolved owing to two specific reasons:

(i)   Stiff competition, and

(ii)   An impatience to deliver results or create sales.

These compelling reasons make the ground battlefield operators restless if they cannot keep pace with their competitors.

It is difficult to clearly say what constitutes an ethical practice and what does not. Except for some exceptional cases, I would say, more often than not, there is no such thing as an unethical practice. If a company is unable to match the practice of its competitor, it is likely to label the competitive action as an 'unethical practice'. The reason could be lack of resources, or lack of skills, or capabilities or strengths, or failure to initiate changes to innovate.

Sometimes a competitor deliberately spreads a rumor about its so-called achievements. Often, these are heard and not seen, and are meant to scare away competition. An organization that is not confident of its strength gets taken in by such rumors, and withdraws even before the fight begins. There is this story (again, it could be a rumor only) of a company that claimed to have spent Rs.40 lakh on a single conference at Delhi. Now, it is really not possible to verify such a claim. The weak and unconfident competitor will develop cold feet. Does it also have to match or surpass this amount of Rs.40 lakh? But one thing is clear: those who have resources and capabilities and are willing to take risks and innovate, will win. And few will call their practices unethical.

It is very important to give added value to the customers. If some of these practices add value to the products, there is nothing wrong. Experience says everything is fair in love, war, and marketing as there are practices and practices and practices.

A few of them are at the borderline of ethical and unethical practices. For example, linking prescriptions to rewards and incentives. Some do it cleverly; others do it blatantly. Take the tactic Cipla once tried for one of their products. It promised the first dose free along with the printed prescriptions which they gave to the doctors. The remaining doses were to be bought by the patients. The patients also found it a good incentive. The doctors were hooked and the company saved sample cost. Clever really! But what would you say to a company giving away Videocon washing machines on the kind of support they get from the doctors? The product manager possibly knew the sales and stock figures of washing machines better than his own product, because he was keeping a tab on the availability of washing machines all over the country. Well, as we said earlier, practices differ. You decide what is good for you, and what is right or wrong.

In practice, on the games field, there are all types of players. And there are a few rules to be followed. You have to plan your strategies, tactics, and use your skills the best way you can. If you are inhibited by your accumulated biases and morals, you will not be able to respond quickly enough and you will lose.

So, how do you cope with the changing rules of the game? There are some issues you must resolve before deciding and designing your strategies to counter the so-called unethical practices. We will now look at some of these issues.

- The intrinsic quality, merit and personality of the MR disseminating information about the product to the doctors. The confidence and assertiveness, with which he handles himself in the clinic and the training given to him, are all important. What you need to ask is: 'How do I want my MR to be perceived by the doctors?' And then decide on the kind of inputs you need to provide him.
- The kind of backing we need to give to the MR in terms of innovative promotion inputs, the positioning of the product, and other efforts needed, so that the doctors take him seriously.

- The quality planning of each brand along with an understanding of the needs of promotion for them. A new anti-cancer drug may require the education of both doctors as well as patients. In essence, what you need to ask is: 'How do I evolve a customer-driven marketing strategy?'
- True, commercialism has entered the domain of pharmaceutical marketing. But is not the degree of commercialism dependent on how you make the doctors perceive you? If you initiated the practice of rewards or incentives to doctors, it is but natural they will have elevated expectations.
- There are other ways too. There are still several unfulfilled needs of doctors which you can satisfy innovatively.
- Finally, what you need to ask yourself is: 'What are my strengths as an organization?' 'How long can I survive in this unending cut-throat game that can only yield short-term gains?' If you do anything consistently over a long period, your customers will perceive you in that light and their expectations will also be in accordance. Your product should be your source of strength. If your product is good, and you are able to give it adequate backing and innovative promotional support, you will win in the long run.

So, look at your strengths, and find out innovative ways to match those practices that will drain away your resources. Go to your customers and find out what they really need. Natco is one company that did an excellent job in identifying the needs of cardiologists who wanted a few article updates of those published in prestigious international journals every month. The company arranged for this and distributed photocopies of the articles. Their value-added service to the customer was appreciated. Innovation is the key.

INSTITUTIONALIZING THE STRATEGIES — STRUCTURAL ISSUES

We have seen earlier that with the help of objectives and policies, we can operationalize the strategies; but institutionalizing the strategies requires the existence of structures and systems. Old structures are collapsing. The concept of one national sales manager with a team of zonal managers, and a group of front-line and second-line managers carrying the company promotion only through MRs is on its way out.

Each organization is trying to find out formal and informal ways of developing structures. These formal or informal structures then develop systems, which, in turn, have to serve the communication needs to nourish the organization and ensure its effective functioning.

There are *three* major issues which affect the level of implementation in terms of structure:

1. Formal and/or informal structures
2. Product- or market-related structures
3. Responsibility-centered structures

1. **Formal and Informal Structures**

   (i) *Formal structures*

   (a) *More than-one-boss-syndrome:* The role of the front-line manager is obviously very crucial for successful implementation by the field force. However, if the field force has to report to different sets of managers for its different functional activities, its cohesiveness and efficiency are bound to be affected adversely. There are organizations where the field representatives report to the sales manager for their sales activities, the marketing manager when it comes to product promotion, and the finance or distribution manager in the context of outstandings and collections. TOMCO is an example where the implementation level deteriorated because marketing was not in unison with the field force.

   This also leads to several departmental problems. This is not to say that this kind of structural demarcation and reporting pattern does not work. In some cases it can, provided there is a strong awareness of the strengths and weaknesses of such structures, and the leader is capable of coordinating and classifying the conflicts.

   (b) *Flat structure:* Cipla had been engaged in a major restructuring of its organization. It was trying to make its organization flatter in terms of hierarchy, and was also attempting a new concept of coordination as against the earlier concept of reporting.

Such structural adjustments and changes are sometimes necessary to ensure successful implementation.

(c) ***Flexi-time structure:*** A few organizations have found out that if they bifurcate the working hours, they can increase the concentration of promotion on selected doctors. As a result, flexi-time teams have been appointed to work in the morning hours and other teams are assigned for the evenings and calling on consultants. A majority of such promoters are girls in metro towns, or those who have implemented this concept earlier. This system has been working so well for a few organizations that they now always launch any new product through flexi-time promoters.

(ii) ***Informal structures:*** Wockhardt started promoting their one 'hospital product' through a set of promoters who, though trained and managed by company managers, were on the payrolls of either distributors or an outside agency. This type of an additional set of promoters for a focused work in hospitals did provide rich dividends to the organization.

2. **Product- or Market-Related Structures**

   (i) ***Product-related:*** Kramer, a speciality division of Kopran was trying to carve out a niche in the market. It was to set the organization in a different way so that the doctors could perceive the difference in promotion. At four centers—metro cities—four to five product officers were appointed and their exclusive job was to follow up those products which had a major stake for the organization. This additional infrastructure of 20 to 25 product officers was created at six to eight headquarters to comb the speciality. Even Ethnor once tried to segregate its MRs to promote Raricap Syrup and tablets separately to different sets of doctors. While the difference in the approach was perceptible, it also created some confusion in the market. So you need to be careful with product-related structures.

   (ii) ***Market-related:*** Charak identified the potential of Ayurvedic products in UP and decided to penetrate the state with the help of more than 35 to 40 MRs. The entire structure was market-related. All hospital products and equipment companies have designed their structures on the basis of markets.

3. Responsibility-Centered Structure

Natco and Stangen restructured their zones making them profit-centers. A pool of products and the resources to make these products successful were available with the head office. Each sales manager had liberty to choose the products, choose the promotion mix, and the cost attached to it to generate a given profit ratio. The responsibility to generate profit was thus squarely placed on the regions or zones.

You need to strengthen any given structure by developing the necessary norms through administrative supports.

SYSTEMS

Whatever structural foundations you lay to develop your marketing organization, you need to also develop the feedback and marketing information system. These systems must help to generate adequate information which can help managers and the management control and support the events and activities of the marketing department and the field staff.

Systems can be formulated and institutionalized in the following areas:

1. Activities of the marketing and field staff, product management group, and distribution personnel
2. Results of the field staff
3. Cost of the field staff
4. Promotional efforts
5. Strategy implementation by the field staff
6. Database generation for marketing efforts
7. Activities and results of distributors/C&F agents/depots
8. Cost of distribution
9. Special campaigns feedback
10. Special problems/opportunities feedback

The systems can provide information which can be used to develop a proactive stance.

CASE

Operation Greenstorm—The Story of a Successful New Product Launch[1]

1. Introduction

The time was April 1993. The task was the introduction of a new product—Dettol Plaster in Mumbai, the home ground of the most formidable competitor, Band-Aid. The challenge—win a 20% share in the regular segment of the medicated market.

A little background. After about 18 months of test marketing the product, the management decided to go national in 1993. The test market results, while meeting minimum acceptance standards, were not replicable uniformly as Mumbai was the single-largest metro-market with Band Aid's market share hovering between 90 and 95%.

2. Operation Greenstorm

While a detailed list of time-bound marketing objectives were set (in terms of awareness, trial, repeat buying, etc.), the management decided to explore the critical success factors in field operation as a few preliminary investigations in the wholesale and retail markets seemed to point out that our selling distribution strategies could give us significant competitive advantages. The management set out three months before launch to understand the distribution, trading terms and strengths/weaknesses of competition in detail. What were these?

- The dominant market leader in Mumbai was 'pull' led. Hansaplast, the second brand in rank nationally, was weak in Mumbai, but in several upcountry markets it had more than 25% share with strong trade incentives and distribution thrust. A detailed study of such winning actions of Hansaplast was drawn up from markets in Madhya Pradesh.
- Band-Aid had a strong wholesale focus.
- The retailer has a strong role in recommending the product.
- Merchandising display activities in the category were few.

---

[1]*This case has been contributed by Mr. AmitavaChatterjee, Former Marketing Manager, Reckitt Benckiser, India.*

- *Pan/Bidi* outlets were a good dispensing medium for the category, but were not under direct/planned coverage of competition.
- The retail margin, though officially at 28% were between 25% and 30% through the year; but the perceived value of the promotions had gone down.
- Given: the continuity of schemes.

This gave birth to the design of Operation Greenstorm, whose mission was the single-minded exploitation of distribution opportunities in the field to carve out a 20% share in the regular segment. While the management knew that there would be advertising support, in the heart of hearts, they knew that Dettol branding in the medicated dressings category would find quick acceptance with the trade and the consumer, given its strong equity and heritage.

Operation Greenstorm became a bold expression of the strategy of focus, designed with the objective of providing maximum man-power with other distribution resources, to build both width and depth so that, in a period of three weeks to a month, Dettol Plaster would be available and displayed in all chemists/other key outlets in all retail markets of Mumbai. Commencement of announcer press advertising coupled with retailer recommendation would leverage offtake much faster, enabling them to build a beachhead and giving competition less time to react. The key success factors of the mission were:

- Secrecy of plans (given common distributors)
- Shift implementation
- Quick build up of width through effective/rapid redistribution
- Measurable targets/objectives for each man in terms of sell-in, width, selective depth, stock covers, and merchandising/displays
- Each man did his task (at the center)
- Teamwork and therefore daily review for eight days

The management decided to mobilize the entire strength of the western region, including the 20-member team of MRs and supervisors who promoted other ethical brands to doctors and chemists and had a strong control on the chemist distribution network. At the launch conference of April 5, 1993, a team of approximately 100 mangers, supervisors, and representatives met at the launch conference for the launch briefing. The highlights were:

- 26 teams with Phase 1 and Phase 2 objectives (15 days total) were formed for coverage of the retail trade only
- Active participation by the distributor—in several teams the distributor himself went on selling
- Focus on Dettol Plaster only
- A, B, C coverage and self-in plan; 35 outlets were targeted per day/team
- Productivity norms with incentives for Phase 1 and Phase 2
- Display norms for selective large outlets to build in six-week-eight-week depth planned for every route with the objective of bouncing back any competitor reaction
- A special PET jar for more than 200 ship purchases to get counter displays and generate impulse trial purchases and dealer push
- Conversion of schemes into 'gifts' to increase perceived value of offer
- A daily evaluation of achievement v. objectives.

The actions were meticulously implemented and each man's commitment to his personal task led to a superforce-multiplier effect:

- At the end of Phase 2 the team had covered 7000 outlets against the objective of 8500. The coverage in A class was on target and the shortfall was mainly in B and C outlets.
- They had already adopted new outlets for the brand where competition hadn't gone. The *pan-bidi* outlets evoked very positive responses.
- Productivity was over 75%. Among chemists, productivity was 100%. In the large 20% chemists segment, the gift schemes were well accepted and two months of retail stock was built up. This prompted the chemist to push Dettol Plaster further, on the one hand, and deny Band-Aid on the other. Thus, consumer offtake commenced even before advertising.
- Megabrand displays of Dettol (both antiseptic liquid and medicated dressings) in leading chemists across. South Mumbai and the Western and Central suburbs gave a redistribution edge in the retail segment.

- Queries started flowing from wholesalers to whom the team sold without any discounts. Prices in the retail market remained stable, and trade incentives worked.

The distribution and market share results were beyond expectation. The challenge was won by the team single-mindedly, showing how team effort well-orchestrated in implementation and used with great force in a short span of time worked effectively in accomplishing the mission. Most interestingly, budgets were surpassed in four months, and the other representatives from outside Mumbai took this learning and accomplishment to their own states, namely Maharashtra, Madhya Pradesh, and Gujarat.

CASE 2

Innovations in Distribution Policy[2]

Although distribution in India is an important function, in the pharmaceutical industry it is generally regarded as a supportive and subsidiary activity. Pharma distribution systems have been traditional in respect of planning for the future with little or no innovations except for a few companies like Sanofi, Sarabhai, Sandoz and Pfizer who have successfully innovated in the past.

In 1983, Sandoz decided to make changes in the methodology of giving discounts to carrying and forwarding (C&F) agents through a simple innovation. Instead of paying a direct percentage on sales to C&F agents, the payment was made on the basis of case lots. Each case lot weighed approximately 12 to 15 kg and they paid Rs.8 to Rs.10 to C&F agent on each of these. As a result, Sandoz reduced the cost of operations by 1.2% of the total turnover. You can imagine the quantum of savings this amounts to for an organization with a large turnover.

Unfortunately, such innovations are not being carried out in all organizations. The outlook towards distribution as a whole still remains traditional. Can't we think differently and approach distribution innovatively?

---

[2]*This case has been contributed by MrGautamKantharia, Former Consultant and C&F agent of Glaxo (Veterinary Division)*

Objective

To help organizations determine the best distribution policy for their operations all over India taking into consideration the comparative financial/nonfinancial (service) benefit analysis of distribution systems like C&F, depot and superstockists. One such study was conducted a few years back to highlight the issues.

Scope and Limitations

Scope: The study can be used as a guideline or reference to calculate the cost—benefit comparison for specific organizations with its own data. An organization can develop a specific need-oriented system.

Limitations: The results of the study would widely differ for organizations having high and low turnovers. Hence the figures will have to be modified to suit individual organizations. There is no readymade single answer for all of them.

Assumptions

For the purpose of this study, the annual turnover of the organization is considered to be Rs.12.0 crore per year:

- One-month inventory of finished goods is assumed
- Inventory is valued at the ex-factory cost price (65% of trade price)
- Interest is calculated at 18% per annum
- Depot rent has been calculated at an average of Rs.4.50 per square foot
- Credit period (receivables) is taken as 45 days
- Deposits from superstockists are not considered as it has cash-flow implications, and companies pay less for outside investment
- Octroi and insurance are considered to be 1.10%
- The customer service level at C&F is assumed to be at 85% to 95%, from the depot also 85% to 95%, and from superstockists 80% to 85%.
- The consignment approach is not considered as it is only a way to finance working capital. As soon as the bill is raised, a central sales tax (CST) of 4% is applicable.

Parameters of Comparison

The following parameters were considered for comparative cost-benefit analysis.

- Inventory-carrying cost
- Operating and administrative cost
- Freight and forwarding cost
- Insurance and octroi
- Interest on receivables
- Commission
- Discount to trade
- Impact of interstate tax
- Staff and personnel liability (long-term) industrial relations problems and associated cost
- Customer service level cost
- Location of factories as reflected in transportation cost
- Information and feedback for decision making
- Sales turnover of the organization:
  (a) low turnover, and
  (b) high turnover
- Necessity of liaison office/sales office for non-distribution functions

Table 10.1 Comparative Cost-Benefit Analysis

		C & F	Branch/Depot	Super stockist
Financial				
1.	Inventory-carrying cost	0.97%	0.97%	-
2.	Operating & administrative cost	-	1.25%-1.5%	-
3.	Freight & forwarding	0.08%-1.2%	0.08%-1.2%	1.25%-1.5%
4.	Insurance & octroi	1.10%	1.10%	1.10%
5.	Interest on receivables	2.7%	2.7%	2.7%
6.	Commission	1.5%-2.0%	-	-
7.	Discount to trade	5%	5%	10%-12%
8.	Impact of interstate tax	Nil at this 11.35%-12.9%	Nil at this 11.10%-12.47%	Nil at this 19.05%-19.30%
Non-Financial				
9.	Staff & personnel liability, (long-term) IR problem & associated cost	Nil	Possibility	Nil

Table 10.1 *Contd...*

		C & F	Branch/Depot	Super stockist
Non-Financial				
10.	Customer service level cost (opportunity loss)	85%-95%	85%-95%	80%
11.	Location of factories as reflected in transportation cost	-	-	Affects transportation cost
12.	Information & feedback for decision making	Whatever company wants	Whatever company wants	Apprehensive
13.	Sales turnover of organization (a) low (b) high	Favorable Favorable	Not-Favorable Favorable	Favorable Favorable
14.	Necessity of liaison office/sales office for non-distribution functions	No additional benefits	Benefits	No additional benefits

It is up to the organization to decide on which mode of 'middlemen' it should follow. Ideally, in India, if you want, you can follow all systems simultaneously. In a few states, depending on the sales turnover, you can operate through a C&F agent, a few through depots/branches, and also through stockists. It has been observed that maximum benefit is derived from operating through all types of 'middlemen'.

LEARNINGS

Operationalization of any strategy depends on how an organization formulates its objectives and important policies which govern the behavior of those who implement.

Policies have an inbuilt advantage in achieving the following *seven* major changes:

1. Uniform code of practice and behavior
2. Automatic decision making
3. Continuity of decisions
4. Effective communication
5. Protection from pressure of exegenics
6. Indirect control over independent actions
7. Counteracting resistance to strategies
8. Successful implementation

Four types of policies always exist in the organization which knowingly or unknowingly help people follow a certain pattern of behavior. These can influence the degree of implementation.

1. Field sales policy
2. Distribution and trade policy
3. Pricing policy
4. Promotional policy

All these policies help the field staff keep us their morale in the face of competition, and also help them adhere to a uniform code of conduct to implement the strategies.

Tactics also assumes importance in operationalizing strategies. Innovation has a big hand in the right use of tactics.

Once you operationalize your strategies, you must look at the structures and systems of the organization as they help in institutionalizing the strategies.

CHAPTER **11**

Core Sales Execution

There is this story of a cabinet maker who had become very successful. He now had 110 people working for him, and had just won a contract with a bag chain of retail stores which would more than double his output for the next five years. He saw that he would have to give up his rather informal 'village' atmosphere, and regroup his people into divisions and hierarchies at city. While he was thinking about the problem, a delegation of his workers came to him. 'We like it the way it is,' they said. 'We don't want this factory to grow any bigger. If you want to grow, why don't you start another factory for this new business?'

And so was this group philosophy and strategy born. No factory had more than 110 workers. A new factory opened every year, and then every five or six months about 25 per cent growth was sustained overall. Each factory made its own line of products and ran itself, asking the man at the center only for new capital.

But eventually he had 23 factories. How long could this go on? The pressures for rationalization were getting stronger. His factories were beginning to compete with each other for business and cutting their margins (his margins) to beat each other. The demands for funds were getting progressively larger—he needed more control over cash inflows if he was to provide cash outflows. The economics of centralized purchasing of services such as accounting and advertising were becoming more and more obvious.

And he still wanted to grow. This is what gave him excitement. The old problem was here again. What should he do? If he rationalized, he might ruin the whole spirit of the factories, offend his workers and feed opportunity to the competitors, and build up an unwieldy and unwanted central organization. But could he resist his own need and the apparent logic of greater consistency and control?

It was difficult for him to implement the same strategy, which had been so successfully working for so many years. It became important to study the organization structure and other prerequisites of implementation before deciding on a 'change in strategy'.

In the end, he worked out a suitable structure but kept the vigor and morale of his people and divided his empire. He no longer has his fingertips on each enterprise, only on three lieutenants. He has lost something, in terms of power or control perhaps, but his organization retains its vigor and its enterprise—and its informality and flexibility to be competitive.

IMPLEMENTATION

Basically, implementation is compliance to given instructions by those who finally have to implement the strategies. These instructions may come from the management, the marketing team, or other superiors. They may also emerge from the company's marketing strategies. For instance, you may identify a few selected activities to be followed on neurosurgeons for a specific product. Implementation is also dependent on the discipline of the entire marketing team, inclusive of the sales force. It is easier to coordinate a given set of activities at the head office level with the marketing team, than exercise control over the events taking place in the market. The field force is usually on its own, and in constant interaction with the environment and competitors, which makes the issue of implementation all the more challenging.

PREREQUISITES TO IMPLEMENTATION

1. Correctness of the Customer Database

A scientifically designed, marketing-oriented customer database can help implementation and lead to dramatic dividends, especially when used in conjunction with well-directed strategies. Using the power of a good customer database, you can gain a greater share of the market, and thus enhance the consumer's loyalty to your company's products.

There are *five* important ways a good database can be developed:
1. By conducting a 'census of doctors' who are relevant.
2. By classifying doctors in A, B, C categories for identification of potential.
3. By developing equipotential areas and clusters of doctors.
4. By ensuring these doctors are not missed out in coverage.

5. By updating or correcting the list every year and developing a more accurate 'response list.'

Once you put in these efforts, all media can be used to reach out to your customer segment easily.

2. Quality and Skills of Front-Line Managers

From my experience in training and development for over three decades now, I have observed that companies who have enhanced the quality and skills of their front-line managers have gone far ahead of others in terms of implementation and are able to achieve satisfactory results.

When we speak of quality of front-line managers, we refer to their ability to achieve results. The MRs in many organizations have hardened attitudes and a high turnover. Dealing with the MRs and their varied demands, and sometimes stubborn and casual attitudes, the front-line managers have sadly lost their market orientation. A lot of behavioral inputs may have strengthened them with techniques, but they have lost their focus on the task at hand—'making MRs work.' Many have been reduced to becoming 'aides' or 'helpers' of the MRs, or have been hopelessly sandwiched between MRs and the management.

It is crucial at this moment to empower them. Only then can you inject life into this powerless world of front-line managers and galvanize them into action. This is the job of the second-line manager and the management. Only when front-line managers feel secure and powerful can they focus their energies on their task, and help organizations implement their plans. This requires robust leadership and can come through continuous training and development, which can provide front-line managers the confidence to effectively deal with their MRs and exhibit quality leadership. Front-line managers need to acquire qualities of assertiveness, and analytical and diagnostic abilities.

The values of doctors, MRs, retailers, wholesalers, and stockists are also changing. Front-line managers require skills to cope with these changes. They obviously cannot interact effectively with 'entrepreneurs'. They need to learn how to better their relations with those they work with. It is a continuous process, and the faster it is begun, the better it would be for your organization.

Let us take just one example of Reckitt Benckiser (South) (Consumer Division). In 1993, on the parameter of performance of targets, and meeting bottom-line and top-line targets, it was the last zone in the country. The then General Manager, MrAnish Gupta, took the initiative and decided to restructure the filed force. And while restructuring, he also decided to clarify the roles of all managers and sales representatives, and equip them with relevant skills to deal with market and organizational issues. The market for Robin Blue—their major brand—was dropping, and the motivation levels of the MRs were also at low ebb. Training was used as an HRD intervention through continuous follow up of individual and group action plans. Also, the general manager introduced two new products and ensured that the morale of the field force was kept high through competence-building processes combined with other managerial actions. Over a one-year period, the South zone closed sales with the achievement of both targets and profits. It was thus determination of the General Manager to develop quality and skills of the field force which took them to high levels of implementation and commitment.

3. **Credibility of Organizational Strategies**

   When a company does not have a track record of having achieved success through implementation of its strategies, the field force is only partly enthusiastic to these efforts. Weaknesses in the administration, poor product management inputs, office politics, or inadequacies in the various managerial functions—be it in R&D, finance, production, or marketing—can give rise of feelings of indifference and apathy among the MRs.

   The best way to ensure implementation in such situations is to clear the mess at the headquarters, and strengthen the home base with proper systems and structures. Many organizations want to go ahead with big, ambitious plans, but cannot support their field staff from the head office. Many field staff complain of non-receipt of promotional materials, poor salaries, and inadequate training.

   Much depends on what kind of success the MRs achieve. Those who get results develop faith in the strategies of their organization; those who do not get results with original strategies try their own and lose faith in those of the organization. It then becomes very difficult to convince them of the efficacy of the methods developed by the head office. If you wish to change this situation, you need well-analyzed and thought-out strategies that will get the support and confidence of your front-line managers.

Otherwise, it becomes difficult to get results from the front-line managers, who sometimes tend to empathize with the MRs and go along with them. Over a period of time, they become indifferent to strategic inputs.

Organizations who suffer from this kind of indifference need participation of the field staff at the time of developing strategies. They also require proper headquarter or head office systems to back up the strategic inputs.

4. **Flexibility of Converting a Marketing Communication Strategy into a Sales Strategy**

Many managers at the head office are under the mistaken impression that if they rigidly adhere to their communication strategy and other in-clinic activities, they will achieve cent per cent results. Things don't happen this way. Unless front-line managers are fully conscious of these strategies and are allowed to adopt them to their specific situations, no implementation plan can succeed. Managers at the head office live in a world of their own. When they work with MRs and go out into the field they are generally in for a surprise. It is only then that they get to know of involuntary deviations from the carefully planned strategy.

What is the solution? Obviously, MRs cannot be let loose in the physician's clinic to do whatever they want. At the same time, they cannot be treated as robots and their initiative be stamped out. It is a catch-22 situation. How then do you manager implementation?

Here are some guidelines you can try:

- Get your front-line managers to participate in developing strategic communication
- Present the entire product-related communication in the way the product management team designed it be—there is merit in a canned presentation. It is complete, it is power-packed with visuals and clever words, and can help influence doctors and retailers.
- Allow, each MR in a group to develop a 'closer' for each product. These will depend on the local competition, their

ambition, the doctors' profile, his needs, and his patients' needs. All MRs can then later own them.

- Each MR can be at liberty to deviate from the suggested closers but not from the text.

Try the above. I am sure you will get results.

5. **Rules to Observe while Working on Markets**

The changing rules of the market and environment of MRs have a significant impact on implementation.

Consider this. You are on army commander and the battle lines have been drawn. Your battalion has been fully equipped with missiles and hi-tech ammunition, and is ready for battle. But suddenly you learn that the enemy plans to use chemical weapons. Your entire battalion, though otherwise fully equipped and confident, gets shaken. They do not know how to cope with the new environment.

The case with your field force is similar. Practically every day the MR needs to be instilled with confidence to face the rapidly changing environment. There are *three* rules that can be observed.

(i) **The clarity rule**: Clarify exactly what you wish your MRs to do irrespective of changes in the competition. The instructions should be specific, measurable, observable, and if necessary, qualified. But ensure that there is 'clarity' as to what needs to be done *every* month. Plan in advance. Each MR must know what he should be doing at least for the next two months.

(ii) **The soundness rule:** Besides being clear in your instructions, you must ensure that front-line managers are skillful in implementing them. The front-line managers must feel convinced that the communication strategies are sound, and that the MRs will find themselves at home with them.

GSK has followed a practice that has worked for them wonderfully well. Whenever their front-line managers work with the MRs, before going out to the field, on the first day, the front-line manager details the entire marketing communication strategy on each product to the MR. This reinforces the soundness of planned activities in the MR's mind. You may or may not follow the GSK policy, but it is important to ensure that your front-line managers know and are able to skillfully implement that strategy.

(iii) ***The partnership rule:*** Strategy is no one's personal property. It is to be shared and jointly owned with front-line managers and MRs at the battlefield stage, and through the product management team, with entire organization at the head office. It should be a growing and mutually rewarding partnership. The following precepts are very important for the partners to keep this partnership healthy.

- Give and take feedback even if it is bad and unpleasant.
- Truth prevails in communication.
- Rewards are shared as per the stakes.

Organizations which can ensure the above can inculcate the attitude of partnership in not only their MRs, but also their stockists and retailers, will be successful. In fact, all important systems—the operational system, marketing information system, etc.—and factors such as quickness of dissemination of information, must be properly tuned so that MRs can view the organization with pride and call it their very own.

SOME COMMON STRATEGIC OPTIONS FOR IMPLEMENTATION

All strategies are principally concerned with numbers, speed, perfection, surpassing quality, intellect, and surprise.

Strategy of Numbers

'If you can't beat them or outrun them, then overwhelm them' is one way of stating the numbers strategy. In war, the superiority of numbers is well recognized. The forces that are inferior numerically must compensate for their weakness by the use of other strategies. However, if the opponent is able to match these plans of action as well, numbers will win out in the end.

The strategy of numbers applies in business also. Many companies have followed this strategy to comb the metro-city markets enmass. After a cycle meeting or briefing session, a team is retained for a day or two to attack the market and call on the doctors of that city collectively. The results they bring are usually fantastic. More than one MR calls on the doctors at a time and presents the products.

Strategy of Speed

One classic answer to numbers in military and sporting endeavors has been speed. Smaller but faster groups often win over larger but less mobile adversaries. Speed is of some use in marketing also, but should not be over-rated. Over-stretched, it can be a very bad strategy. There is a different between selling and war or sport. There is always a limit established in a battle of either a military or sporting nature. Neither can go on endlessly, and speed can be of great use in the short run. But when it comes to selling, its just not possible to maintain the same speed indefinitely with no effect on performance. Also, as MRs get older, they tend to slow down. The leader must be willing to adopt a policy whereby optimum utilization is ensured and the people are deployed as per their competence. Restructuring and realignment are equally important to maintain speed. Speed is of use in special campaigns lasting for just one to two months. All attach and expand their energies in these two odd months to get results. This a good strategy for new product launches.

The launch of a new product requires speed of actions on the part of the marketing team. If you do not launch in time, your competitor will, and score over you in the minds of doctors.

Strategy of Perfection

It is seldom wise to sacrifice perfection for speed or numbers. In war, neither is of much use against an army that executes its tactics with perfection, fights with know-how, and is proficient in its use of arms and weaponry. Similarly, perfection in product, personnel, or performance is much desired in business also. Whatever is done should be done right. In the management of a sales force, perfection should be the basic strategy in most instances. It makes little sense to make all effort to call on a doctor without perfecting the detailing strategy.

Strategy of Intellect

Some degree of intellect is required to carry out any strategy, but some organizations place a premium on intelligence. Evidence of this strategy in action is an emphasis on both technical and marketing research. The executive who employs intellect as a basic strategy may think, 'May be we are few in number, and may be we don't execute plans as well as they should be done, but atleast we will be in the right market at the right time with the right product.'

The difference between the strategy of intellect and one of perfection is marketing is that often a 'smart' action is something less than perfect. Perfection may cost more than the market will pay. In other activities, the executive hopes to solve problems with applied intelligence. This is a good strategy, and one that cannot be ignored by any manager.

Surpassing Quality

Stangen surpassed everybody when it lowered the price of Norfloxacin. But the doctors were unaware of Stangen as it was a new company then. They had apprehensions about quality. To rule out these apprehensions, the entire field force promoted the 'quality' of Stangen products by showing them invoices of Stangen selling bulk drugs like ranitidine to GSK UK holdings. Thus they could surpass all competitors. But a strategy of this kind is not at all easy to implement. It involves years of research, and the cost of producing a product of the required quality may be very high.

Strategy of Surprise

Surprise can be of tremendous advantage in war or sports, but it is of little use in business. It is difficult to surprise competition, since industrial secrecy is almost impossible to maintain. Even if tight secrecy is possible concerning some move, not much is usually gained by attempts to surprise competition.

What did Stangen really get from their efforts to reduce the price of Norfloxacin? It compelled leading competitors like Cipla and Ranbaxy to reduce their prices.

Nevertheless, there is often a need for secrecy about business decisions and contemplated actions. A firm's plans are of its most vital assets. The intention may not be to surprise but to maintain a competitive advantage.

IMPLEMENTATION THROUGH THE FIELD FORCE

Allocation and Deployment of Field Force

A crucial question confronting companies today, and one that will be even more important tomorrow, is how many MRs should an organization have? How should the field force time be distributed over the different products in the company's portfolio?

Companies often take a pragmatic view with respect to these types of allocation decisions. 'We know we might be spending 50% too much, but we don't know which 50%.' Over a period, companies need to adopt one of the following approaches.

It is relatively very difficult to take a decision in allocating the efforts of MRs to ascertain what is optimum. To improve these decisions, there is a relatively new method, which could be called 'turbo-driven'. It has been used successfully by a number of large pharmaceutical companies abroad including Novartis, GSK, and Bristol-Myers Squibb. Let us study this method.

This particular method starts with the premise that managers will make decisions that are in line with their company's policy and objectives. The approach starts out from a S-shaped response function as illustrated in Figure 11.1 in the case of the field force; similar curves can be used for the other communication media.

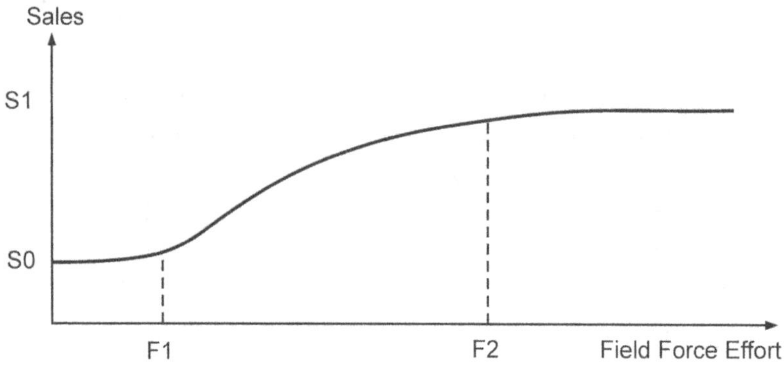

Figure 11.1 Field Force Response Function

This rather general S-shape implies that for any product even with no field force effort there will be some sales (S0). A minimum field force effort (F1) is necessary to make an impact.

If more field force time is allocated to a product, the sales will rise fast up to a point (F2) from where the field force impact on sales will still increase but at a decreasing rate. Finally, whatever be the field force effort for a product, sales can never exceed saturation sales level S1. In more formal terms, this curve can be expressed as:

$$S = S0 + (S1 - S0)\left(\frac{FF^{\alpha}}{\beta + FF}\right)$$

where   S = sales
             S0 = minimum sales without sales effort
             S1 = maximum sales with sales effort
             FF = field force effort (expressed in the number of MRs, or in terms of number of MR contacts).
             α = sales with half sales effort
             β = sales with 50% greater sales effort

The four parameters of the model (S0, S1, α, and β) can then be estimated, based on the manager's experience. Suppose a company wants to decide how many MRs to put on a specific product for the next year, managers who are familiar with the product and its market position will be asked five questions to help calibrate the parameters of the field force response function.

They will be asked to think about next year's situation for their product, and then consider the following possibilities:

What will be the sales if no field force effort is allocated to a product? The answer to this question will give 'S0'.

What will be the sales if half the present field sales effort is allocated to a product? The answer will give 'α'.

What will be the sales if the same effort as being made at present is allocated to a product? We will use this as a reference condition.

What will be the sales if 50% greater effort is allocated to a product? This will give 'β'.

What will be the sales at the saturation level? The answer to this question will give 'S1'.

Usually, several managers familiar with the product are asked to respond to these questions separately. Later, the answers are compared and discussed, and a reasonable level of consensus is arrived at. This interactive process can be time-consuming. On the positive side, it forces managers to quantify their intuitions and defend their opinions in the open. Furthermore, it involves managers in the process, and increases the chances of acceptability of the resulting decision.

Once the response curve is specified, contribution and cost figures can be added to the sales estimates, and the optimal sales force can be determined via a sensitivity analysis.

Consider a product 'Hypo T'. Let us calculate the values on an imaginary basis per territory.

> $S0 = 50$ units → Sale is dependent on prescribing doctors. Even if there is no representation by an MR, the sales remain at this level.
> $\alpha = 68$ units → The level of sales when 50% of the time MR is not allocated.
> Reference = 100 units → Sales trend of the last few years.
> $\beta = 390$ units → Trend of sales during bonus offers and other campaigns—50% greater efforts.
> $S1 = 200$ units → Average sale dependent on the total sale of major brands (competitive) and their strengths.

Suppose there are 200 MRs and they make at least six calls promoting 'Hypo T' per day. This would work out to a total of 3,60,000 presentations per year. Sales for this product at the moment are Rs. 30,00,000; the gross profit it generates is around 35%, i.e. Rs.10,50,000.

Solving the equations, it will be clear to you that for a sale of 157 to 160 units per month, you conceptually do not need more than 50 MRs with the same coverage and frequency. Thus, you can lessen the calls by four and ask the MRs to make two effective calls every day to generate this value. This method provides a thumb-rule calculation for the required number of field force.

A Harvard Business School case on Syntex provides the following example (Syntex case study 1983). Let me take the data for only one of the products of Syntex—Naprosyn.

Sales Effort for Naprosyn					
No. of calls	**Half**	**Present**	**50% more**	**Saturation**	
Sales of Naprosyn	47%	68%	100%	126%	152%

47% refers to the consensus opinion of Syntex managers that if in the following year no field force effort were to be assigned to Naprosyn, it would reach a sales level of 47% of the previous year's sales level. If 50%

of the present efforts were assigned to Naprosyn, the sales would reach 68% of the previous year's sales level. The present level of sales is taken to be 100%. If 50% more efforts were assigned to Naprosyn, the sales would reach a level of 126% of last year sales. Finally, the saturation level is dependent on the total market; and it would reach 152% of previous year's sales.

Allocation of efforts were as follows:

Allocation of Efforts to Naprosyn	Optimal number of MRs	Presentations	Slaes (US $)	Gross Profit (US $)	Net profit (US $)
	265	9,75,964	3,09,37,624	25,09,06,061	23,61,76,981

Along with Naprosyn, Anaprox, Norinyl 135,Norinyl 150, Lidex, Synalar, and Nasalide were also detailed.

Based on these inputs the sales-response functions for the seven products were calculated, and subsequently, taking into account the profit margins of the seven products, the sales force level that would maximize profits was derived. This gave the optimal number of sales force size as 751 MRs. In the previous year, the number of MRs had been 433. In the case of Syntex, increasing more than 300 MRs at a time was difficult owing to other managerial issues like availability, training, supervision, and management of such an increase. Finally, it was decided that the company would increase the number of MRs, but not dramatically.

ROLE OF MEDICAL REPRESENTATIVE IN IMPLEMENTATION

What would you view as competitive assets? A strong balance sheet? A leadership position in the market? A higher market share in the operating product group? Higher growth rates in the operating markets? Whatever it may be, in the ultimate analysis it is your sales force that can prove to be a definite organizational strength or a debilitating weakness—an asset or a liability.

Just as it takes several years for any organization to generate deep-rooted credibility and status among its customers, it takes an equal amount of time, if not more, to develop a strong sales force. In some cases the sales force may gradually develop by itself provided there are good and effective front-line managers available. The latter too require years of training on the job to become truly effective individually. Organizational success depends on close-knit team operations. Managers take considerable time to develop team thinking and to learn to work together as a team. Because it is they who have to evolve and implement planned sales programs. Don't you think these factors alone can bring amazing results?

The sales force is a very important medium for communicating with customers. And it is definitely more dynamic, more active, than say, advertising; it is a live medium. But it takes time to train and develop the sales force to represent the organization effectively. Thus, though the response time of an effective sales force is slightly longer than that of advertising, its impact is more predictable and longer lasting. Organizations who are solely dependent on their sales force for their sales force for their business have to obviously bank almost totally on the quality of their sales personnel. A committed team of motivated individuals who can effectively translate the company's strategies into results in the market place is vital for an organization's success.

In ethical marketing you have little flexibility in changing the media mix. Sometimes you may not have any other alternative but to develop the sales force. If necessary, you may need to change the strategies and structure of the organization. In fact, the field staff cost is usually fixed. Hence its proper deployment becomes very crucial.

Alembic in 1984-85 restructured its field staff to derive optimum utilization. They felt that it was basically the mobility of their field staff which was the issue. It segregated people into different categories, and those who were considered mobile, were given intensive field jobs, while others were given depots or branches to look after. It was a major internal restructuring exercise. Similarly, the introduction of Megacare gave a chance to the younger lot, while many young MRs were also recruited. Both these exercises changed the complexion of the Alembic field staff.

The sales force, then, is an important available human resource, and can potentially affect the implementation as well as organizational budget. A strong sales force which has good relations with its customers is a definite asset. However, a weak or non-existence sales force with poor customer relations is a pronounced liability.

Thus, as it stands today, the sales force plays a crucial role in the success of an organization. True to its name, a sales force generates a tremendous amount of force, power or energy which can either take the business ahead or ruin the organization. But this human energy needs to be channelized properly. If the sales force morale is maintained at a high level, they can reach newer and higher dimensions. The morale of an individual may not necessarily affect group or team morale. On the other hand, inspired group morale can percolate down to the individual level.

1. ***The medical representative:*** The MR and his 'technology' of communication have been more or less stagnant since the last three decades. Neither he nor his methods have undergone any radical transformation. However, the values and attitudes of this vital medium have changed. At the same time, this medium now has more constraints and also some limitations.

   Imagine for a moment that you are marketing soap or detergent products and not pharmaceutical formulations. To communicate to your customers you would probably choose a combination of different media. Your choice may depend on the profile of your customer segment. TV has been the major media for many products, aided by other media like radio, hoardings, magazines, etc. You still would have a tough competition on TV as more than 15-20 advertisements of the same commodity would have crowded and captured 'prime time'. You would have carefully chosen your message, used an effective script and presented it in a way that the visual impact remains embedded in the minds of customers.

   The medium used would have been expensive, and yet there would have been no guarantee that it could provide adequate exposure to your product or give it a perceived identity. You would have got only around 15 to 30 seconds to exhibit your products. Although your customer would be part of a captive audience, he could switch you off. And today, he has the choice of many channels. Where would you project your message?

   Let us now look at ourselves, pharmaceutical marketers. We are so input-oriented that we concentrate on MRs and hardly on doctors.

   The time available to our MRs is more than a product gets on television. In fact, they are better off as their messages and product presentations do not get cluttered with other types of commodities in a given time. They probably visit doctors who often have 10 to 15 MRs waiting for them. On TV, you hardly get 15 to 20 seconds while with the MRs as a medium, you may get 1 to 3 minutes. Further, the MRs create a personal rapport and is therefore better for your purposes than TV, provided the MRs are matured and motivated. (If they aren't, it can be worse.)

Can a MR per se product results? Can a MR per se guarantee prescriptions? Like any medium, the coverage, frequency, exposure of products, wastage, the liveliness of the presentation, and the persuasion and the situation of each decideris equally important to control. Are we seriously looking at our MRs as a medium? If we aren't, don't you think its time we did? Howe are we controlling this medium? Are they really under our control, or have we fully left them on their own to product results? Do we have parameters to measure their output?

Let us consider that an MR generates sales worth Rs.2,50,000 per month after working for five years in an area. How do you compute his efficiency? This output results from around 250 doctors. So, the average productivity per doctor comes to around Rs.1000 per month.

It is usually seen that four to five major products contribute at least 80% of the total sales. This makes it around Rs.200 per month per product. If we consider an average price of Rs.20 for each product, it would mean that assorted ten products or ten units of a product are sold per month. This also means that one unit of one brand is sold in every three days. Doesn't this appear terribly low, after continuous exposure of your medium for those four to five products? But this is what normally happens. However, the law of averages means there are a few handful of doctors who prescribe every day while many do not prescribe at all. Should we still continue to invest on these doctors through this medium? All of us need to address this issue more commercial-mindedly. Each MR must earn his ROTI (Return of Time Invested) every day.

Overdependence on detailmen has led many organizations to frustration. And also to incur heavy cost in the bargain, as it usually happens with any medium. We may not have any other effective medium so far. Do we really see a 'future' with this medium, when the constraints are unlimited and values are changing? It is unfortunate but true that everyone in most pharmaceutical organizations from the managing directors to the front-line managers is totally dependent on detailmen for results. Many organizations have failed to generate even breakeven volume after 20 years of development. But still the management continues to put its faith in this human medium. Can there be a commitment which will ensure sufficient brand share through this medium? Are we merely dependent or are we over dependent on it?

2. ***Orientation for Success:*** The role of the MR has undergone rapid changes. Today, the MR must know what the physicians are prescribing. He must collect and put together information about the profiles and prescription habits of the physicians in his territory. He must book and ensure that the goods are made available, and then regularly interact with the physicians to persuade them to prescribe the brands he is promoting. Till the prescription is taken up, and even later, he must regularly follow up with them and then convert them in 'brand loyal' doctors. Thus, MRs must take their share of responsibility for both demand creation and demand fulfillment.

At the same time, MR must ensure that the share of the brand and market grows year after year. Hence the survival of an organization depends a lot on how committed and motivated its MRs are. And on how they are able to extract the most from their time by proper planning and management of their territories, and get results.

There is yet another category of customers—the retailers—who also must be influenced. Thus, the job of MR requires commitment, energy and a willingness to work hard without any supervision. It is a proactive demanding role, not a passive accepting one. If the MRs are oriented for success and you are able to communicate the strategies down the line, your battle is won.

But things are not as easy as they sound. As it stands today, this medium of detailmen has several constraints and limitations. First, since this is the only major medium of communication and implementation, there is considerable pressure on the MRs to get results. Other media like journal advertising are not developed as much for ethical brands. Second, physicians also pose problems; they are unwilling to give more time to the MRs, and are reluctant to receive more than one or two persons from one organization. The values of customers, doctors and retailers are today different from those in the past. The MRs have accordingly had to adapt to the changing requirements.

In such circumstances, the role of a front-line manager has become very crucial. It is his responsibility to raise the morale of his team as a whole, and maintain a high motivation level of his individual MRs.

ROLE OF THE MANAGEMENT IN DEVELOPING FIELD FORCE MORALE

'Morale' by itself is quite difficult to define. You can perhaps experience it and 'feel' it. Most of you who have worked in teams would have experienced this 'feeling'—you at once get to know how high or low the morale is in an organization. And it is this 'feeling' which conveys the image of the organization to the outside world, to the customer. If you observe closely, you will be able to identify some parameters by which you can judge the morale of the field force:

1. *Availability of MRs:* It has been observed by all managers that to recruit new MRs is becoming difficult year after year. On the one hand, there is no awareness of this profession, and on the other, there is no qualifying examination where students can appear and qualify themselves for the job. Although it is technical selling, many organizations have already lowered their parameters of selection. They recruit any graduate or sometimes even undergraduates. Many become desperate to fill up vacancies and ignore the quality for recruits, as all of them look for achievement of targets. When such a selection takes place, the turnover rate of MRs increases. There are many organizations who virtually 'reinvent' their organizations every third year as they have a people turnover of more 30 to 40%. Within three years the organization's cost of recruitment, induction and training gets doubled. The industry needs to deal with this issue of getting the right quality of MRs collectively; otherwise the incoming competence will be difficult to identify.

   Although the pharmaceutical industry is one where an MR has the potential to become the marketing chief, the total morale-building process has been gradually vitiated.

   It is also possible that since the ration of MRs to called-on doctors by any medium-size company is becoming 1:1, the doctors tend to neglect the presence of the MRs. Over a period of time, imparting prestige for MR selling of pharma products has become a challenge.

The Cipla experience of sending courier mail and samples would not have worked at all, had there been an impact of face-to-face selling. The success of the Cipla experiment has really forced everyone to rethink about the utility of MRs as a solitary medium. Over the last few years many organizations are considering augmentation of the MR role through other media or trying to identify alternative media. However, the fact of life is that there are fewer talents available when we need them.

2. ***Extensive turnover:*** A graduate who starts as an MR changes his job for monetary prospects or better perceived promotional prospects, or for improved service conditions. A few organizations become labeled 'training grounds', and hence MRs join these organizations with the express purpose of changing later. This excessive turnover can lead to continuous gaps in the frequency of representation. When the customer does not see the same MR more than two or three times, he may wonder why people are leaving the company. The MR is thus not able to build any long-lasting rapport with the customers. Business suffers. This phenomenon is seen more in metro cities. This is a definite sign of low morale, ineffective front-line management, or poor organizational image.

3. ***Tendency to make excuses:*** If factors like bank delays or postal delays in receiving instructions are made a big issue regularly, then it is a sure indication that the morale of the MR is low.

4. ***Withdrawal from the job:*** As the sales force does not work under one roof and does not have close supervision, poorly motivated individuals tend to shy away from work. Precious time is frittered away. This is the first barrier to productivity.

5. ***Effect on other colleagues:*** Even one disgruntled member in the sales force can have a negative influence on the others. The entire group can become apathetic and indifferent—a disease no organization can afford to ignore.

6. ***General disgruntled feeling about the management:*** When the sales force perceives a series of managerial actions to be incongruent, it feels separated from the management. It starts talking in terms of 'we' and 'you', as if the objectives of the

management and those of the sales force were different. This is the first dividing line drawn between MRs and the management.

7. ***Unsatisfactory sales performance:*** Continuing unsatisfactory sales performance takes away the involvement of the sales force, which is the first demotivating factor for successful MRs.

8. ***Rationalizing self-failure:*** Depending on the average age of the sales force, they start rationalizing their self-failure, putting the blame on extraneous factors. The first sign of lethargy.

9. ***Propagation of inferiority complex:*** Amidst tough competition, they give up. They feel inferior, and become ineffective; the first sign of defeat.

10. ***Dual pressure on profits:*** If the fixed expenses of the sales force are unfortunately coupled with low turnover, it brings a dual pressure on the profits of the organization.

Surely, you would have noticed a few or all such signs either in yours or someone else's sales force. Next time you observe these indications, act before it is too late. There can be many reasons for such reactions from the sales force.

Lack of communication, either verbal or written, can lead to lack of contact, and consequently, lack of understanding between those who manage and the sales force. Many marketing chiefs try to exercise their control without direct contact or communication with the sales force. Feedback becomes extremely difficult in such organizations. In India, because of our cultural inheritance, we have an inter-dependent nature. In one of our traditional games, Kho-Kho, you are not supposed to get up unless touched or pushed by your team members. We tend to lie back unless somebody urges us to go ahead. Lack of proper communication may bring about a rift in understanding each other's objectives and means.

On the job, in the field, or sitting at the desk, managers are faced with several decision-making situations every day. Often, unintentionally, operating managers make commitments which have financial implications—unnecessary commitments which ultimately cannot be fulfilled. Operating managers start doubting their own authority, and question their accountability. They tend to feel they also are just conveyor belts of the directions of the higher management. This attitude percolates down to the sales force. If all this happens, there is obviously something wrong somewhere.

Operating managers must be able to project a 'fair and firm' image. If they are not able to display good managerial qualities, the sales force loses confidence in them. Once this happens, the sales force is bound to become apathetic and indifferent.

Results also play their part, sometimes, on the decisions of the management. Imagine a situation where three or four products launched in succession do not become successful in spite of a lot of marketing effort. Or existing products start losing market share. The net result is that the sales force begins to think that the decisions of the management have been all wrong. They perceive the difference in the marketplace between themselves and their more successful competitors.

Similarly is the case when the success of the sales force goes unnoticed by the management. This lack of recognition can be quite disheartening. It is not that every MR must be given a promotion every time he shows good results. But there can be other incentives. Sometimes, it is the sheer 'thrill' of achieving, the challenge, which acts as the motivating factor. Organizations need to understand this. Every representative is an individual in his own right, and needs recognition of his work. He should be able to get the feeling that his talents are being fully utilized. Otherwise, he will be frustrated.

There can be other causes of frustration. The skilled fighter requires an enemy and a place to fight. The skilled fighter requires an enemy and a place to fight. A skilled sales force too requires good strategies and potential territory to show results. Members of the sales force grumble over territories, quotas, compensation, and the like. A poor territory may, over a period of time, waste and frustrate a good salesperson. Unachievably high quotas year after year can make the salesperson indifferent. And poorly formed compensation plans may make the sales force angry and agitated.

Whatever be the reason, and these do differ from organization to organization, morale is a key factor. The mental state of the individual members of the sales force plays a pivotal role in the success of any organization.

Herzberg's theory lays stress on the role of 'hygiene factors' in the motivation of workers. According to the theory, factors such as a well-lit office, and welfare facilities like canteens, could definitely have a positive influence on the performance of workers. In our context of the pharmaceutical sales force, morale appears to be the key element.

CASE

Leadership Culture and Effective Implementation— Cadila's Strength[1]

Let us compare the strengths of the leading pharmaceutical companies in India—GSK, Ranbaxy, and Cadila. What do we have? Cadilaover the years has been successful in retaining its edge through its marketing capabilities. Whenever these capabilities have fallen short, Cadila has had to either give up the chase, or close its divisions.

Cadila (Formulations) has been a successful division which has grown seven times over in the last couple of years. It has also extended and diversified into six major divisions. From 1988, it started with Alidac, Hospital Products Division, Cosmetics and Oncocare. In 1992, it diversified into another marketing company—Zieta. Today, Cadila is forging ahead with the backup of a consistent team which has grown with Cadila since 1982.

Consistent Leadership

Success has come with hard work and consistent team effort. A special, unique type of group leadership of four members has evolved in such a way it became a winning combination in the pharmaceutical industry.

The sudden demise of the company's Chief Executive (Marketing), Mr. Singhada in 1988, forced the mantle of leadership on the young shoulders of a deputy. For the survival of the organization, it was clearly evident that he needed all possible support. From 1982, the team of four, including the deputy, all in the formative years of their career, decided to forge a close bond and provide a unique, informal leadership. While there was no formal leader among them, yet leadership was assumed by one.

---

[1]*This case has been contributed by Interlink Marketing Consultancy Pvt. Ltd., Mumbai.*

This unique leadership established the base of an 'informal culture' with formal responsibilities. An expressive photograph of this foursome still adorns the cabins of their offices in Ahmedabad to serve as a symbol of what healthy culture, team work and mutual understanding can achieve. It is not that there were no differences among the group, but there was healthy respect for each other's opinions.

An open, informal and yet performance-oriented culture which prevails in Cadila the speed and drive to augment relationship and achieve success. Policies like promotions from within helps increase involvement in the organization and keep the hopes and interests of the employees alive. Sincere, hard work remains as the core basis for the organization's success. The leader's role is related to leading victories on the marketing battlefield. This consistency of leadership found recognition in the form of the prestigious Vijay Shree Award instituted by the International Friendship Society of India being conferred on the leader—Mr. Ganesh Nayak.

This Cadila leadership case is an example of how consistency of principles, policies, style, and leadership can make for better implementation of strategies. If there are changes at the top every few years, and strategies are changed mid-stream, the effect will surely be felt at the implementation level, and the smooth rhythm of the field force will be disturbed. Cadila has retained its implementation edge because of its unique and unchanging leadership.

LEARNINGS

Strategy without its implementation is merely a concept. The test of every strategy is in its successful implementation.

There are *five* prerequisites for the process of implementation:

1. Correctness of customer database
2. Quality and skills of front-line managers
3. Credibility of earlier organizational strategies
4. Skills to convert marketing strategy into sales strategy
5. Following the ground rules of the market

These pre-requisites, if followed properly, can make the implementation process stronger in terms of its impact in the marketplace.

A few strategic options can be adopted while implementing any decided strategy. These options provide a quality differentiation to any strategy. There are *six* available options:

1. Strategy of numbers
2. Strategy of speed
3. Strategy of perfection
4. Strategy of intellect
5. Surpassing quality
6. Strategy of surprise

Depending on the nature of the market, competition, and product, you can choose any one or more of these options and weave them into your strategy.

In the pharmaceutical industry, all of us try to implement our strategies through the field force. It is important to decide on the following *three* issues for better implementation:

- Allocation and deployment of the field force
- Role of MRs
- Role of the management in developing the morale of MRs

Preparation and continuous follow-up are key factors for achieving a high degree of implementation.

CHAPTER 12

Marketing Finance

The Great Indian epic, *Mahabharata*, is replete with incidents where strategic interventions and decisions have led to a desired outcome. At times, the plans and strategies were so well laid that the impact of such decisions became a foregone conclusion.

Like Krishna for the Pandavas, the opposing camp of the Kauravas had Shakuni, the maternal uncle of Duryodhana, as their master strategist. He meticulously designed the strategies, and implemented them to the last detail, thus ensuring that the expectations of his camp members were fully met.

In order to seize the empire for the Kauravas, Shakuni devised a devious strategy involving a game of dice. In the rules of the game to be played by the two rival camps, the complete assets of each side were to be pledged, with the winner taking it all.

To ensure victory for the Kauravas, Shakuni's tactics were to manufacture specially loaded dice that would favor them and to against the Pandavas. Naturally, the Pandavas lost all their assets and their share of the empire. But it did not end there, and soon the Pandavas and their wife, Draupadi, had been enslaved by the Kauravas; the Pandavas had to submit to the cruel decree of the Kauravas that they leave the capital city of Hastinapur for twelve years. After completion of the twelfth year, they were to remain in disguise for another year. If identified during this one-year period, they would have to go back to another 12 years of banishment.

Ethics and morality apart, Shakuni's ingenious plan and implementation were perfect. In his mind, Shakuni had already been able to measure the impact of his operations even before the first round of dice had been thrown. Thus, from the point of evaluation of Shakuni's basic operation, it was more than cent per cent achievement. In our context, is it possible for us to evaluate our marketing operations before taking our vital marketing decisions? Can we identify certain specific parameters that can help us evaluate our operations by studying its impact on the results? This is what we will try and explore in this chapter.

THE IMPORTANCE OF A STRATEGIC MARKETING IMPACT REVIEW (SMIR)

While much work has been done on the evaluation of marketing strategy on the basis of the Profit Impact on Market Strategy (PIMS) database in US and UK, in India this has rarely been tried. At most, attempts have been made to evaluate marketing efforts, and the consequent results. If the results are positive, we feel satisfied, but if we do not get the desired outcome, we at once put the blame on the strategy, making it a scapegoat.

While developing a suitable framework, it is important to understand the distinction among a marketing plan, a marketing audit, and evaluation of the marketing results, also known as strategic marketing impact review (SMIR).

A *marketing plan* is a yearly exercise in which the implementation of the marketing strategy is detailed.

A *marketing audit* is a comprehensive analysis of the whole marketing system, including the marketing strategy, the marketing tactics, and the marketing organization. It is done far less frequently than a marketing plan, and less frequently than a SMIR.

A SMIR is focused on the marketing strategy and decisions of the company. Usually the marketing manager of the company is responsible for its nature and contents, and also its completion. More specifically, a SMIR is periodic, systematic and objective evaluations of a company's marketing decisions to enable the top management accomplish essentially two tasks:

1. Evaluate the impact of past strategic marketing decisions and operations
2. Provide a basis for future strategic marketing decisions and operations

The first step to a successful SMIR is that it should be action-oriented, either to diagnose the current strategic marketing position, or to make an impact on strategic marketing decisions for the future. The purpose of a SMIR is not merely to generate more data which would make decision making even more difficult. Finally, a SMIR has to be seen in an evolutionary process. A lot of time and effort will be required the first time it is done. Subsequent SMIRs, however, can build on the first, and therefore, should be faster and easier to accomplish. The ultimate goal is to develop a standardized procedure that can be easily updated and adjusted to changes in the company, the products, and the general environment.

COST-BEHAVIOR ANALYSIS FOR A SUCCESSFUL SMIR

To introduce a SMIR in any organization, the first step is to work out a method of studying the *behavior of existing costs*. The purpose of cost-behavior analysis is essentially to generate, and subsequently provide, financial and quantitative data to decision makers to improve the quality of marketing decisions. The following important techniques of cost-behavior analysis can provide meaningful data to aid marketing policies.

(i) *Marginal cost analysis:* Marginal costing is an important factor in generics. And price becomes an important criterion for those who buy generics. Thus, while marginal cost analysis helps in the pricing of all types of products, it may be more applicable to price-sensitive products.

(ii) *Relevant cost analysis:* Whether it is the introduction of a new product, or making a change in the packaging of an existing product, or dropping an existing product, the relevant cost analysis is useful in all cases. It can affect the entire variable cost and part of the fixed cost of the organization. This behavior can be studied every year while working out a proper product mix.

(iii) *Cost-Effective analysis:* There are two types of cost-effective techniques:

To achieve the decided objective at much lower cost. For instance, there could be a method to cater to remote interior areas through sub-stockists, instead of appointing a new stockist, in cases where it is difficult to get a financially sound party.

To maximize the sales of a product within a budgeted cost of sales, the various activities can be taken up in such a way that they provide synergy and help to get more sales. You could also experiment with different media.

(iv) ***Opportunity cost analysis:*** This can help you to decide whether you should concentrate on one or more than one product with one doctor. If you concentrate on only one product, what would be the opportunity loss/gain in relation to each of the two cases? This gives an added dimension to maximizing the time spent by an MR on a doctor.

(v) ***Differential cost and incremental revenue analysis:*** When we compare two specific strategies, and thereby two sets of activities to be performed, we must identify the differential cost and differential revenue to justify that expenditure:

- To make one extra call, the MR gets an incentive, say Rs.X. You must be able to justify the additional cost by way of incentive to gain this increase in revenue.
- Suppose, one strategy revolves around concentrating on 20 core doctors, and the other depends on direct mailing to 2000 doctors. Once again the incremental cost and revenue need to be analyzed before making your choice between the two alternative strategies. This technique always helps in deciding the alternative activity or operational decision which maximizes cost and revenue.

(vi) ***Cost-benefit analysis:*** This technique helps in allocating the resources to the various marketing avenues. It is generally useful in deciding on the following issues:
- New product launch
- Manufacture, or obtain a loan-license facility
- Processing of the product
- Extraordinary promotional campaigns

If you integrate these techniques while reviewing your strategic decisions, it can provide an insight into:
- Customer profitability and productivity
- Product costs and profitability
- Total cost impact on incremental value
- Business appraisal

This insight can help you minimize your risks by taking adequate steps and investing efforts.

CONCEPTUAL FRAMEWORK OF A SMIR

SMIR can be conducted in four different stages:

1. Planning
2. Assessing strategic business units (SBUs)
3. Evaluating strategic performance and options

Stage 1: Planning for the SMIR

The first step in this stage is to set the sales and contribution objectives.

(i) ***Sales objectives:*** When we specially set any sales or marketing objective, such as the forecast for the year, there is always a risk associated with it. Suppose there are three outcomes of forecasts on basis of three different strategies. We can calculate the impact of risk as follows:

Table 12.1 Evaluating Impact of Risk

Sales Forecast-Strategic Alternatives	Probability of Success	Rate of Return
A	0.05	30%
B	0.65	18%
C	0.30	9%
	1.00	

Observing the risk of getting just 9% return if alternative C becomes a reality, we can re-examine alternative C and modify its probability of success. In addition, the well-known Bayesian approach can be used to evaluate the risk under uncertainty to set these objectives.

Besides the sales target, you can also decide to take up market share as an objective for products and industry ranking for the organization.

(ii) ***Contribution objectives:*** Profit planning and budgeting are inter-dependent aspects of marketing. Table 12.2 gives the performance of an organization for its five groups of products for a particular year.

Table 12.2 Comparative Performance for Major Product Groups of an Organization

		(Figures in Rs. million)	
Product Groups	**Sales**	**P/V Ratio**	**Contribution**
A	10	30%	3
B	5	40%	2
C	11	50%	5.5

Table 12.2 *Contd...*

			(Figures in Rs. million)
Product Groups	**Sales**	**P/V Ratio**	**Contribution**
D	4	60%	2.4
E	7	30%	2.4
Total Domestic	37	40.5%	15
Total Exports	3	33.3%	1
Total	40	40%	16
Fixed cost (including interest)		8	
Pre-tax profit		8	
Tax at 38.5%		3.08	
After-tax profit		4.92	

For the following year, the management has laid down the following objectives:

(a)   Growth in total sales by 20%

(b)   Export sales be at least Rs.50 million

(c)   ROI at least 30%

(d)   Equity dividend rate be stepped up from 15% to 20%

(e)   Dividend policy—Retention of 20% of after-tax profit before distribution of any dividends

(f)   Working capital requirement not to exceed 30% of the sales

(g)   The capital structure to be as follows:

	Rs. In million
Equity share capital	12
5% preference share capital	4
Reserves	10
Institutional loan @ 10%	30

(h)   50% of the working capital financed by internal sources

(i)   Product D may not grow more than 10%; product B has shortage of raw materials

(j)   Fixed costs for this year estimated at Rs.10 million

(k)   Due to escalation of costs, across the board reduction *P/V* ratio expected by 10%.

Let us highlight the salient aspects and work out the ROI:

1. Contribution Objectives

		Rs. million
5% preference dividend		0.2
20% equity dividend		2.4
Total dividend		2.6

Table *Contd...*

		Rs. million
At dividend policy 80% after the profit		3.5
At 66.33% tax rate		9.7
Fixed cost	100.00	
Add interest on incremental working capital	0.60	10.06
(interest at 10% on Rs.0.6 million only)		
Total contribution required		19.81

2. Minimum Sales Objectives

		Rs. million
Total sales (40% + 20%)		48.0
Export Sales		5.0
Minimum domestic sales		43.0

3. ROI

		Rs. million
Working capital = Max. 30% of 48		14.4
Outside financing of working capital		7.2
Owned and loan capital		30.0
Total investment		37.2
R.O.I @ 30%		11.16

As a result, a contribution objective of Rs.20 million, a total sales of a Rs.48 million, and an ROI of Rs.11.16 million will provide the justification for the profit-related objectives.

You must have also realized that it is essential to integrate the organizational financial health with the marketing objectives.

Stage 2: SBU Assessment

For analysis and review, it is useful to define a strategic business unit (SBU), such as a zone, and then work out the cost relationship with the zonal activities and the results achieved in that zone.

(i) *Key market parameters:* The parameters are given in Table 12.3. In India, it will be difficult for an average company to provide information for on the market value and the number of patients treated. However, certain data on the basis of sample size can be ascertained. The basic objective is to enable the management assess the past and future attractiveness of the market.

Table 12.3 Key Market Indicators

	t-5	t-4	t-3	t-2	t-1	t	t+1	t+2	t+3
1. Market value (Rs)									
2. Growth of market value (Rs)									
3. Market value/total pharma									
4. Market value (%)									
5. GP/market value (%)									
6. R_X (No. written)									
7. No. of patients treated									
8. Total promotional spend									
9. Total market value (%)									

t denotes the present time, and this table can be worked out in months or years for the purpose of evaluation. It is not possible to trace the information for five years, information of three years can still indicate the trend.

(ii) ***Patients:*** Patient behavior can be analyzed focusing on the following parameters:

- Size of the patient pool and patient categorization
- Perceptions and expectations of patients regarding the available therapies
- Role of patients in the therapies (decider, influencer, user)

An analysis of the behavior of patients provides the marketing strategist a better understanding of their perceptions, attitudes, etc.

(iii) ***Customers:*** It includes the analysis of prescribers, influencers, referrals, and other support people. Thus, prescribers span the whole range of general practitioners, specialist doctors, and hospital prescribers. Influencers include patient organizations, government agencies, word-of-mouth, one-time patients and prescribers, etc.

(iv) ***Segments:*** The first step is to specify rationally the current segmentation system. Next, alternative segmentation schemes should be proposed and evaluated in regard to:

- Homogeneity with respect to the needs within the segment
- Economic viability
- Identifiability
- Selective reachability

For each segment identified, a set of key indicators needs to be specified:

- Size and growth rate for the planning horizon
- Major competing products
- Promotional intensity (heavy, medium, light)
- Prescriber type and the key benefits being looked for

(v) *Competition:* The following competitive issues should be clearly analyzed to provide the marketing strategist with a clear view of the competitive threats and opportunities:

- Identifying competitors and competing brands
- Market share evolution of competitor(s) and competing brands
- Brand-switching matrix
- Relative importance of the product(s) to the competitor(s); this could be approximated by estimating the share of this product's sales in the total sales of the competitor
- Areas of vulnerability of the competitor(s)
- Areas where the product is vulnerable to the competitor(s)
- Expected new competitive products (with expected launch dates)

(vi) *Differential advantage:* For a clear analysis, you will need to specify the differential advantage of the products in the market, and those expected to come out into the market in the near future.

(vii) *Environment:* Important anticipated changes in the environment during the strategic planning horizon have to be made explicit. Such environmental changes can, for example, include government policies, customer education, pressures for generics, pressures from customer groups, pricing, parallel importing, and so on.

Stage 3: Assessing Strategic Marketing Performance and Options

Performance evaluations can be internal and external. The internal performance evaluation is based on the targets set for the marketing performance within the company. External performance evaluation is based on more global and broadly defined targets. Each of these is discussed in turn below.

(i) *Inside the company:* The most common type of objectives used by pharmaceutical companies are set in terms of profits, growth, and market share. The ultimate 'bottom line' test of product performance is profitability, which reflects the market viability of the product and its ability to compete. Profits can be measured in absolute or relative terms. Return on investment (ROI) is probably the most commonly used profit indicator. It refers to the efficiency and effectiveness of the product management strategy, i.e. the extent to which the scarce resources invested on the product management have been used to generate value. Profitability objectives are sometimes difficult to use in the pharmaceutical industry at the subsidiary (country) level. Indeed, because of the complexities of the transfer pricing systems dictated by headquarters, real profits are often ambiguous. Often, in those subsidiaries the only viable performance indicators are sales, market share, and growth.

Growth objectives as measured by the evolution of sales, market shares, and profits are good indicators of the current and long-term business health of the PM. Market-share objectives focus attention on the PM's competitive position.

(ii) *Conceptual framework of relevant data*
- Market share (%)
- Relative Market Share (%)
- New product sales (%)
- Relative market penetration index
- Marketing expenditure to sales (%)
- Receivables to sales (%)
- Value added to sales (%)
- Investment to sales (%)
- Investment to value added (%)
- Capacity utilization (%)
- Potential to invest in R&D (index)

Two major parameters need to be further emphasized while evaluating the strategic stance:

1. Relative quality
2. Customer satisfaction

In effect our decisions have a direct relevance to the variable cost of the organizations. Simple 'trade offers', samples, field staff cost, training, gifts and other promotional material can cost a fortune. However, through innovation and experience curve, the cost can be brought down. Both budgets abd marketing costs need to be monitored for better profitability.

ROMI (RETURN ON MARKETING INVESTMENT)

All over the world, it has been seen that instead of ROI, ROMI (Return on Marketing Investment) is used. Basically, ROMI addresses the question of making choices regarding the allocation of resources. Promotion and brand portfolio requires resources to build brand assets. Brands are usually evaluated and are capable of generating funds for the company. As we know brands add value to marketing activities.

Standardized ROMI matrixes are absolutely essential for pharmaceutical companies. Many high potential and heritage brands, products never receive even essential marketing investment unless compelled. As a result, no measurable impact can be generated. In comparison to many industries the kind of promotional percentage spent in pharma industry on returns sometimes results into net losses. In pharmaceuticals, we are engaged in field force arms race which is different from other industries to generate and fulfill the demand.

While conducting ROMI, best practices are emerging in pharma industry all over the world. The models which are available align themselves to strategic goals and activities which support those goals. Similarly, drivers of ROMI directly connect to bottomline measures. Soft ROI such as customer appreciation, awareness intention etc. is difficult to measure but not impossible to quantify in ROMI frame-work.

ROMI Challenges

In totality ROMI captures the impact of marketing program on external market dynamics. There are many challenges for measuring ROMI in a global environment. India is not an exception. All over the world inclusive of India you find following challenges to measure ROMI:

- Management's failure to recognize the need
- Number of products on promotion with a span of few minutes of in-clinic performance
- Multiple events: A promotional chain makes it difficult to isolate the contributions of single effort
- Objectivity of profiling, targeting, inputs and results

- Variable accountability: accurate knowledge of the causal relationship on incremental activity in prescribers clinic
- Causal relationship establishment of prescriptions
- Getting enough data: setting up testing to measure against controls
- Lack of industry standards/approaches on how to measure or build measurement
- Limited budget and resources
- Creating the will (internally) to do it.

Techniques and Tools for ROMI

- Campaign Measurers
- Marketing Mix Analytics Using Historical Data
- Marketing Mix Analytics Using Analogue Data
- Internal Marketing Database Tracking Combined with Analytics
- Predictive Analytics Using Validated Current Market Perception Data
- Physician Detailing Effect
- Brand Optimizers

SALES & MARKETING RETURN ON INVESTMENT (SAMROI)

In India, we need to consider SAMROI (Sales & Marketing Return on Investment).

SAMROI and its Future

Sales & Marketing ROI is a mix of quantitative and qualitative measures as many aspects affect Returns such as vacant territory management, reach of untapped markets, field force strategy, secondary sales, expiries, bonus offers, commercial deals, competitive tactics in the territory potential of key customers, new drivers, barriers etc.

To ensure that you can still measure Returns, you need to define Returns on what? On Territory? Or on doctor? Or on MR?

Let's get a few components of SAMROI.

Return on Field Force Implementation

All these studies provide an objective analysis at the inputs and optimisation of inputs. As we involve filed force to implement these marketing activities, we need to standardise the process of *"call"*, "repeat call", major calls, minor calls, profiling, targeting and measuring output per physician under clinical performance, their standard and motivation of field force with prioritisation of objective of each sale needs to be defined.

These *qualitative dimensions* will strengthen implementation. Besides, sales force activities, CRM activities are in high demand in India. In order to derive good results from CRM following steps need to be followed.

Return on CRM

We need to make sure that sales staffs are accurately tracking each actual sale in CRM system, by converting opportunities into closed orders, with accurate order values.

In addition to normal CRM entries, make sure your CRM has standard fields to capture the following data:

- Lead source
- Campaign
- Market segment
- Sales Region
- Win /Loss
- Reasons for Win / Loss
- Competitor

Return of Promotion

It is important to ensure that Return on Promotional expenses are planned / measured and controlled on time to time basis.

Return of Field Force Efficiency

Field Force efficiency is becoming an important issue which directly affects the structure, cost of structure, cost of attrition, designing of territory, productivity of each territory and hence per person productivity needs to be planned, measured and ensured that the growth is kept in view.

It's a Herculean task, yet it needs to be taken up on the **front deck** than to keep it in backburner and work on budgets. If not done, it may be a perpetual way to remain non-quantified to measure the return on sales & marketing investment.

Marketing's Worth

There is ever increasing competing pressure in the world of marketing today. With digital advertising and social media marketing, the traditional mass-marketing models are facing a threat. As a result it is important to have approaches that make the marketing investments count in this complex and competing environment. With growing importance of new kinds of media and mobile communications, the Return on Investment (ROI) has become a challenge for the organizations.

Growing financial pressure and a challenging economic environment are compelling marketers to explore new-media tools along with measuring their impact through new analytic approaches. Many marketers are making progress through these initiatives.

Influence on Consumers

Digitization has influenced consumers in a big way along with influencing their purchasing decisions. They have become more informed about considering products by reading online reviews and comparing prices. In stores, these very consumers search for deals and drive hard bargains. They also become reviewers and demand an everlasting relationship with products and brands. Even with heaps of data and research, companies cannot answer the fundamental question of how the consumers are influenced.

Traditional advertising methods are declining because the consumers regard the reviews read on the Internet as more objective. Thus, for any organization it is important to construct a marketing allocation model that included both the importance of the consumer and the cost-effectiveness of different interaction points. This can enable sharper decisions about the marketing mix, both by geography and specific product situations.

Sometimes the companies do realize the importance of touch points but do not understand the true value of their effects or how to influence them. The solution is to have a research that gets to the heart of the consumer's decision journey. This work should highlight the touch points and messages that actually influence consumer behavior.

In today's dynamic world, how consumers interact with the company's evolution would help in making marketing investments cost-effective thus, influencing purchasing decisions.

Well Informed Marketing Judgment

Marketing is a combination of facts and judgments. It is important to have confidence in one's judgment on spending and messaging. It is essential as well as difficult to make a rational investment for additional marketing approaches.

The rapidly changing marketing environment makes it difficult for the marketers to integrate all the information for improving judgments as well as implement smart marketing changes. The solution for this is to formulate a hypotheses regarding the impact of changes to the marketing mix right at the beginning and then seek analytical evidence.

It is very important to know and remember that data and analytics can only remain useful as the expertise one brings to bear and that good judgment will always remain a hallmark of good marketers.

Managing Financial Risks

Targeting and hitting the correct audience with the right message at the right time is a sign of successful communication. Today influencers can shift swiftly and there is little experience with the marketers with respect to the kind of message that works, when to apply the particular message and above all whom to influence. Obtaining the desired sales results from a given amount of marketing spending has become difficult, that is, the risk of Return on Investment (ROI) has increased.

Spending on new media is a bet that companies are compelled to make. But at the same time managing the risk from these spending is critical and thus, marketers shouldn't be shy about raising this issue. Thoughtful scenario planning and cross-functional participation can make these discussions on managing risks more rich and rewarding at the same time.

Coping with Added Complexity

The internal environment becomes complex along with the external marketing environment. Marketers today have access to dozens of communication approaches with the number growing rapidly. This has given rise to both internal and external specialists with expertise and experience. It is thus, critical to manage this exponential growth in marketing complexity.

To start with one will need to have specialists. Secondly, one will need someone to integrate marketing efforts across channels and focus on the bottom line. Last but not the least one will need absolute clarity in the processes, roles and responsibilities throughout the company as well as externally.

The complexity thus, needs to be addressed on a comprehensive and dedicated way.

Metrics to Track Options

Many usually imperfect ways exist today to measure the most established marketing forms. No single metric can evaluate the effectiveness of marketing investment. One needs to have a way to track progress and hold marketers accountable.

Even with no single way of measuring ROI for different channels, marketers can move toward an apples-to-apples way of comparing returns across media.

Having said that, metrics are rarely perfect. Yet the amount of data that is available today makes it possible to find metrics and analytic opportunities that take advantage of one's insights, provide evidence and lay foundation for sophisticated approaches to track ROI.

STRATEGIC OPTIONS

In order to arrive at the strategic options we need to first evaluate the operating performance and then alone decide on the options. The options will depend on the specific needs of the marketing operations. The two prime ratios that drive return on total assets are:

- Sales to total assets ratio
- Margin on sales percentage

Marketing managers must concentrate on these two drivers in order to arrive at the strategic options to improve performance. However, these ratios cannot be operated directly. Each of them is dependent on a whole series of detailed results from widely separated parts of the operation. The other cost ratios that affect organizational performance include: sales to total assets, sales to accounts receivables and sales to inventories.

Drivers of the Sales to Total Assets Ratio

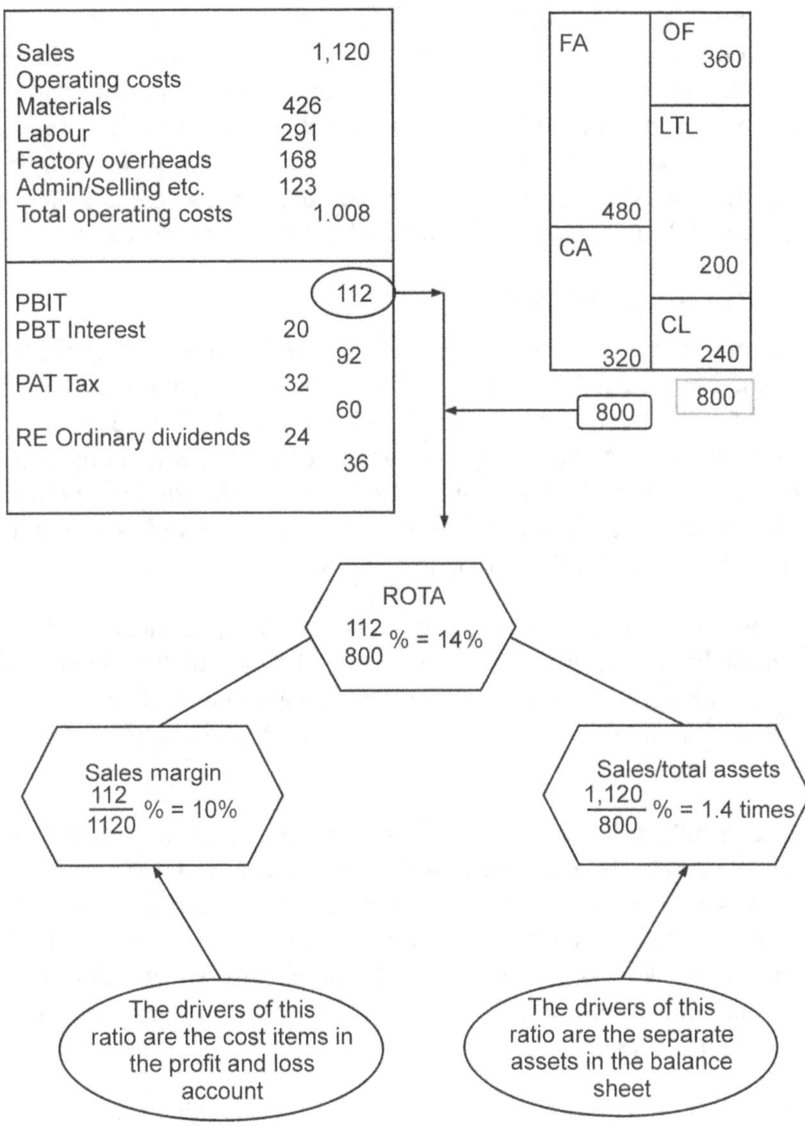

Figure 12.1 *Components of Sales to Total Assets Ratio*

This ratio may be broken down into its component parts. We identify the main groups of assets straight from the balance sheet and we then express the ratio between each group and the sales figure as shown in Figure 12.1.

On the basis of these operating issues and the need for better marketing performance, you can choose the relevant ratio as options to correct the performance. You can benchmark these ratios with suitable companies, and improve the performance through innovative practices in sales, selection of new products (yielding better gross margins), understanding the performance of non-performing assets such as inventory, debtors, etc. action plans can be drawn accordingly.

Drivers of Margin on Sales

If the management wishes to improve its margins, then one or more of the cost percentages must fall. For instance as per Figure 12.2, if the material cost percentage can be reduce by two points, from 38% to 36%, then, other thing, being equal, the margin percentage would improve by two points to 12%. This margin of 12% would then combine with the sales to total assets ratio of 1.4 times to give an improved return on the total assets of 16.8% (12% multiplied by 1.4).

These cost ratios allow managers to plan, budget, delegate responsibility and monitor performance of the various functional areas under control. They can quantify targets for all areas, and calculate the effect of a variation in any one of the subsidiary ratios on the overall performance.

The results achieved by different managers, products, zones, and divisions can also be compared, and the experiences of the best passed on to the others to help them improve. We must recognize, however, that there are operating factors that the model does not cope with. The variables of selling price, volume and product mix, which have such a powerful impact on profit, are not easily distinguished from other factors in the model.

As a marketing chief you may not be exercising direct control over materials and labor, yet as the CEO you will need to ensure that there is no loss of productivity at the factory nor an increase in wastage so that adequate funds are available in the competitive areas of business such as marketing. A ratio of 11% of the cost of administration/ selling to sales turnover is definitely too low; this is usually the case in laid-back companies.

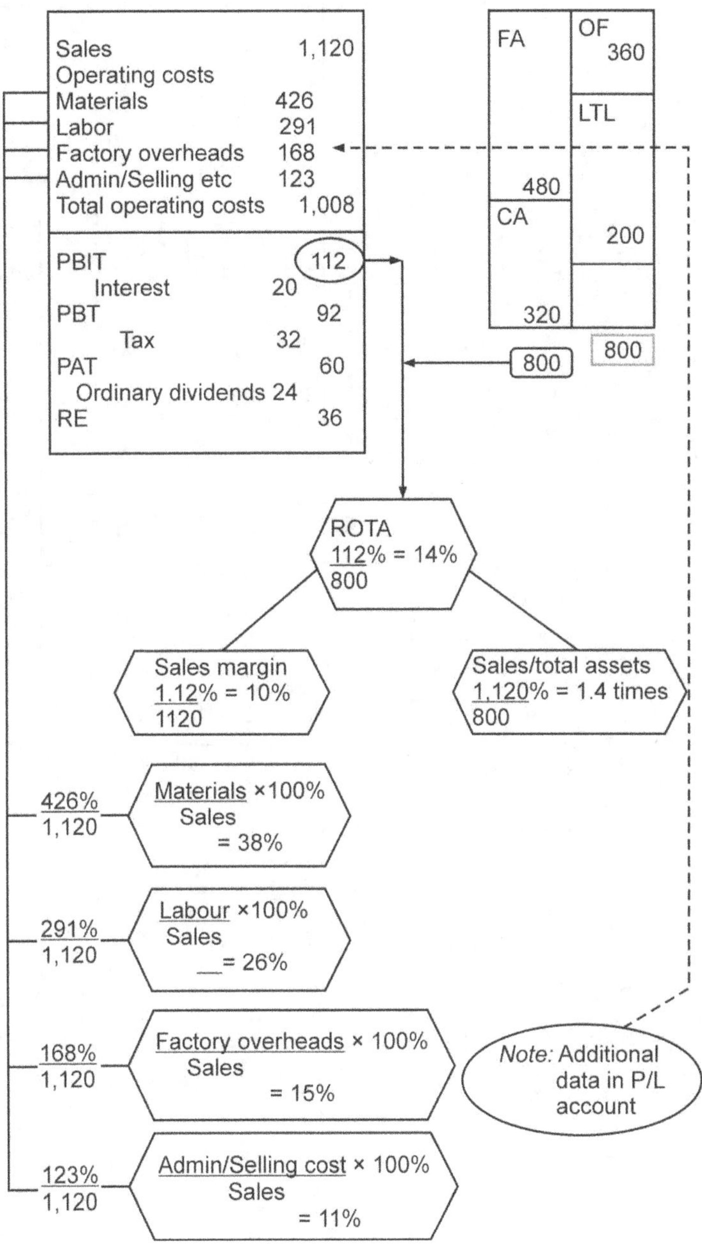

Figure 12.2 Components of Margin on Sales

Sales to Total Assets Ratio

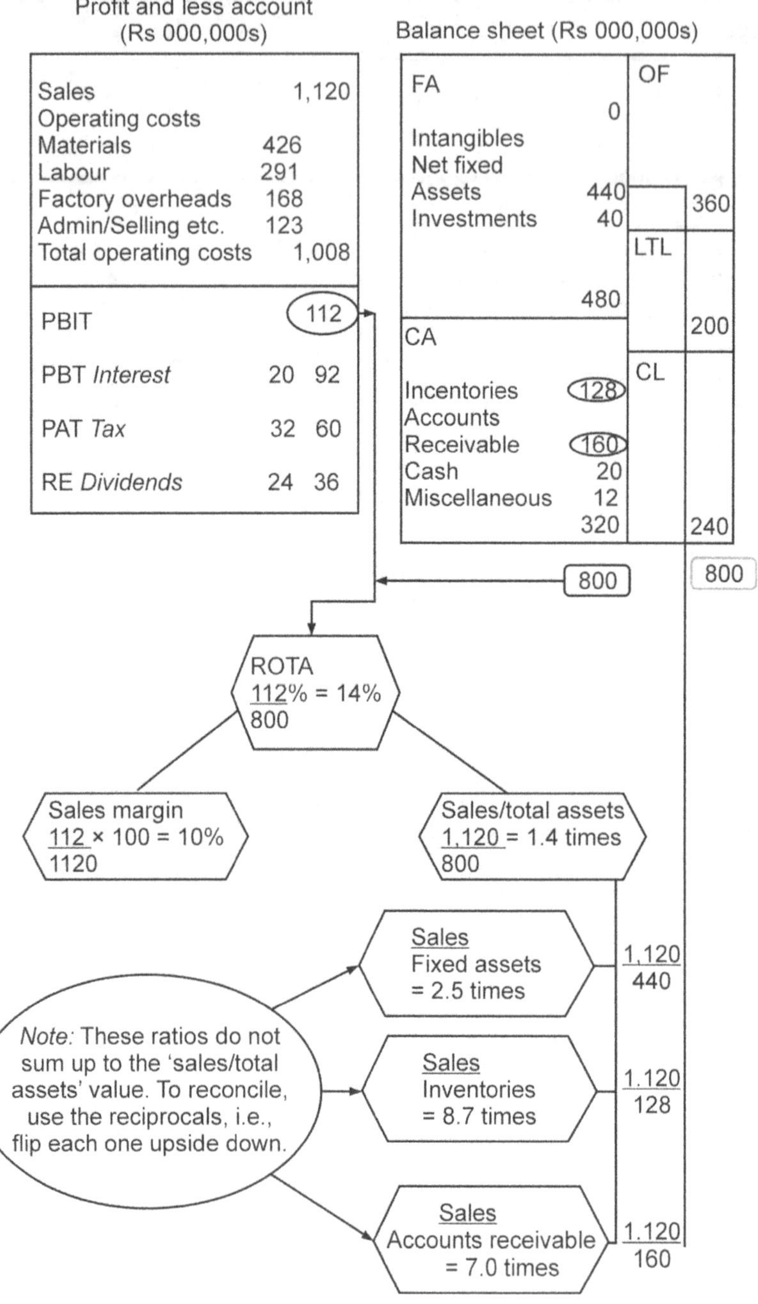

Figure 12.3 Components of Sales to Total Ratio

The three major asset blocks in all enterprises are:

- fixed assets
- inventories (stocks)
- accounts receivables (debtors)

The value of each of these in relation to sales is shown in the subsidiary boxes in Figure 12.3. The ratio for fixed assets is 2.5 time (from sales of Rs.120 million divided by fixed assets of Rs.440 million). Note that the sum of these separate values does not agree with the sales to total assets ratio as did the sales margin on the other side withhe operating costs. This is because they are expressed differently. The link will become clear if you take the reciprocals of the values.

The figure shows the importance of managing the balance sheet as also profit and loss account. For instance, if the total assets can be reduced from Rs.800 million to Rs.700 million, then the sales to total assets ratio would move up from 1.4 to 1.6 times. The effect on the return on total assets would be to increase it from 14% to 16%. Ifin addition, the margin was increased by 1% to 11%, then the new return on total assets would be almost 18% (11% x 1.6 times). The original value of 14% is an average value, whereas a return on total assets of 18% represents an excellent performance.

Production managers can work with finance and marketing departments to quantify targets for stock holdings and accounts receivables. The impact of an increase in fixed assets caused by a major capital investment project can also be assessed in profitability terms.

Drivers of Sales to Accounts Receivables Ratio

This ratio is commonly expressed in terms of day's sales and the method of calculation is shown in Figure 12.4. Instead of the formula we have been using here sales over accounts receivables, the alternative is to show accounts receivables over sales and multiply the result by 365. The answer represents the average number of days' credit customers take before paying off their accounts.

This ratio is often referred to as 'debtor days' or the 'collection period'. The concept of the number of days outstanding is easy to understand. The number is very precise, which means that a slippage of even a few days is instantly identified. Also, figures can be compared with the company's normal terms of trade and the effectiveness or otherwise of the credit control department can, therefore, be monitored.

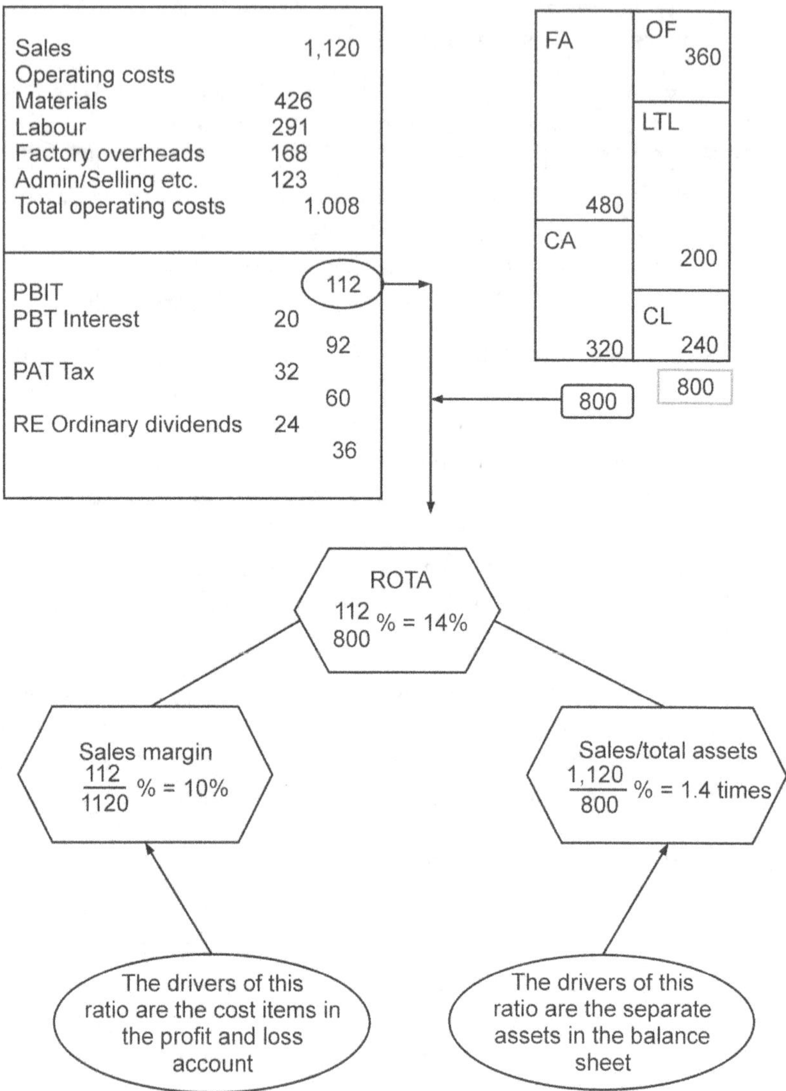

Figure 12.4 *Components of Sales to Inventories Ratio*

Drivers of sales to Inventories Ratio

This calculation is similar to the one above and is also known as inventory days. The ratio may, therefore, be linked to purchases or material usage, whichever gives the most useful guidance.

Besides the financial analysis and implications, there is another aspect-brand valuation-which needs discussion.

BRAND VALUATION

Financial evaluation and accounting procedures for brand have become subjects of considerable debate, as can be seen by the numerous articles which have been published on the subject. The debates are becoming international as they concern the financial information of large multi-national corporations holding brands which are strong or are presumed to be. However, from one country to other differences exist between accounting procedures for brands and their place on the balance sheet. This can greatly affect the interpretation of the health of these companies.

The first people to reveal the monetary value of brands were financial analysts. They were not any old analysts, but were those of hostile companies who were trying to take over companies with brands or of companies fighting to buy firms that were found to have, after careful examination, either modest net assets or negative net assets when accumulated debts are taken into account. Recent times have seen a huge increase in mergers and acquisitions with new norms. Initially, acquisition prices were determined by the financial results of the target company. The norm was to pay eight to ten times its profits. If the firm possessed brands, it was believed that their effects were already incorporated in the profits. Brand value was considered to be included in the earnings, and it was thought that if a company made a loss, its brand was worth very little. This explains why companies that were in financial difficulty were bought for virtually nothing.

The notion of value is ambiguous and a source of several misunderstandings. It is important to understand that there is no single value for a brand; in fact there are several because the valuation will be different on its aims. There are eight ways to look at brand valuation.

- The value of liquidity in the case of a forced sale
- The book value for company accounts
- The value needed in order to encourage banks to lend the company money
- The value of losses or damage to the worth of the brand
- The value in order to estimate the price of licenses
- The value for management control which depends on the behavior encouraged in managers

- The value for the partial sale of assets
- The value in case of a takeover or a merger and acquisition

It is necessary to include brands on the balance sheet? This question is already out of date. Acquired brands must be included, whether it be in consolidated accounts or company accounts. Created brands may be included. The accounting framework which allowed for the capitalization of a part of R&D expenses also gives an adequate answer to those who ask about the capitalization of commercial expenses. Nevertheless, for the moment, those in favor of inclusing created brands on the balance sheet have been kept quiet.

There are five ways to valuate the brand:

- Cost-based Brand Valuation Methods
- Valuation by Replacement Costs
- Valuation by Market Price
- Valuation by Potential Earnings
- Multi-criteria Valuation of a Brand's Potential

All of these are self-explanatory except the last one. Let's see how it works.

	Brand	
	A	B
Awareness (percent of people who know the brand)	50	40
Trial/ prescription (proportion of those people who know the brand who have already bought or used it)	40	35
Re-prescription (proportion of initial users who continue to use it)	20	40
Rate at which it is prescribed (compared to the market average)	110	100
Availability (percent of people who can easily find the brand)	70	20
Prescription utilization share (equivalent to the market share)	3.1	1.1
Potential (with 100% awareness and 100% RN/RV retail presence)	8.8	14

As a result, you can value Brand A or Brand B on the basis of the last method.

From the above you would have realized the importance of financial analysis of the business to develop suitable options for marketing strategy and marketing operations. The importance of brands is undoubtedly an organizational priority and organizations can be effective by increasing their brand equity. Organizational health is dependent on various factors: the accuracy of sales and marketing forecasts; timely investments in human resources and innovation; monitoring of debtors and creditors; etc. these strategic decisions can be taken by the marketing chief using the tools of financial analysis given above. However, in the words of Peter Drucker:

In the final analysis,

Management is practice

Its essence is not knowing...but doing

Its test is not logic...but results

Its ultimate authority is performance.

LEARNINGS

To formulate and implement a methodology for evaluation of impact of strategic marketing, you need the following five-step approach:

- Cost-behavior analysis
- Planning for SMIR
- Product market assessment
- Strategic performance
- Strategic options

It is also essential to have a conceptual framework of a SMIR in place with different stages like:

- Planning for the SMIR
- SBU Assessment
- Assessing Strategic Marketing Performance and Options

All over the world, it has been seen that instead of ROI, ROMI (Return on Marketing Investment) is used. ROMI addresses the question of making choices regarding the allocation of resources. Drivers of ROMI directly connect to bottom line measures.

Sales & Marketing ROI is a mix of quantitative and qualitative measures as many aspects affect returns such as vacant territory management, reach of untapped markets, field force strategy, secondary sales, expiries, bonus offers, commercial deals, competitive tactics in the territory potential of key customers, new drivers, barriers.

Components of SAMROI

- Return on field force implementation
- Return on CRM
- Return of Promotion
- Return of field force efficiency

With growing importance of new kinds of media and mobile communications, ROI has become a challenge for the organizations. Many marketers are making progress through:

- Influence on consumers
- Well informed marketing judgement
- Managing financial risks
- Coping with added complexity
- Metrics to track options

In order to arrive at the strategic options it is important to arrive at drivers of return on total assets viz.

- Drivers of the sales to assets ratio
- Drivers of margin on sales
- Sales to total assets ratio
- Drivers of sales to accounts receivables ratio
- Drivers of sales to inventories ratio

The notion of brand valuation is ambiguous and hence, it is important to understand that there is no single value for a brand, there are several because the valuation will be different on its aims.

The importance of brands is undoubtedly an organizational priority and organizations can be effective by increasing their brand equity.

Bibliography

1. Andrew, Kenneth (1980). *The Concept of Corporate Strategy*, rev. edn. Richard D. Irwin Inc.

2. Ansoff, Igor (1977). *Business Strategy*. Penguin Books Ltd.

3. Ansoff, Igor (1979). *Strategic Management*. John Wiley.

4. Bartlett, C.A., Ghoshal, S (1989). *Managing Across Borders. The Transnational Solution*. Boston, Mass: Harvard Business School Press.

5. Beckwith, Harry (1977). *Selling the Invisible*. Warner Books.

6. Bono, Edward de. (1994). *Tactics: The Art and Science of Success*. William Collins.

7. Bonoma, T. (1984). *Managing Marketing: Test, Cases and Readings*. Free Press.

8. Bonoma, T. (1985). *The Marketing Edge: Making Strategies Work*. Free Press.

9. Broadstreet, Dun V. (1971). *Successful Sales Management*. W. Foulsham& Co. Ltd.

10. Brown, Linden (1990). *Competitive Marketing Strategy*. Thomas Nelson.

11. Buzzel, R.D.(1983, January). 'Is Vertical Integration Profitable?' *Harvard Business Review, Vol. 61, No. 92*, 102.

12. Buzzel, R.D. and Gale, B.T. (1987). *The PIMS Principles- Linking Strategy to Performance*. Free Press.

13. Capra, Fritjof (1990). *The Turning Point*. Simon & Schuster.

14. Chandler, A.D. (1962). *Strategy and Structure*. MIT Press.

15. Christensen, Roland, C., Andrews, K.R. and Bower, J.L. (1978). *Business Policy: Text & Cases*. Richard D. Irwin Inc.

16. Clansewitz, Carl von. (Reissued 1986). *On War*. Penguin Books.

17. Corstijeus, Marcel. (1997). *Marketing Strategy in the Pharmaceutical Industry*. Chapman & Hall.

18. Cross, Robert G. (1998). *Revenue Management*. Brozaway Books.

19. Dasgupta, P. and Sengupta. (1987). *Pharmaceutical Marketing*. Allied.

20. Day, George S.; Shocker, Allan D.; and Srivastava, Rajendra Kumar (1979). 'Customer-Oriented Approaches to Identifying Product Markets.' *Journal of Marketing*, 43(4), Research Collection Lee Kong Chian School Of Business.

21. Ding, Min; Eliashberg, Jehoshua and Stremersch, Stefan (2013). Innovation and Marketing in the Pharmaceutical Industry: Emerging Practices, Research, and Policies. Springer.

22. Drucker, Peter F. (1954). *The Practice of Management*. Harper.

23. Drucker, Peter F. (1973). *Management: Cases, Responsibilities, Practices*. Harper & Row.

24. Drucker, Peter F. (1977). *People and Performance: The Best of Peter Drucker on Management*. Heinemann.

25. Drucker, Peter F. (1985). *Innovation and Entrepreneurship*. Harper & Row.

26. Ellis, Patrick (1992). *Who Dares Sells*. Thorsons.

27. Fletcher, K. and Hart, W.S. (1990). 'Marketing Strategy and Planning in the UK Pharmaceutical Industry: Some Preliminary Findings.' *European Journal of Marketing, Vol. 24, No. 2,* 55-68.

28. Gabor, A. (1977). *Pricing: Principles and Practices*. Heinemann Education Books.

29. Gaitonde, D.W. (1987).*Disciplinary Proceedings*. Durga Enterprise.

30. Gaudilliaere, Jean-Paul (2015). The Development of Scientific Marketing in the Twentieth Century: Research for Sales in the Pharmaceutical Industry. Pickering & Chatto Publishers.

31. Goldacre, Ben (2012). *Bad Pharma*. Fourth Estate.

32. Green, P., Tull, D. and Albaum, G. (1985). *Research for Marketing Decisions*. Prentice Hall.

33. Griffith, Winter H. (1985). *Complete Guide to Prescription and Non-Prescription Drugs: Side Effects, Warnings & Vital Data for Safe Use*. HP Books Inc.

34. Gumpert, David E. (1985). *The Marketing Renaissance*. John Wiley & Sons Inc.

35. Handy, Charles (1991). *Gods of Management*. Business Books Ltd.

36. Holden, Peter (1992). *Marketing Communications in the Pharmaceutical Industry*. Radcliffe Professional Press.

37. Humble, J.W. (1967). *Improving Business Results*. McGraw-Hill Inc.

38. Katsanis, Lea (2015). Global Issues in Pharmaceutical Marketing. Routledge Press.

39. Kay, John (1993). *Foundations of Corporate Success: How Business Strategies Add Value*. Oxford University Press.

40. Kelly, Joe (1974). *Organizational Behavior*. Irwin Inc.

41. Khandwalla, Pradip N. (1984). *Fourth Eye: Excellence through Creativity*. Wheeler Publishing.

42. Kharbande, O.P. (1988, January 7) 'Strategy is the Crux'. *The Economic Times*, Mumbai, Maharashtra.

43. King, William R. (1967). *Quantitative Analysis for Marketing Management*. McGraw-Hill Inc.

44. Kiranshankar, Kodiyalbail (1973). 'What the Medical Profession Expects from Medical Detailmen.' *PhD Thesis*, Manipal University.

45. Kotler, P. (1986).*Marketing Management*. Prentice-Hall.

46. Kotler, P and Keller, K.L. (2015). *Marketing Management, Global Edition*. Pearson.

47. Kuczmarski, Thomas D. (1988). *Managing New Products*. Prentice Hall.

48. Lamb, Charles W., Hair, Joseph F. and McDaniel, Carl (2004). *Marketing: 7th Edition*. South-Western, Cengage Learning.

49. Levitt, Theodore (1965). *Marketing Myopia*. Harvard Business Review.

50. Levitt, Theodore (1986). *The Marketing Imagination*. Free Press.

51. Levitt, Theodore (1965, November-December). 'Exploit the Product Life-Cycle.' *Harvard Business Review*, 81-94

52. Lidstone, J. (1987). *Marketing Planning for the Pharmaceutical Industry*. Gower.

53. Luck, David J. and Ferrel, O.C. (1979). *Marketing Strategy and Plans*. Prentice Hall.

54. Lynn, Matthew (1991). *Merck vsGlaxo: The Billion Dollar Battle*. Heinemann.

55. MacCrimmon, Kenneth R. and Wehrung, Donald N. (1986). *Taking Risk: The Management of Uncertainty*. The Free Press.

56. Makens, James C. (1985). *The Marketing Plan Workbook*. Prentice Hall.

57. Matsushita, Kōnosuke (1988). *Not for Bread Alone*. PHP Institute Inc.

58. Mazze, Edward M. (1970). *Introduction to Marketing: Readings in the Discipline*. Chandler.

59. McDonald, Malcolm (1992). *Strategic Marketing Planning*. Granfield.

60. McGee,John and Thomas, Howard (1986).'Strategic groups: Theory, research and taxonomy.' *Strategic Management Journal*, Volume 7, Issue 2, Pages 141–160, DOI: 10.1002/smj.4250070204

61. McLuhan, Marshall (1964). *Understanding Media*. Routledge and Kegan Paul Ltd.

62. *Medical Marketing & Media*, May 1992, September 1992, January 1993, October 1992, November 1992, April 1992, August 1992, June 1992, December 1992, August 1993, April 1993.

63. Nabhi (1986). *The Consumer Protection Act 1986.*

64. Nain, Ashok (1997). *Professional Valuation Practice*. Tata McGraw-Hill Pub. Co. Ltd.

65. Naisbitt, John (1984). *Megatrends*. Warner Communications Co.

66. NMIMS (1989). *Product Mix Strategy for Bulk Drug Industry*.

67. Ohmae, Kessichi (1990). *The Borderless World*. McKinsey & Co., William Collins Co. Ltd.

68. Olives, Wolff (1990). *Guide to Corporate Identity*. The Design Council.

69. Palkhiwala, N.A. (1994). *We The Nation*. UBSPD.

70. Porter, Michael E. (1979, March-April). 'How Competitive Forces Shape Strategy.' *Harvard Business Review*, 137-145.

71. Porter, Michael E. (1980). *Competitive Strategy*. The Free Press.

72. Porter, Michael E. (1985). *Competitive Advantage*. The Free Press.

73. Porter, Michael E. (1990). *The Competitive Advantage of Nations*. Macmillan.

74. Rao, Subba (1990). *Pharmaceutical Marketing in India: Concepts, Cases, Strategy*. Panther.

75. Ries, A. and Trout, J. (1986). *Positioning: The Battle for Your Mind*. Warner Books.

76. Rodgers, F.G. (1986). *The IBM Way*. Harper & Row.

77. Rollins, Brent L. and Matthew Perri III (2013). Pharmaceutical Marketing. Jones & Bartlett Publishers.

78. Russel, Thomas J. and Lane, Ronald W. (1990). *Kleppner's Advertising Procedure*. Prentice Hall.

79. Sarma, Vishnu (1993). *The Panchatantra*. Penguin.

80. Schendel, Dan and Channon, Derek (March-April 1986, May-June 1986, July-August 1986,September-October 1986, November-December 1986). *Strategic Management Journal*, Vol. 7, No. 2; Vol. 7, No. 3; Vol. 7, No. 4; Vol. 7, No. 5; Vol. 7, No. 6. A Wiley-Interscience Publication.

81. Seldin, Donald W. (1977). 'The Medical Model: Biomedical Science as the Basis of Medicine.' *Beyond Tomorrow*. Rockfeller University Press.

82. Sengupta, Subroto (1990). *Brand Positioning: Strategies for Competitive Advantage*. Tata McGraw- Hill.

83. Serge, Peter M. (1993). *The Fifth Discipline*. Century.

84. Shapiro, Benson P. (1977). *Sales Program Management: Formulation and Implementation*. McGraw-Hill Inc.

85. Shapiro, Lovelock and Star, Davis (1949). *Problems in Marketing*. McGraw-Hill Inc.

86. Shaw, Steven J., Willenborg, John F. and Stanley, Richard E. (1980). *Marketing and Management Strategy*. Prentice Hall.

87. Shiva, Vandane (1991). *Biotechnology and the Environment*. Third World Network.

88. Slatter, Stuart (2014). Competition and Marketing Strategies in the Pharmaceutical Industry. Routledge.

89. Smith, Mickey C. (1985). *Principles of Pharmaceutical Marketing*. Lea & Febiger.

90. Smith, Mickey (2007). *Pharmaceutical Marketing*. Pharmaceutical Products Press.

91. Smith, Mickey (2014). *Principles of Pharmaceutical Marketing.* Taylor & Francis.

92. Stanrapp, Collins Tom (1988). *Maxi-Marketing: The New Direction in Advertising, Promotion and Marketing Strategy.* McGraw-Hill Inc.

93. Still, Richard R., Cundiff, E.W. and Govani, A.P.N (1988). *Sales Management: Decisions, Strategies & Cases.* Prentice Hall.

94. Sun, Tzu (1983). *The Art of War.* Dell Publishing.

95. Taylor, James W. (1985). *Competitive Marketing Strategies.* Modern Business Reports.

96. Tofler, Alvin (1991). *Powershift.* Bantam Books.

97. Vyas, Jay Narayan and Shah, Gitesh (1992). *Pharmaceutical Data Book.* Saket Communications Center.

98. Weintraub, Scott; Lewis, R.J., McHugh, Joanne; Zan, Roger; Sitler, Brad (2015). Results: The Future of Pharmaceutical and Healthcare Marketing. Advantage Media Group.

99. Whitney, John O. (1992). *Taking Charge.* Warner Books.

100. Wilkie, W.J. and Cohen, J.B. (1977). *An Overview of Market Segmentation: Behavioural Concepts and Research Approaches.* Cambridge, Massachusetts: Marketing Science Institute, Report Number 77-105.

101. Wilkie, William L. and Pessemier, Edgar A. (November, 1973). 'Issues in Marketing's Use of Multi-Attribute Models.' *Journal of Marketing Research,* 10, 428-41.

102. Willsmer, Ray L. (1975). *Directing the Marketing Effort.* Staples Press Ltd.

103. Wison, Richard M.S., Gilligan, Colin and Pearson, David J. (1992). *Strategic Marketing Management: Planning, Implementation and Control.* Butterworth-Heinemann Ltd.

104. Wouk, Herman (1978). *War & Remembrance.*Pocket Books.

Webliography

1. Pharma 2020: Marketing the future, Marketing the future - Which path will you take?
   http://www.pwc.com/gx/en/industries/pharmaceuticals-life-sciences/pharma-2020/pharma-2020-marketing-the-future-which-path-will-you-take.html [Accessed: 25th August 2016]

2. Manish Panchal, CharuKapoor and MansiMahajan, February 17, 2014. Success strategies for Indian pharma industry in an uncertain world, Mumbai, http://www.business-standard.com/content/b2b-chemicals/success-strategies-for-indian-pharma-industry-in-an-uncertain-world-114021701557_1.html [Accessed: 25th August 2016]

3. Persuading the Prescribers: Pharmaceutical Industry Marketing and its Influence on Physicians and Patients, Fact Sheet, November 11, 2013. Prescription Project, The Pew Charitable Trusts Research & Analysis,http://www.pewtrusts.org/en/research-and-analysis/fact-sheets/2013/11/11/persuading-the-prescribers-pharmaceutical-industry-marketing-and-its-influence-on-physicians-and-patients [Accessed: 25th August 2016]